P9-BJB-251

Childhood Epilepsies: Neuropsychological, Psychosocial and Intervention Aspects

WILEY SERIES ON
STUDIES IN CHILD PSYCHIATRY

Series Editor
Michael Rutter
Institute of Psychiatry
London

The First Year of Life
Psychology and Medical Implications of Early Experience
Edited by
David Shaffer and Judy Dunn

The Clinical Psychiatry of Adolescence
by Derek Steinberg

Longitudinal Studies in Child Psychology and Psychiatry
Practical lessons from research experience
Edited by
A.R. Nicol

Treatment of Autistic Children
by Patricia Howlin and Michael Rutter

Childhood Epilepsies: Neuropsychological, Psychosocial
and Intervention Aspects
Edited by Bruce P. Hermann and Michael Seidenberg

Further titles in preparation

Childhood Epilepsies: Neuropsychological, Psychosocial and Intervention Aspects

Edited by
Bruce P. Hermann
Baptist Memorial Hospital, Memphis TN, USA
and
Michael Seidenberg
Chicago Medical School, Chicago IL, USA

JOHN WILEY & SONS
Chichester · New York · Brisbane · Toronto · Singapore

Library of Congress Cataloging in Publication Data

Childhood epilepsies.

(Wiley series on studies in child psychiatry)
Includes bibliographies and index.
1. Epilepsy in children. I. Hermann, Bruce P.
II. Seidenberg, Michael. III. Series. [DNLM: 1. Epilepsy
—in infancy & childhood. WL 385 C5357]
RJ496.E6C45 1989 618.92′853 88–33849
ISBN 0 471 91270 0

British Library Cataloguing in Publication Data

Childhood epilepsies: neuropsychological,
psychosocial and intervention aspects.
1. Children. Epilepsy
I. Hermann, Bruce P. II. Seidenberg,
Michael
618.92′853

ISBN 0 471 91270 0

Typeset by Inforum Typesetting, Portsmouth
Printed and bound in Great Britain by Anchor Press Ltd, Colchester, Essex

Contents

List of Contributors

STANLEY BERENT, PhD	*Department of Psychiatry, University of Michigan Medical Center, Ann Arbor, MI 48109, USA*
CHRISTINE CULL, PhD	*The David Lewis Centre for Epilepsy, Warford, Near Alderly Edge, Cheshire, SK9 7UD, England*
DAVID CLEMMONS, PhD	*Epilepsy Center, Department of Neurosurgery, University of Washington, Seattle, WA 98104, USA*
JADE DELL, MRE	*Center for Urban Affairs, Northwestern University, 2046 N. Sheridan Rd., Evanston, IL 60201, USA*
F.E. DREIFUSS, MD	*Department of Neurology, University of Virginia Medical Center, Charlottesville, VA 22908, USA*
M. ANDREW DUBOIS, PhD	*Department of Psychology, Chicago Medical School, 3333 N. Green Bay Rd, North Chicago, IL 60064, USA*
MICHAEL FERRARI, PhD	*Department of Individual and Family Studies, University of Delaware, 228 Alison Hall, Newark, DE 19716, USA*
ROBERT FRASER, PhD	*Epilepsy Center, Department of Neurosurgery, University of Washington, Seattle, WA 98104, USA*
BRUCE HERMANN, PhD	*Epi Care Center, Baptist Memorial Hospital, 899 Madison Ave, Memphis, TN 38146, USA*

ALLAN MIRSKY, PhD	*Laboratory of Psychology and Psychopathology, National Institute of Mental Health, NIH, Bldg 10– Room 4C 110, Bethesda, MD 20892, USA*
ERNST RODIN, MD	*Epilepsy Center of Michigan, 3800 Woodward Ave, Detroit, M 48201, USA*
J. CHRIS SACKELLARES, MD	*Epilepsy Program, Department of Neurology, University of Michigan Medical Center, Ann Arbour, MI 48109, USA*
NANCY SANTILLI, RN	*Epilepsy Center, Department of Neurology, University of Virginia Medical Center, Charlottesville, VA 22908, USA*
DAVID SCHOTTE, PhD	*Department of Psychology, Chicago Medical School, 3333 N. Green Bay Rd, North Chicago, IL 60064, USA*
MICHAEL SEIDENBERG, PhD	*Department of Psychology, Chicago Medical School, 3333 N. Green Bay Rd, North Chicago, IL 60064, USA*
DAVID TAYLOR, FRCP, FRCPsych	*Department of Child and Adolescent Psychiatry, Jesson House (RMCH), 78 Manchester Rd, Swinton, Manchester M27 1FG, UK*
MICHAEL TRIMBLE, FRCP	*National Hospitals for Nervous Diseases, London, UK*
STEPHEN TONELSON, PhD	*Epilepsy Center, Department of Neurology, University of Virginia Medical Center, Charlottesville, VA 22908, USA*
STEVEN WHITMAN, PhD	*Center for Urban Affairs, Northwestern University, 2046 N. Sheridan Rd, Evanston, IL 60201, USA*
ALLEN WYLER, MD	*Epi Care Center, Baptist Memorial Hospital, 899 Madison Ave, Memphis, TN 38146, USA*
JANUSZ ZIELINSKI, MD	*Epilepsy Center of Michigan, 3800 Woodward Ave, Detroit, MI 48201, USA*

Series Preface

During recent years there has been a tremendous growth of research in both child development and child psychiatry. Research findings are beginning to modify clinical practice, but to a considerable extent the fields of child development and of child psychiatry have remained surprisingly separate, with regrettably little cross-fertilization. Much developmental research has not concerned itself with clinical issues, and studies of clinical syndromes have all too often been made within the narrow confines of a pathological condition approach with scant regard to developmental matters. The situation is rapidly changing but the results of clinical–developmental studies are often reported only by means of scattered papers in scientific journals. This series aims to bridge the gap between child development and clinical psychiatry by presenting reports of new findings, new ideas, and new approaches in a book form that may be available to a wider readership.

The series includes reviews of specific topics, multi-authored volumes on a common theme, and accounts of specific pieces of research. However, in all cases the aim is to provide a clear, readable and interesting account of scientific findings in a way that makes explicit their relevance to clinical practice or social policy. It is hoped that the series will be of interest to both clinicians and researchers in the fields of child psychiatry, child psychology, psychiatric social work, social paediatrics, and education—in short all concerned with the growing child and his problems.

This sixth* volume differs from its predecessors in taking a specific set of medical conditions, the epilepsies of childhood, as its focus; however, it adopts the same clinical–developmental perspective. Epilepsy is a relatively common problem in childhood affecting some 5–9 children in every 1000. The medical management involves a careful appraisal of the particular type of epileptic fit being experienced, together with investigations for possible underlying medical conditions. However, the epilepsies are of particular interest from a psychological perspective for several rather different reasons. They are associated with an increased risk of educational and psychiatric difficulties; the drugs used

* One early title, *Out of School*, edited by Lionel Hersov and Ian Berg, is now out of print.

to treat them may have both beneficial and harmful effects on behavioural and cognitive functioning; the sudden loss of consciousness that takes place in a fit causes frightening overtones for both the child experiencing it and the family witnessing it; and public attitudes to epilepsy involve elements of prejudice and stigma. This volume brings together research and clinical approaches in order to consider the meaning of this complex array of psyche–soma interactions and to devise practical ways of helping children suffering from epilepsy. The book brings out well the immense variability that lies behind the diagnosis of 'epilepsy'. In many cases, the outlook for normal life and development is excellent and the main need is to ensure that everyone appreciates that epileptic children need not, or should not, be treated differently (beyond the need to take regular medication). At the other extreme, there are some children in whom the epilepsy is associated with an assortment of handicaps and in which the control of the epileptic seizures constitutes a considerable medical (and sometimes surgical) challenge. The book provides a clear account of the key research findings that need to guide clinical practice and goes on to describe how experienced clinicians of different professional disciplines tackle these important problems.

MICHAEL RUTTER

Preface

The past two decades have witnessed a relative explosion of interest in epilepsy. Special centers designed to treat patients with epilepsy have proliferated, the classification of epileptic seizures and the pertinent diagnostic and treatment procedures have been sharply refined, and there is a reawakening of interest in the surgical treatment of epilepsies. In general, awareness of this long neglected disorder has been heightened. While there is still much that needs to be done, the improvements in the medical care of people with epilepsy have been significant.

Conversely, interest in the treatment and prevention of the psychosocial problems which often accompany epilepsy has lagged. As pointed out by the National Commission for the Control of Epilepsy and Its Consequences in the United States, and the Reid Report in Great Britain, the psychosocial difficulties associated with epilepsy represent significant problems, sometimes of a greater magnitude than the siezures themselves.

Nowhere is this truer than for children and adolescents with epilepsy. It is a cruel fact that the majority of epilepsy begins in childhood and adolescence, a time when these youngsters are in the process of acquiring knowledge and developing the cognitive and social skills which will serve them the rest of their lives. Hence, the onset of epilepsy in childhood or adolescence can have particularly pernicious effects on the quality of the child's life, as well as on the larger family unit.

Several excellent texts on childhood epilepsy have been published recently. While extremely comprehensive in their attention to medical issues, most of these volumes have devoted considerably less attention to the psychosocial characteristics of childhood epilepsy. It is in this context that the current text was conceived.

In this volume we have brought together a collection of clinicians and researchers from a variety of disciplines in order to address the issue of childhood/adolescent epilepsy from a psychosocial perspective. This collection of presentations will reflect the current status of the field in a number of ways. Some topic areas are moderately developed and are highly quantitative in approach, others are less well developed and are largely descriptive in nature. Some topics are clinical in approach and assessment, others are theoretical and experimental. Most areas of research are still attempting to identify the causes of specific psychosocial problems and, therefore, the important issues of significant issues which clinicians from a diversity of disciplines will face when working with children/adolescents with epilepsy.

This text was assembled so as to address four content areas. First, there are two introductory chapters which address medical issues and the relationship of neuropsychology to the medical management of childhood epilepsy (*Dreifuss*; *Berent and Sackellares*). A later contribution by *Zielinski* discusses in part some special diagnostic and treatment issues pertinent to multiply handicapped children with epilepsy. These chapters will provide a state of the art description of some medical aspects of epilepsy which should be of value to non-neurological physicians and clinicians from other disciplines who need to update their understanding of the childhood epilepsies.

Second, several chapters address the general topic of neuropsychological functioning in children with epilepsy. This is a heterogeneous area with presentations covering the prognosis of cognitive functions (*Rodin*), the neuropsychological effects of epilepsy (*Seidenberg*), academic achievement (*Seidenberg*), the effects of epilepsy anticonvulsant drugs on cognitive function (*Cull and Trimble*), and the relationship between absence/petit mal epilepsy and disturbances in attention (*Mirsky*).

Third, several contributions examine the effects of epilepsy on behavioral and social adjustment (*Taylor*; *Hermann, Whitman and Dell*) as well as the effects of epilepsy on the family system (*Ferrari*).

Fourth, we were committed to exploring the ways in which the psychosocial problems of childhood epilepsy could be treated or prevented; hence the final section examines intervention procedures. Contributions address vocational intervention (*Fraser and Clemmons*), the use of behavioral procedures as an adjunct in the attempt to improve seizure control (*Schotte and DuBois*), surgical approaches to the treatment of childhood epilepsy (*Wyler*), special concerns when working with children with epilepsy with other developmental disabilities (*Zielinski*), and the role of comprehensive epilepsy centers (*Santilli and Tonelson*).

It is our sincere hope that this volume will help to: (1) assist clinicians to improve the quality of care which they provide to children/adolescents with epilepsy and their families; (2) identify significant gaps in our understanding of the psychosocial complications of the childhood epilepsies, thereby helping to delineate problems and issues that need further empirical investigation; and (3) call greater attention to the significant psychosocial problems of childhood epilepsy and the importance of investing research time and monies to the development of treatment and prevention programs.

BRUCE P. HERMANN
MICHAEL SEIDENBERG
December, 1988

Chapter 1

Childhood Epilepsies

Fritz E. Dreifuss

Three-fourths of epileptic seizures begin prior to 18 years of age and the childhood age group is additionally vulnerable to seizures other than due to epilepsy. The etiologies of epilepsies in childhood differ from those in adult life. The preponderance of seizures fall into the syndromes representing idiopathic or primary epilepsies and many of these are characterized by primary generalized seizures.

The effects of anticonvulsant drugs are different in children not only by virtue of different metabolism but also because of their side-effects on cognitive function during the vulnerable ages of knowledge acquisition. During childhood a person's coping skills are developed and biopsychosocial aspects of epilepsy in childhood are of great consequence, including the opportunity for prevention.

During the past decade there have been advances in knowledge concerning diagnosis as well as the natural history of the epilepsies of infants and children. These have resulted in upgraded classifications of epileptic seizures as well as epileptic syndromes (Commission on Classification, 1981, 1985). The seizure is the observed phenomenon of epilepsy. In addition the syndrome consists of an etiology, a natural history, a family history and a prognosis. The seizure therefore is only a small part of the condition, though the seizure type determines which particular anticonvulsant drug is the drug of choice for its management. The syndrome will determine whether or not medication is necessary, and if so how long it is likely to have to be continued. The syndrome will also determine consideration of other treatment modalities and has genetic implications.

For this reason this chapter will include discussions of epileptic seizures which are commonly manifested in childhood as well as a more detailed description of the epilepsies. As most epileptic syndromes of childhood are age-dependent the organization of this chapter follows a chronological order, though some syndromes may cover a wide range of ages.

Childhood Epilepsies: Neuropsychological, Psychosocial and Intervention Aspects
Edited by B. Hermann and M. Seidenberg

CLASSIFICATION OF EPILEPTIC SEIZURES

1. Partial (focal, local) seizures

Partial seizures are those in which, in general, the first clinical and electroencephalographic changes indicate initial activation of a system of neurons limited to part of one cerebral hemisphere. A partial seizure is classified primarily on the basis of whether or not consciousness is impaired during the attack. When consciousness is not impaired, the seizure is classified as a simple partial seizure. When consciousness is impaired, the seizure is classified as a complex partial seizure. Impairment of consciousness may be the first clinical sign, or simple partial seizures may evolve into complex partial seizures. In patients with impaired consciousness, aberrations of behaviour (automatisms) may occur. A partial seizure may not terminate, but instead progress to a generalized motor seizure. Impaired consciousness is defined as the inability to respond normally to exogenous stimuli by virtue of altered awareness and/or responsiveness.

There is considerable evidence that simple partial seizures usually have unilateral hemispheric involvement and only rarely have bilateral hemispheric involvement; complex partial seizures, however, frequently have bilateral hemispheric involvement.

Partial seizures can be classified into one of the following three fundamental groups:

A. Simple partial seizures (consciousness not impaired)
   1. With motor symptoms
   2. With somatosensory or special sensory systems
   3. With autonomic symptoms
   4. With psychic symptoms

B. Complex partial seizures (with impairment of consciousness)
   1. Beginning as simple partial seizures and progressing to impairment of consciousness
      (a) With no other features
      (b) With features as in A.1–4
      (c) With automatisms
   2. With impairment of consciousness at onset
      (a) With no other features
      (b) With features as in A.1–4
      (c) With automatisms

C. Partial seizures secondarily generalized

II. Generalized seizures (convulsive or nonconvulsive)

Generalized seizures are those in which the first clinical changes indicate initial involvement of both hemispheres. Consciousness may be impaired and this impairment may be the initial manifestation. Motor manifestations are bilateral. The ictal electroencephalographic patterns initially are bilateral, and presumably reflect neuronal discharge which is widespread in both hemispheres.

A. 1. Absence seizures
   2. Atypical absence seizures
B. Myoclonic seizures
C. Clonic seizures
D. Tonic seizures
E. Tonic–clonic seizures
F. Atonic seizures

III. Unclassified epileptic seizures

This includes all seizures that cannot be classified because of inadequate or incomplete data, and some that defy classification in hitherto described categories. This includes some neonatal seizures, e.g. rhythmic eye movements, chewing and swimming movements.

Seizures are categorized as either partial or generalized. Partial (focal or localization-related) seizures arise in specific loci in the cortex which carry with them identifiable signatures, either subjective or observational, and these may range from disorders of sensation or thought to convulsive movements of a part of the body, which may become generalized. Simple partial seizures are those in which consciousness is preserved. These arise from six-layered specific symptoms to be discerned. At other times they spread quite rapidly and become more elaborate in their manifestations and ultimately may generalize. Complex partial seizures are those in which consciousness is impaired, and they may follow on simple partial seizures or may begin as complex partial seizures with impaired consciousness at the onset. With impairment of consciousness any activity manifested during the seizures occurs in the form of automatisms. The implication of complex partial seizures is that these involve in their elaboration elements of the limbic system, thus leading to early bilaterality of dysfunction. This may involve temporal or frontal lobe structures.

Generalized seizures involve large volumes of brain from the outset, and are usually bilateral in their initial manifestations and associated with early impairment of consciousness. They may range from absence seizures characterized only by impaired consciousness to generalized tonic–clonic seizures in which widespread convulsive activity takes place. Myoclonic seizures, tonic seizures, and clonic seizures may also occur as generalized attacks.

DEFINITIONS

A. Partial seizures

Simple partial seizures

1. *With motor signs*. Any portion of the body may be involved in focal seizure activity depending on the site of origin of the attack in the motor strip. Focal motor seizures may remain strictly focal or they may spread to contiguous cortical areas producing a sequential involvement of body parts in an epileptic 'march'. The seizure is then known as a Jacksonian seizure. Other focal motor attacks may be versive with head turning to one side, usually contraversive to the discharge.

When focal motor seizure activity is continuous it is known as epilepsia partialis continua.

2. *With autonomic symptoms*. Symptoms such as vomiting, pallor, flushing sweating, piloerection, pupil dilatation, borborygmi, and incontinence may occur as simple partial seizures.

3. *With somatosensory or special sensory symptoms*. Somatosensory seizures arise from those areas of cortex subserving sensory function, and they are usually described as pins-and-needles or a feeling of numbness. Occasionally a disorder of proprioception or spatial perception occurs. Like motor seizures, somatosensory seizures also may march, and also may spread at any time to become complex partial or generalized tonic–clonic seizures. Special sensory seizures include visual seizures varying in elaborateness and depending on whether the primary or association areas are involved, from flashing lights to structured visual hallucinatory phenomena, including persons, scenes, etc. Like visual seizures, auditory seizures may also run the gamut from crude auditory sensations to such highly integrated functions as music. Olfactory sensations, usually in the form of unpleasant odors, may occur.

Gustatory sensations may be pleasant or odious taste hallucinations. They vary in elaboration from crude (salty, sour, sweet, bitter) to sophisticated. They are frequently described as 'metallic'.

4. *With psychic symptoms (disturbance of higher cerebral function)*. These usually occur with impairment of consciousness (i.e. complex partial seizures).

Dysmnesic symptoms: a distorted memory experience such as distortion of the time sense, a dreamy state, a flashback, or a sensation as if a naive experience had been experienced before, known as deja-vu, or as if a previously experienced sensation had not been experienced, known as jamais-vu, may occur.

Cognitive disturbances: these include dreamy states; distortions of the time sense; sensations of unreality and detachment, or depersonalization.

Affective symptomatology: sensation of extreme pleasure or displeasure, as well as fear and intense depression with feelings of unworthiness and rejection may be experienced during seizures. Unlike those of psychiatrically induced depression, these symptoms tend to come in attacks lasting for a few minutes. Anger or rage is occasionally experienced, but unlike temper tantrums, epileptic anger is apparently unprovoked, and abates rapidly. Fear or terror is the most frequent symptom; it is sudden in onset, usually unprovoked, and may lead to running away.

Illusions: these take the form of distorted perceptions in which objects may appear deformed. Distortions of size (macropsia or micropsia) or distance may occur, depersonalization, as if the person were outside the body.

Structured hallucinations: hallucinations may occur as manifestations or perceptions without a corresponding external stimulus and may affect somatosensory, visual, auditory, olfactory, or gustatory senses.

Complex partial seizures

Automatisms: these are described as 'more or less coordinated adapted involuntary motor activity occurring during the state of clouding or consciousness either in the course of, or after an epileptic seizures, and usually followed by amnesia for the event. The automatism may be simply a continuation of an activity that was going on when the seizures occurred, or, conversely, a new activity developed in association with the ictal impairment of consciousness' (Gastaut, 1973). They may occur in complex partial seizures as well as in absence seizures. Postictal epileptic automatisms may follow any severe epileptic seizure, especially a tonic–clonic one, and are usually associated with confusion.

Generalized seizures

Absence seizures

The hallmark of the absence attack is a sudden onset, interruption of ongoing activities, a blank stare, possibly a brief upward rotation of the eyes. Usually the patient will be unresponsive when spoken to. In some, attacks are aborted when the patient is spoken to. The attack lasts from a few seconds to half a minute, and evaporates as rapidly as it commenced. In addition there may be mild clonic components, occasionally changes in postural tone—either an increase in tone usually affecting the extensor muscles or a decrease in tone in which there may be a loss of posture or relaxation. Occasionally this may cause the person to fall. As previously noted, automatisms may occur as a complication of absence seizures, particularly when these are prolonged.

Myoclonic seizures

Myoclonic jerks (single or multiple) are sudden, brief, shock-like contractions which may be generalized or confined to the face and trunk or to one or more extremities, or even to individual muscles or groups of muscles. Myoclonic jerks may be rapidly repetitive or relatively isolated. They may occur predominantly around the hours of going to sleep or awakening from sleep. They may be exacerbated by volitional movement (action myoclonus). At times they may be regularly repetitive.

Atonic seizures

A sudden diminution in muscle tone occurs which may be fragmentary, leading to a head drop with slackening of the jaw, the dropping of a limb or a loss of all muscle tone leading to a slumping to the ground. When these attacks are extremely brief they are known as 'drop attacks'.

EPILEPTIC SYNDROMES*

The epilepsies may be classified according to seizure type and EEG findings—for example partial or generalized, or according to etiology—that is, into idiopathic or symptomatic. Or they may be anatomically localized, for example into frontal lobe, rolandic, occipital, or temporal epilepsies and finally they may be classified according to precipitating factors. Age of onset may be of importance, as may certain diurnal influences (Table 1.1).

Table 1.1
International classification of epilepsies and epileptic syndromes

1.	*Localization-related (focal, local, partial) epilepsies and syndromes*
1.1	Idiopathic (with age-related onset) At present two syndromes are established, but more may be identified in the future: —benign childhood epilepsy with centrotemporal spike —childhood epilepsy with occipital paroxysms

* (Commission on Classification, 1981; Roger *et al.*, 1985)

Table 1.1
International classification of epilepsies and epileptic syndromes

1.2	Symptomatic This comprises syndromes of great individual variability which will mainly be based on anatomical localization, clinical features, seizure types and etiological factors (if known)
2.	*Generalized epilepsies and syndromes*
2.1	Idiopathic (with age-related onset—listed in order of age) —benign neonatal familial convulsions —benign neonatal convulsions —benign myoclonic epilepsy in infancy —childhood absence epilepsy (pyknolepsy) —juvenile absence epilepsy —juvenile myoclonic epilepsy (impulsive petit mal) —epilepsy with grand mal (GTCS) seizures on awakening Other generalized idiopathic epilepsies, if they do not belong to one of the above syndromes, can still be classified as generalized idiopathic epilepsies
2.2	Idiopathic and/or symptomatic (in order of age) —West syndrome (infantile spasms, Blitz–Nick–Salaam Krampfe) —Lennox–Gastaut syndrome —epilepsy with myoclonic–astatic seizures —epilepsy with myoclonic absences
2.3	Symptomatic
2.3.1	Non-specific etiology —early myoclonic encephalopathy
2.3.2	Specific syndromes —epileptic seizures may complicate many disease states Under this heading are included those diseases in which seizures are a presenting or predominant feature
3.	*Epilepsies and syndromes undetermined, whether focal or generalized*
3.1	With both generalized and focal seizures —neonatal seizures severe myoclonic epilepsy in infancy —epilepsy with continuous spike waves during slow-wave sleep acquired epileptic aphasia (Landau–Kleffner syndrome)
3.2	Without unequivocal generalized or focal features All cases with generalized tonic–clonic seizures where clinical and EEG findings do not permit classification as clearly generalized or localized-related, such as in many cases of sleep-grand mal
4.	*Special syndromes*
4.1	Situation-related seizures (Gelegenheitsanfälle) —febrile convulsions —seizures related to other identifiable situations such as stress, hormonal, drugs, alcohol, sleep deprivation, etc.
4.2	Isolated, apparently unprovoked epileptic events
4.3	Epilepsies characterized by specific modes of seizure precipitation
4.4	Chronic progressive epilepsia partialis continua of childhood

DEFINITIONS

The important dichotomies in the Classification of Epileptic Syndromes are into syndromes which are characterized by seizures that have a localization-related or focal element and those that are generalized, and between epilepsies which are idiopathic or primary and those which are symptomatic, secondary or lesional. Thus, localization-related (focal or partial) seizures may be seen as idiopathic or symptomatic syndromes.

Idiopathic localization-related epilepsy includes benign childhood epilepsy with centrotemporal spikes, childhood epilepsy with occipital paroxysms and other benign childhood syndromes including benign partial epilepsy with affective symptoms.

Benign childhood epilepsy with centrotemporal spikes is a syndrome of brief simple partial hemifacial motor seizures frequently having associated somatosensory symptoms which have a tendency to evolve into generalized tonic–clonic seizures. The onset with male preponderance is between 3 and 13 years, and recovery before ages 15 to 16. Genetic predisposition is frequent. The EEG shows blunt high-voltage centrotemporal spikes often followed by slow waves, activated by sleep and tending to spread and/or shift from side to side.

Benign partial epilepsy of childhood with occipital paroxysms is a condition described by Gastaut (1982), and is characterized by seizures beginning with visual symptoms (amaurosis, phosphenes, illusions or hallucinations) which are often followed by a hemiclonic seizure or automatisms. The appearance of migraine headache is quite frequent. Electroencephalographically paroxysms of high amplitude spike wave or sharp wave or rhythmically recurring occipital posterior temporal rhythms are noted when the eyes are closed.

Benign partial epilepsy with affective symptoms is seen in small children whose ictal symptomatology is characterized by fear, the patient often running to the mother and clutching her, then becoming limp or confused with automatisms of chewing or swallowing, laughing or salivation, pallor or sweating as frequent phenomena. Electro-encephalographically, temporal or frontotemporal sharp waves are frequent during the attacks. The prognosis is usually quite benign. The majority of localization-related epilepsies belong in the symptomatic category whose prognosis is that of the underlying lesion and whose manifestations are characteristic of epilepsy originating in the anatomical regions under consideration.

Syndromes characterized by predominantly generalized seizures also vary according to whether the etiology is idiopathic or symptomatic. Generalized idiopathic epilepsies in order of age include:

Benign neonatal familial convulsions. This rare form of neonatal syndrome begins on the third day of life and is dominantly inherited. The seizures are usually self-limited.

Benign neonatal convulsions without a familial element occur on about the fifth day of life, and again the syndrome is of short duration.

Benign myoclonic epilepsy in infancy is a condition characterized by brief bursts of generalized myoclonus with EEG findings of generalized spike wave activity occurring during the early stages of sleep. These seizures are quite easily controlled and the prognosis is that of a benign self-limited condition.

Childhood absence epilepsy (pyknoleptic petit mal) is a syndrome occurring in children of school age with a strong genetic predisposition in persons who have made normal intellectual and developmental progress. The characteristic seizure type is absence occurring many times each day, the EEG shows bilateral synchronous symmetrical three per second spike wave activity with a normal interictal background. The prognosis is for spontaneous resolution in teenage and good response to medication (Drury and Dreifuss, 1985).

Juvenile absence. In this condition absence is less frequent, occurring perhaps two or three times a week with onset in early adolescence in a person who has made normal intellectual and neurological development. Frequently these persons also have myoclonic seizures. Response to therapy is less dramatic than pyknolepsy, and the prognosis may not be as favorable for terminal remission.

Juvenile myoclonic epilepsy is a condition appearing around puberty, characterized by seizures with bilateral, single or repetitive, irregular myoclonic jerks, predominantly in the upper extremities. Because of preponderance of early-morning seizures many patients complain of dropping breakfast utensils. There may be a dominant heritable component. The myoclonus is frequently interspersed with generalized tonic–clonic seizures and it may be the latter that bring the patients to medical attention. Absence seizures may also occur. Attacks are characteristically precipitated by sleep deprivation, noncompliance with medication and by alcohol. The electroencephalogram frequently shows rapid generalized irregular spike wave and polyspike wave activity, and many of the patients demonstrate photic sensitivity. Response to the appropriate anticonvulsants is good (Janz and Christian, 1957; Asconape and Penry, 1984).

Epilepsy with generalized tonic-clonic seizures on awakening is a syndrome very reminiscent of juvenile myoclonic epilepsy in its characteristics, except that it arises at a somewhat later age and is less often associated with myoclonus. The genetic predisposition and precipitating factors are as with juvenile myoclonic epilepsy.

Some epileptic syndromes consist of seizure types which may be localization-related or generalized. These include:

West syndrome (infantile spasms). Infantile spasms are characterized by a specific seizure type, arrest of psychomotor development and hypsarrhythmia on the EEG. The spasms may be flexor or extensor and they may be jack-knife spasms or head nods. While the onset is usually between 3 and 8 months, while response to ACTH is usually good, and while the seizures may commence on a background of normal development, there is a second less benign form of the disease in which the spasms are preceded by an abnormal neurological development. There is evidence of structural neurologic disease beginning early in life, as evidenced by psychomotor retardation, neurological findings, radiological signs or the presence of other seizure types, and the etiology may be known as a specific metabolic disorder, a prenatal inflammatory condition, hypoxic ischemic encephalopathy or tuberous sclerosis. In the second variety the response to medication is less good and certainly less persistent, and the prognosis depends on whether the condition is idiopathic or symptomatic.

Lennox–Gastaut syndrome. In this condition children from 1 to 8 years of age are affected. The most common seizure types are tonic axial, atonic and absence seizures with a relatively high frequency and occasional status epilepticus with prolonged stupor.

The EEG has slow and abnormal background interspersed with 1½ to 2½ per second slow spike wave and multifocal abnormalities. In general there is significant mental retardation and the seizures are rather intractable.

Rather similar in appearance, but of much more benign outcome, is epilepsy with myoclonic astatic seizures in which there is frequently a hereditary predisposition and in which the development of seizures is preceded by a normal developmental history. Here myoclonic and astatic seizures predominate, though absence may be seen and status may occur. The spike wave activity on the EEG is frequently more rapid than three cycles per second. While the cause and outcome are variable, they are better, in general, than what occurs in the Lennox–Gastaut syndrome.

Epilepsy with myoclonic absence is a condition clinically characterized by an absence-like syndrome accompanied by severe bilateral rhythmical clonic jerking, and consciousness may not be lost to the same degree as in most cases of absence. The EEG is accompanied by bilateral synchronous and symmetrical three-per-second spike and wave. The age of onset is in the mid-first decade, there is a male preponderance and intellectual deterioration may occur more than one would see with absence of the pyknoleptic variety but less severe than occurs in Lennox–Gastaut syndrome.

Some symptomatic epilepsies which may have features both localization-related and generalized include:

Neonatal seizures. Most neonatal seizures have predominantly focal characteristics. They are often described as subtle because the clinical manifestations are frequently overlooked and include tonic horizontal deviation of the eyes, eyelid blinking or fluttering, sucking, smacking or other buccal–lingual–oral movements, swimming or peddling movements and occasionally apnea. Other neonatal seizures occur as tonic extension of the limbs, multifocal clonic seizures which may begin in one area and migrate to other body parts, or focal clonic seizures much more localized and sometimes hemicorporeal, first on one side and then on the other. Occasionally myoclonic seizures may occur. Tonic seizures and myoclonic seizures have a rather poor prognosis, and the EEG pattern is frequently that of suppression bursts activity.

Severe early myoclonic encephalopathy (Aicardi, 1987). The main characteristics of the syndrome include onset before 3 months of age, fragmentary myoclonus, erratic partial seizures, massive myoclonus or autonomic spasms with an EEG showing suppression bursts activity evolving into atypical hypsarrhythmia. The clinical course is severe with lack of psychomotor development. Familial cases are frequent, suggesting one or several congenital metabolic disorders.

Acquired epileptic aphasia (Landau Kleffner syndrome). This is characterized by an association of an acquired aphasia, multifocal spikes and spike and wave discharges. The seizures are usually generalized convulsions or partial motor seizures, and remit frequently before the aphasia, which is not directly related to the convulsive disorder.

Many childhood seizures are manifestations of specific disorders and these may be classified under special syndromes. These include:

Febrile convulsions. Febrile convulsions are an age-related disorder almost always characterized by generalized seizures occurring during an acute febrile illness. The majority of febrile convulsions are brief and uncomplicated, but a minority may be more prolonged and followed by transient or permanent neurological sequelae, such as the hemiplegia hemiatrophy epilepsy (HHE) syndrome. There is a tendency for recurrence of febrile convulsions in about one-third of those affected. Controversy about the risks of developing epilepsy afterwards have largely been resolved by some recent large studies (Nelson and Ellenberg, 1976), and it seems that the overall risk is not greater than 4 percent. The indications for prolonged drug prophylaxis against recurrence of febrile convulsions are more clearly defined now, and the majority do not require it. Essentially, this condition is a relatively benign disorder of early childhood.

Epilepsies characterized by specific modes of seizure precipitation (reflex epilepsies). In simple forms, seizures are precipitated by simple sensory stimuli (e.g. light flashes). The intensity of the stimuli is decisive, the latency of the response short (seconds or less), and mental anticipation of stimulus without effect. In complex forms the triggering mechanisms are elaborate (e.g. sight of one's own hand, listening to a certain piece of music). The specific pattern of the stimulus, not the intensity, is the desicive factor. Latency of response is longer (in the range of minutes), and mental anticipation of stimulus, even in dreams, may be effective.

Epilepsia partialis continua progressiva. Two types are now recognized, but only one of these two types is included among the epileptic syndromes of childhood, because the other one is not specifically related to this age. The first type represents a particular form of rolandic partial epilepsy, both in adults and children, and is related to a variable lesion of the motor cortex. Its principal features are motor partial seizures, always well localized; often late appearance of myoclonias in the same site where there are somatomotor seizures; an EEG with normal background activity and focal paroxysmal abnormalities (spikes and slow waves); occurrence at any age in childhood and adulthood; frequently demonstrable etiology (tumoral, vascular); and no progressive evolution of the syndrome (clinical, electroencephalographic, or psychological), except the evolutive character of the causal lesion. The childhood disorder, suspected to be of viral etiology, has onset between 2 and 10 years (peak, 6 years) with seizures that are motor partial seizures, but are often associated with other types. Fragmentary motor seizures appear early in the course of the illness and are initially localized, but later become erratic and diffuse, and persist during sleep. A progressive motor deficit follows, and mental deterioration occurs. The EEG background activity shows asymmetric and slow diffuse delta waves, with numerous ictal and interictal discharges that are not strictly limited to the rolandic area.

General comments

In general, idiopathic epilepsies are free of underlying lesional pathology, there is often a positive family history of similar seizure types, and the child has made normal progress to the time of the development of seizures. The seizures are usually self-limited and the prognosis is quite good for favorable response to medication. The medication has to be appropriately chosen for the type of seizure under discussion.

On the other hand the symptomatic epilepsies tend to have an anatomico-pathological substrate: a lesion is frequently at the basis of the problem and there is often a biochemical abnormality which is detectable. Neurological abnormalities are the rule, and associated with this there is abnormal neurological and intellectual development. A family history of seizures other than those under consideration may be present. Seizures are frequent and are not always of the same variety. They are more difficult to control than is the case in idiopathic epilepsy.

These distinctions can thus be applied to nearly all the childhood syndromes. On the one hand there are seizures which are benign, familial and may even require no treatment while, on the other hand, they may be the manifestation of underlying diseases with a severe prognosis. This is true of febrile seizures, of the West syndrome, the syndromes characterized by absence seizures and the syndromes characterized by astatic and myoclonic attacks. Some forms of benign primary epilepsies such as benign febrile seizures and benign partial childhood epilepsies may not require therapy, and others respond well to treatment which may not have to be continued into the indefinite future. Others again respond well, but require continued treatments, such as juvenile myoclonic epilepsy and generalized tonic–clonic seizures on awakening. The establishment of a putative prognosis is one of the more important reasons for classifying epileptic syndromes, and it is upon such a prognosis that the intelligent management of the epilepsy is predicated. Some epilepsies—by virtue of their natural history, the development of kindling, of mirror foci as manifestations of secondary epileptogenesis, of progressive seizure-induced cerebral pathology, or progressive psychosocial invalidism as well as chronic drug effects—manifest as progressive disease (Dreifuss, 1987). It is in such instances that a definitive surgical option might be elected, whereas in the majority of the seizures enumerated above conservative medical management is the treatment of choice.

REFERENCES

Aicardi, J. (1987). *Epilepsy in Children*, Raven Press, New York.

Asconape, J., and Penry, J.K. (1984). Some clinical and EEG aspects of benign juvenile myoclonic epilepsy, *Epilepsia*, **25**, 108–114.

Commission on Classification and Terminology, International League Against Epilepsy (1981). Proposed revisions of clinical and electroencephalographic classification of epileptic seizures, *Epilepsia*, **22**, 480–501.

Commission on Classification and Terminology, International League Against Epilepsy (1985). Proposal for classification of epilepsies and epileptic syndromes, *Epilepsia*, **26**, 268–278.

Dreifuss, F.E. (1987). Goals of surgery. In J. Engel, Jr (ed.), *Surgical Treatment of the Epilepsies*, Raven Press, New York, pp. 31–49.

Drury, I., and Dreifuss, F.E. (1985). Pyknoleptic petit mal, *Acta Neurologica Scandinavica*, **72**, 353–362.

Gastaut, H. (1973). Definitions. In *Dictionary of Epilepsy*. Part 1. World Health Organization, Geneva, pp. 75.

Gastaut, H. (1982). A new type of epilepsy: benign partial epilepsy of childhood with occipital spike-waves. In H. Akimoto, H. Kazamatsuri, M. Seino and A.A. Ward, Jr (eds), *Advances in Epileptology*, Raven Press, New York, pp. 19–24.

Janz, D., and Christian, W. (1957). Impulsive-petit mal, *Journal of Neurology*, **176**, 346–386.

Nelson, K.B., and Ellenberg, J.H. (1976). Predictors of epilepsy in children who have experienced febrile seizures, *New England Journal of Medicine*, **295**, 1029–1033.

Roger, J., Dravet, C., Bureau, M., Dreifuss, F.E., and Wolf, P. (1985). *Epileptic Syndromes in Infancy, Childhood and Adolescence*. John Libbey Eurotext, Paris and London.

Chapter 2

Clinical Monitoring of Children with Epilepsy: a Neurologic and Neuropsychological Perspective

Stanley Berent and J. Chris Sackellares

The early neurologists had little effective treatment for neurological disorders. They therefore focused clinical efforts on the description of signs and symptoms manifest in patients with neurological disease, classification of clinical syndromes, and the study of pathological changes in the nervous system. The only diagnostic tools at their disposal were the patient history and the neurological examination. Neurologists today, despite the number of remarkable diagnostic tools at their disposal, still depend primarily upon methods of history-taking and bedside neurological examinations which were developed and refined in the nineteenth century. Much of our understanding of the clinical and pathological manifestations of neurological disorders remains based largely on astute observations and analyses made by pioneers in the field. This fine tradition of defining and describing neurological conditions has been handed down to the modern neurologist. In relatively recent years, effective treatment and modern diagnostic resources have entered the scene. The modern neurologist is faced with the new task of developing the most effective and efficient means of applying these tools.

No longer is the role of the neurologist confined solely to description and diagnosis. In addition to identifying and characterizing the neurological disorder and its consequences, the neurologist must now formulate appropriate therapeutic interventions and monitor their effects, both positive and negative, on the patient's overall functional ability. With respect more specifically to epilepsy, initial enthusiasm regarding the newfound ability to control seizures with modern medication has been tempered by the realization that, even with the most effective drugs available, seizures cannot be controlled in every person. Further, we have become more cognizant of the potential for excessive

Childhood Epilepsies: Neuropsychological, Psychosocial and Intervention Aspects
Edited by B. Hermann and M. Seidenberg

antiepileptic drug therapy to adversely affect behavioral functions such as motor speed and coordination, concentration and attention, learning and memory, mood and affect. The potential for anticonvulsant medications to interfere with a child's education and development of social skills has become increasingly obvious. One of our present concerns is the impact of epilepsy and its treatment on the child's ability to cope with the disorder itself—problems in adjusting to discrimination by others, whether it be family members, employers, health care givers, or even stemming from the child's own negative self-image. The role of the neurologist has expanded in recent times to include not only the diagnosis and treatment of epileptic seizures, but concern also with the neurological and psychosocial consequences of the disorder and its treatments.

The broader scope of objectives in the management of epilepsy and its consequences is reflected concretely in the findings and recommendations of the Commission for the Control of Epilepsy and its Consequences (1978). The work of this group represented the efforts of many people from diverse specialties and disciplines, and emphasized the need for a comprehensive and multidisciplinary approach to the treatment of the child with epilepsy. This work strengthened the rationale for the continued development of comprehensive epilepsy programs. In addition to attention to basic and clinical research in epilepsy, these programs also focused on the development of models for comprehensive multidisciplinary treatment for patients with epilepsy. Each of these comprehensive epilepsy centers developed treatment programs which built on the strengths of existing personnel and other resources, but each emphasized the importance of comprehensive care and the need to employ professionals from a variety of health care disciplines in order to provide such comprehensive care. No longer must the neurologist view himself as a sole health care provider, instead he must view himself as a member of a health care team. Therefore he must reexamine his role in providing health care to patients with epilepsy and define his unique contributions to the comprehensive care of these patients.

At least in its applied aspects, neurology has a longer history than does clinical neuropsychology. As a profession it derives directly from medicine; whereas neuropsychology stems from the academic tradition of psychology. Applied neuropsychology has a very short history that can be dated in major ways to the 1940s (Benton, 1987). Although from a philosophical point of view neuropsychologists are more likely than neurologists to be atheoretical in their approach to patients, in practice both are likely to refer to a medical model of disease. That is, they are likely to consider disease processes that fit traditional medical models such as trauma, infection, systemic disorder or more recent concepts of unified disease theory. The two approaches are quite complementary and, when interfaced optimally, they greatly potentiate one another in terms of effective patient care. The neurologic exam is systematic and anatomically based. It is exclusive as well as inclusive, diagnostic and localizing in approach. Subjective information is obtained from the patient or his or her parents (e.g. the medical history). Objective observations of the physical examination are then synthesized. The object of this synthesis is to formulate an anatomical and etiological diagnosis. When possible, the neurologist seeks to verify or disprove these diagnostic formulations through independent and objective diagnostic tests. The neuropsychological exam is empirical and quantitative in its approach. It emulates science and is problem- (e.g. question)-oriented. In the neurological exam, quantification is often discrete, allowing for yes-and-no responses with respect to the presence or absence of defined signs or symptoms. In the neuropsychological examination, quantification may be discreet, but it is most often continuous. This distinction in type of quantification contributes to the value these two fields have to one another. Because of this difference, each field can provide feedback to the other, serving as verification as well as criterion-setting for one another. In research, the neurologist–neuropsychologist team can work to expand the diagnostic window in a given disease. In clinical practice this team can create baseline and follow-up plans that will allow for accurate, speedy diagnoses and continued monitoring of patient progress that might otherwise be unobtainable. While the neurologist brings applied anatomy, physiology, pathology, and pharmacology to patient care, the neuropsychologist brings the teachings of traditional psychology in such areas as personality, human development, intelligence, learning and memory, and psychosocial functioning. These topics of human behavior are applied through the procedures of clinical psychology (diagnoses of psychopathology, psychosocial conditions, psychotherapy and other behavioral intervention) together with the principles and procedures for assessment and intervention in the specialized area of brain–behavior relationships.

THE CONCEPT OF 'COMPLAINT'

Both the neurologist and the neuropsychologist are likely to find the concept of 'complaint' helpful in the process of identifying the clinical problem(s) to be addressed. A complaint is a verbalization or indication in some other manner that something is wrong. Complaints are almost always in reference to perceived deviations from normal standards in the realms of comfort, functional efficiency, or orientation to reality (Berent, 1986). Buss (1966) attempted to operationalize these three realms of patient complaint by defining discomfort as a manifestation of somatic pain or the related conditions of anxiety, worry or depression. He called bizarreness a deviation from accepted standards of behavior or from consensually validated reality, as might occur in delirium, hallucination, delusion or altered states of consciousness. Finally, inefficiency is defined as inability to meet the responsibilities of assigned roles. Roles might be occupational or they might be societal. The complaint may be communicated by the patient directly or, as is often the case when a young child is brought to the doctor, the complaint may be voiced for the patient by someone else. When the criteria of complaint are not obvious from the history alone, they may be brought to light in the patient's performance on psychological tests. Whether the patient sees the neurologist first or the psychologist first, the complaint is a sign that something is wrong. The professional then seeks, through examination and referral, to identify the condition (diagnose), to determine the causes (etiologies), and decide on prognostic statements and treatment strategies. Etiology is referred to in the plural because often the abnormal condition results from multiple factors.

While the two approaches, neurological and neuropsychological, are complementary and overlapping in some procedures, they also are quite different from one another in practice. Below we summarize each of these endeavors and present a model of the processes involved in each.

The neurologic process

In the management of childhood epilepsy, the diagnostic and therapeutic goals of the neurologist can be defined as a process that involves separate objectives.

The neurologic process

Diagnosis

Classification

Therapy

Monitoring

Treatment modification

The neurologist must first establish the diagnosis of epilepsy and then accurately classify the patient's seizures. An etiology must be established, and the psychological and social consequences need to be identified. The correct therapy is then instituted and monitored. Finally, treatment must be modified through an ongoing follow-up of patient progress. At any point in this process the neurologist might productively interact with people of other disciplines or specialities in order to reach objectives in the most efficient manner possible. The objective assessments of the neuropsychologist, for example, may be of enormous help in providing quantified observations that contribute to an accurate diagnosis or in monitoring the effects of drug treatment. Neurologists are trained in methods for diagnosis, drug selection and administration of antiepileptic drugs. The modern physician has become more conscious of the need to treat the patient as a whole, and has developed interview skills which are directed toward assessing the impact of the disorder on psychosocial spheres. However, in many cases, he or she relies on colleagues in nursing, psychology, education and social work to provide in-depth and more complete evaluation of the impact of epilepsy upon intellectual and cognitive function, personality development, educational endeavors and the development of social skills. In many cases these professionals may recommend or institute other types of therapeutic intervention, such as individual or family counseling, education regarding epilepsy and its treatment, and defining specific approaches to the child's education. In terms of the neurologist's approach itself, however, the following represents a brief description of the process.

Diagnosis

The initial goal of the neurologist is to determine whether or not the patient is suffering from epilepsy. This objective is complicated by the fact that the characteristic symptoms and signs of epilepsy, the seizures, occur intermittently and unpredictably. Therefore the physician must rely primarily on historical information to establish the diagnosis. The patient's descriptions of attacks are often vague and incomplete. This is not surprising since many seizures result in loss of awareness or impairment of recall of what occurred during the seizure and in the postictal state. In many cases it is essential that the patient's own descriptions be supplemented by descriptions obtained from family members and friends.

The neurological examination is at times of limited value in establishing the diagnosis in epilepsy. Often the examination is normal. However, there may be subtle signs of neurological abnormality which indicate the presence of focal neurological damage. Some seizures, such as *absence seizures* or *myoclonic seizures*, may occur frequently enough to be observed during the examination or may be induced by having the patient hyperventilate. Diagnostic tests such as the EEG are employed to aid in establishing the diagnosis. The interictal EEG often shows paroxysmal abnormalities which may be used to confirm the diagnosis of epilepsy and indicate the seizure type. However, in the interictal state the EEG may be normal, or it may reveal only nonspecific abnormalities. In some cases EEG recordings performed over several hours in conjunction with videotaped recordings of the patient may be required to establish the diagnosis of epilepsy and determine the seizure type. Ambulatory EEG cassette recordings which allow continuous recording of the EEG for several hours to several days may be required in some cases in order to increase the chances of recording interictal or ictal EEG abnormalities.

Classification of seizures

Classification of the seizures is based on the clinical symptomatology during the seizures, the EEG manifestation of the seizures and the interictal EEG.

Accurate classification depends upon careful history taking and judicious use of interictal, and in some cases ictal, EEG recordings. Seizure classification, along with family history, neurological examination and neuroimaging tests, such as the X-ray CT scan or magnetic resonance imaging, are used to establish the diagnosis of a specific etiology or epileptic syndrome. Classification of the seizures and accurate diagnosis of the epileptic syndrome of etiology are required for appropriate choice of antiepileptic drug therapy and to determine the prognosis for seizure control or development of other neurological deficits. See also Chapter 1 in this book, by Dreifuss, for a comprehensive treatment of the topic of classification.

In addition to establishing an accurate diagnosis on which to base rational therapy, the neurologist seeks to estimate the severity of the disorder. One obvious measurement of severity is the frequency and duration of the epileptic seizures. Another measurement of severity is the degree to which the disorder interferes with the child's quality of life. Epileptic seizures may disrupt family, school, and social experiences. Just as importantly having seizures sets the child apart as different, impaired or more dependent than his peers in the eyes of his family, friends, teachers, and in his own eyes. Any assessment of the impact of epilepsy on the child's life and well-being must involve an accurate estimate of the severity of seizures as well as the psychosocial consequences of having epilepsy. The psychosocial consequences of epilepsy in a child are not confined to the child, but may affect the entire family.

Therapy

Appropriate use of antiepileptic drugs usually results in reduction of seizures. In some cases seizures may be completely controlled. In other cases only a reduction in the frequency and severity of the seizures can be achieved. In a minority of cases antiepileptic drugs may be totally ineffective. The drugs of choice for the treatment of specific seizure types undergo constant change as new compounds are introduced and we acquire new information regarding the safety and efficacy of existing drugs. Some of the major drugs currently in use are listed in the Appendix.

In evaluating the impact of any therapeutic intervention one must weigh the benefit against the risk of adverse effects. In the case of antiepileptic drugs the impact of reduction in seizure frequency must be weighed against any side-effects which may interfere with the child's daily function. Seizure control should not be seen as the ultimate objective. Rather, the ultimate goal should be to reduce the adverse effects of epilepsy on quality of life. Seizure control is only one aspect of this goal. It is a means to an end. In recent years evidence has accumulated that the appropriate use of a single antiepileptic drug (monotherapy), in contrast to concurrent treatment with two or more drugs (polytherapy), is most often the best means of achieving optimal seizure control while reducing the incidence of adverse effects such as sedation, psychomotor retardation, and cognitive impairment.

Monitoring

It is the responsibility of the clinician continually to assess and reassess (monitor) the effect of his treatment on the overall function of the patient. One aspect of this monitoring is the effect of drug therapy on seizure control. For this task the clinician relies on periodic interviews with the child and his family. Assessment of seizure control involves obtaining a global assessment by the child and his family regarding the effects of treatment on seizure control. While this overall assessment is important, it is not enough. The global assessment is by definition subjective, and reflects overall satisfaction with the therapy and overall adjustment to the disorder. If the child is doing well at home and at school, the global assessment may be a positive one, even though seizure control is not obtained. On the other hand, if the child is doing poorly at home and at school the global assessment may be negative. Because the global assessment is influenced by factors other than seizure control, it is not a reliable measure of seizure control. For this reason a more objective indicator of seizure control should supplement the global assessment. This can be accomplished by having the patient or his parents keep a seizure diary or log. The seizure diary is used to record each seizure, what it was like, how long it lasted, and the date and time of occurrence. The diary is reviewed during each visit to the neurologist. Entries into the seizure diary can be transferred by the neurologist to a table or a graph along with drug doses, drug plasma levels and side-effects. Review of this graph will quickly provide evidence of the effect of changes in drug or dosage on seizure control and side-effects.

Antiepileptic drug levels must be monitored frequently in children. When treatment fails to improve seizures, or seizures break through periodically, one must be sure that the child is receiving sufficient doses and that medications are being taken consistently. Published dose recommendations represent gross estimates which can be used as guidelines for dosing. Individual children will vary considerably in their dosage requirements due to individual differences in biometabolism and biological responses. By following blood levels one can determine whether a child's failure to improve is due to failure of the dose to yield a sufficient blood level or the resistance of the seizures to adequate blood levels of the drug. If seizure breakthroughs are accompanied by drop in blood levels, then one must investigate the possibility of drug–drug interactions or noncompliance. In some cases drug levels may change due to a change from one brand of the drug to another brand of the same drug which has a different bioavailability or pharmacokinetic property.

Drug level monitoring may also be helpful in detecting the source of side-effects. Drug levels are particularly useful for identifying the cause of side-effects when the child is receiving more than one antiepileptic drug. For example, side-effects which occur after initiating valproic acid in a child already receiving phenobarbital may occur as a result of a rise in the phenobarbital level as a consequence of a drug–drug interaction. Changing the dose of one drug can affect the level of a comedication, even though the dose of the second drug was not altered. A common mistake is to change a drug dose simply because the blood level is above or below the usual 'therapeutic range.' If the seizures are under good control, yet the blood level for the drug is below the 'usual therapeutic range,' it may be unnecessary to increase the dose of the drug. Likewise, if the child is experiencing side-effects, subtle though they may be, reduction in dose should be considered regardless of whether the level is within the 'usual therapeutic range'. Like the dose, the blood level should serve only as a guide to therapy. But the most important guide to therapy is the child's response in terms of seizure control and functional efficiency.

The EEG is an essential tool for the diagnosis of epilepsy in children. The EEG can also be used as a guide to therapy in some instances. If the EEG background is normal prior to drug therapy, excess slowing in the EEG background following treatment with a drug should alert the physician to the possibility that the child may be overmedicated. Unfortunately, assessment of slow activity in the EEG is rather subjective and the amount of slow activity may vary considerably from one child to the other. Therefore, comparison of the most recent EEG with previous recordings may be necessary to detect significant changes. The EEG can serve as a guide to seizure control in generalized absence seizures. If there is persistence of the generalized 3 Hz spike-and-slow wave pattern, either occurring spontaneously or with hyperventilation, it is likely that the child is still experiencing absence seizures. Absence seizures are often brief and consciousness may be only reduced rather than lost. Therefore, history alone may not be sufficient for establishing the presence of absence seizures. Appropriate drug therapy may reduce the duration or severity of the seizures, making them more difficult for the parents or teachers to detect. In some cases it is impossible to distinguish brief pauses or inattentiveness from absence seizures. Thus, the EEG can serve as an invaluable aid to monitoring the effects of therapy on seizure control.

One extremely useful tool for monitoring absence seizures is the 24 hour ambulatory EEG cassette recording. This procedure provides continuous monitoring of the EEG while allowing the child to return home and remain relatively active. By comparing the incidence of generalized spike-and-slow-wave discharges of 3 or more seconds duration to the seizures actually reported by the parents, one can not only obtain an accurate estimate of seizure frequency, but also detect under- or over-reporting of absence seizures. The EEG is not helpful for monitoring tonic–clonic or complex partial seizures. These seizures are quite obvious and parental reporting usually provides sufficiently accurate seizure counts. The interictal EEG findings do not correlate with the degree of seizure control for these types of seizures. The history and neurological examination are useful for detecting adverse effects of drugs on a child's level of alertness, ability to concentrate, and ability to learn. However, these tools are somewhat limited. A careful history may be sensitive to changes in the child's functional ability, but it may not provide definitive proof that the problem is related to the drug. For example, a child's school performance may deteriorate due to emotional problems, difficulty in adjusting to the school environment or intellectual and cognitive problems which are unrelated to the medications. Certain epileptic syndromes such as familial progressive myoclonic epilepsy are associated with dementia as the neurological disorder progresses. In many cases neuropsychological evaluation may be extremely helpful in differentiating between the various causes to the child's decline in school performance—the contribution of antiepileptic drug effects, the neurological condition, psychiatric disturbance, or emotional adjustment difficulties—to name but a few.

The neuropsychological process

Referral

Consultation

Procedure

Report

Interpretive session

Follow-up

The neuropsychological process can be related to the model given above. Clinical practice (evaluation, diagnosis, treatment, etc.) as well as teaching, research and administration, all occur within the context of this model. Here, we will elaborate on the model, explaining each step in turn and relating it to clinical cases as relevant.

Referral

The neuropsychological enterprise works on a referral basis. It is important to keep two things in mind. While a referral for an adult is usually self-intiated, referrals for young children are usually parent- or school-initiated. The neuropsychologist is often an independent practitioner who may well be the first contact for the family, and who may see himself or herself as the primary provider for a given patient. In such cases it is not unusual for the psychologist to initiate the referral to another professional, and this will often be a neurologist.

These technical considerations include *validity* (Does the test measure what it purports to measure?), *reliability* (How consistent are the test results?), availability of relevant normative data (Will the results be generalizable to the present patient population?), and other factors, including the neuropsychologist's unique training background (for further information on this topic the reader is referred to Anastasi, 1968; Cronbach, 1970; Filsov and Boll, 1981). He or she will later interpret the test findings in light of the referral questions and attempt to answer them.

Matarazzo has termed this process 'assessment,' and he has contrasted it with the less complex endeavor of 'testing' (Matarazzo, 1986). Many psychologists do both their own testing and assessment, and all psychologists conduct interviews and do some of the testing. However, testing in this sense is often carried out by technicians who have been specially trained for this purpose and who always work under the direct supervision of a neuropsychologist. These test technicians are sometimes termed '(child) neuropsychology test technicians' or 'psychometricians.' The system that involves these technicians working with and under the supervision of the clinical neuropsychologist is termed the 'professional–technician model.'

Report

There are three aspects of this phase of the process that are of utmost importance. These are accuracy, effectiveness of communication, and documentation. Accuracy relates to the assessment aspects of the procedure phase, but it is also intimately related to effective communication and clear documentation. Accuracy is enhanced when reports are tied to the referral questions. In some ways, limitations on accuracy are set when those questions are formulated. Again, this underscores the importance of the consultative process and the communication that takes place at that time.

Interpretive session

There are many possible facets to this part of the model. On the one hand, an 'interpretive' session may consist of a standard and somewhat traditional interview with the child and/or parent, designed to communicate directly to the patient the major findings of the neuropsychological examination. However, the interpretive session may differ from a traditional interview. It may become a time for further assessment that seeks to address questions previously posed or even those that are newly formed. It may be a time of confrontation, when a resistant patient or parent is counseled about the need for a particular treatment or diagnostic test. The session may become a time of crisis intervention, or it may be extended into several meetings that evolve into brief or even extended psychotherapy. The interview may become a liaison, in some cases, to referral for other resources, often across large geographic distances. While the session is often with the patient, especially when the patient is an adolescent, it may be a meeting with child and parent(s) or even with a larger family unit. The session may be with school personnel, other care givers, or the referring person. The extent of the interpretive session is determined by the needs of a given situation, the original planned strategy, and the competencies of the particular neuropsychologist. For instance, a referral may often request that the neuropsychologist talk to the patient and/or their family about the need for psychotherapy, and to offer that treatment if it seems warranted. In some cases the neuropsychologist may possess the necessary background and training to offer these services. In other cases he or she may elect additional professional consultation for the patient.

In the interpretive setting the neuropsychologist helps the child and family define questions they each may have about the examination, the reasons for the examination and related topics. Together, they then address these questions. It is good practice to meet with the child and each family member alone before meeting with them as a group, as there are often things that need to be said, or that can only be said, in privacy. In all cases, however, one must retain a realistic perspective with regard to limitations on that privacy. For instance, the neuropsychologist would never promise not to tell the parent about an admission of some behavior that might be dangerous to the child or to another. It is good to remember the idea that confidentiality is a process and its content is worked out in negotiation and agreement. During the interview the person may reveal misconceptions about the nature of the illness and/or fears related to the particular condition. There are many fears and misconceptions that derive from what can be termed the 'existential' reality in which the patient functions. Some of these fears are common to many patients, having more to do with the predictability of the situation in combination with the limited number of alternative responses than to individual peculiarities. This idea was discussed in an earlier work (Berent, 1986). Nevertheless, for anyone working with children with epilepsy it is important to keep these phenomena in mind. For example, the child with epilepsy often fears the recurrence of a seizure, even when it may have been years since one occurred. In another instance the child may agonize under a misconception that another seizure will be terminal. A teenage girl may harbor an unspoken fear that her future children will be damaged because of her epilepsy. Horowitz (1982) has listed some themes that occur in the thinking and feeling of persons who are facing serious life events. Several themes common to patients with epilepsy are:

1. *Fear of repetition (fear of having another seizure)*. A patient reported difficulty in sleeping. In fact this person engaged in late-night conversations, heavy coffee consumption, and a variety of other behaviors that were designed to prevent sleep. At first the patient seemed unaware of

their contribution to sleeplessness. The patient suffered from nocturnal seizures and behind these behaviors, the patient came to realize, was a fear of going to sleep and having another seizure.

2. *Shame*. A teenage girl reported an incident in the cafeteria at school. Following a generalized convulsion she regained consciousness to find her 'friends' laughing and mimicking her contortions. This young lady was so mortified that extensive counseling was required before she could return to school. The same patient verbalized a sense that her seizures were a punishment for 'bad' behavior. Although she was unable to specify the bad behavior, she seemed certain that her parents were disappointed in her for not being a 'better' person and bringing the seizures to an end.
3. *Anger*. Although at times irrational, the patient (or family) often seems to need to blame someone for the situation in which they find themselves. The anger is at times displaced, and this may explain some instances of litigation that appear to be otherwise unfounded. On a more subtle level, such anger may be involved in (passive–aggressive) noncompliance with the prescribed treatment regimen, missed appointments, behavior problems at school, and the like.
4. *Fear of stigmatization*. There is frequently a resistance to identifying with other patients, or of being identified by others with them. This may manifest itself in not wanting to sit in the waiting room or to take part in educational or self-help groups, or it may have the more serious consequence of not taking medications properly. It is as if patients want to avoid any activity that reminds them, or others, of their epilepsy.
5. *Concerns about loss of self-control*. In some cases the patient may feel that he or she is likely to do or say something that may be perceived by others as inappropriate. It is worth mentioning that the fears here listed, though relatively common, are not irrational. One 13-year-old patient, for example, tended to wander postictally. On several occasions she was found, still confused and disoriented, miles from her home.
6. *Resentment over dependency*. Reminders of lack of independence can be numerous and range from denial of a driver's license to reluctance about letting the patient cook, babysit, or otherwise tend to their needs or the needs of others. Not only does this situation lead to a constellation of dependency behaviors with their own consequences, but the well-meaning parent also stirs feelings of resentment in the child through the protectiveness.

As pointed out by Weiner (1982), the symptoms of disease themselves constitute a major change in the person's life. These symptoms may also directly affect the mechanisms that are needed for effective coping and adaptation and at a time when stress is heightened. A lowered intelligence level also, not uncommon in childhood epilepsy, may interfere with adaptive function (Menolascino, 1970). Many children with lowered intellectual ability or other cognitive dysfunction become aware of their limitations and, as a result, suffer from lowered self-esteem and depression (Edgerton, 1967). In addition, the consequences of symptoms may complicate acquisition of social skills important to effective coping and adaptation. In turn, poor socialization may add to the normal stress of parenting, and this may lead to parental responses towards the child that are less than ideal.

A sensitive and empathetic approach during the interpretive session will often bring these phenomena into the open where they can be addressed in a caring and effective manner. Aside from direct responses aimed at remediation, the information obtained at this time will be used to further formulate diagnostic impressions and to develop treatment strategies. In the case of children these strategies may include recommendations that involve the parents directly in the treatment process. It is in this area perhaps that one of the big differences between adult and child clinical work emerges. Perhaps children are more dependent than adults, or perhaps there is more money and therefore more resources for children, or it may be a combination of such factors. Nevertheless, in working with children the professional may find that many more people are involved than with adults, and whether they are parent or agency, school or clinic, any participants in this network may be in need of some remedial intervention themselves. Such remediation may range from a need for current information to psychotherapy. The interpretive session is the place where these needs can be identified and dealt with.

Follow-up

The first step in the follow-up stage is to complete a *progress note*. A progress note is placed in the patient's chart along with completed test forms and related materials. It is a record of the interpretive process and should contain a summary of what transpired in the interview. All participants should be listed along with revised impressions, recommendations made, and patient and parent reactions. When pertinent the progress note can be made more formal and sent to the referring person as a supplement report. Often formal action is not necessary, and the note can be maintained in the neuropsychologist's office file and kept as a continuing record of the patient's progress over time. Any new contact regarding the patient will be accompanied by an additional notation in the patient's progress note. This note will be consulted before future patient contacts and will serve as a reminder of actions to be taken. It is not at all unusual for years to pass before a patient is seen again. In such cases the progress note proves invaluable. Nor is it unusual for the neuropsychologist to 'see' (sometimes by way of telephone calls) the child and/or the family numerous times in the interim between formal examinations. Every case will be different. Nevertheless, it is fairly routine with children that, once seen, they are likely to be followed either more or less actively for long periods of time.

A formal repeat neuropsychological examination is often prescribed. When this occurs, the model just described is reactivated and its processes begun again. Before the exam date, the consultation takes place. New factors about the case are presented and discussed, and a new or revised set of questions is formulated. If documentation has been appropriately completed the consultation goes smoothly, even when the professionals involved are new to the case.

Whenever a neuropsychological examination occurs, even if it is a repeat, a formal report should be written. When a repeat, the assessment analysis should include comparison of performance against the baseline examination and explanations in the report with regard to differences that are observed.

APPENDIX: COMMONLY USED ANTIEPILEPTIC DRUGS

Drugs for partial seizures: carbamazepine, phenytoin, phenobarbital, primidone.

Drugs for generalized tonic–clonic seizures: carbamazepine, phenytoin, valproic acid, phenobarbital, primidone.

Drugs for generalized absence seizure: ethosuximide, valproic acid, clonazepam.

Drugs for myoclonic seizures: valproic acid, clonazepam.

ACKNOWLEDGMENTS

Sincere gratitude is extended to V. Joy Berent, Martha Sevetson and Kathy Stoddard for their expert reading and editorial advice. We wish also to thank Anne Burke, BA; Bruno Giordani, PhD; and Shirley Lehtinen, MA.

REFERENCES

Anastasi, A. (1968). *Psychological Testing*, 3rd edn, Macmillan, New York.

Benton, A.L. (1987). Evolution of a clinical speciality. *Clinical Neuropsychologist*, **1**, 5–8.

Berent, S. (1980). Psychological assessment in epilepsy: a case illustration. In B.M. Kulig, H. Meinardi, and G. Stores (eds), *Epilepsy and Behavior*, Swets and Zeitlinger, Amsterdam, pp. 25–29.

Berent, S. (1986). Psychopathology and other behavioral considerations for the clinical neuropsychologist. In S. Filskov and T. Boll (eds), *Handbook of Clinical Neuropsychology*, Vol. 2, Wiley, New York, pp. 279–304.

Buss, A.H. (1966). *Psychopathology*, Wiley, New York.

Cronbach, L.J. (1970). *Essentials of Psychological Testing*, 3rd edn, Harper & Row, New York.

Edgerton, R.B. (1967). *The Cloak of Competence: Stigma in the Lives of the Mentally Retarded*, University of California Press, Berkeley.

Filskov, S.B., and Boll, T.J. (1981). *Handbook of Clinical Neuropsychology*. John Wiley, New York.

Horowitz, M.J. (1982). Psychological processes induced by illness, injury, and loss. In T. Millon, C. Green, and R. Meagher (eds), *Handbook of Clinical Health Psychology*, Plenum, New York, pp. 53–67.

Lazarus, A. (1966). *Psychological Stress and the Coping Process*, McGraw-Hill, New York.

Matarazzo, J.M. (1986). Computerized clinical psychological test interpretation: unvalidated plus all mean and no sigma. *American Psychologist*, **41**, 4–24.

Menolascino, F.J. (1970). *Psychiatric Approaches to Mental Retardation*, Basic Books, New York.

Weiner, H. (1982). Psychological factors in bodily disease. In T. Millon, C. Green and R. Meagher (eds), *Handbook of Clinical Health Psychology*, Plenum, New York, pp. 31–52.

Wechsler, D. (1974). *Manual for the Wechsler Intelligence Scale for Children—Revised*, Psychological Corporation, New York.

Chapter 3

Prognosis of Cognitive Functions in Children with Epilepsy

Ernst Rodin

GENERAL OVERVIEW

When one reviews the literature on cognitive functions in children with epilepsy one is impressed with the heterogeneity of the material which inevitably reflects itself in the conclusions being drawn. Epilepsy can essentially be subdivided into two large groups—one which is associated with brain damage of varying degrees as a pre-existing or concomitant condition and the other where spontaneously recurring seizures are the only manifestations of the illness. The literature by-and-large tends to recognize these differences and classifies patients who fall into the first group as symptomatic or acquired epilepsy, and those in the second as idiopathic. Although this is a time-honored division it is not necessarily entirely accurate for scientific studies, and can account for variances between investigators. For instance, a patient who has suffered a mild blow to the head by falling off a swing, and who develops seizures some time thereafter, may be regarded as having symptomatic–post-traumatic epilepsy, when in fact the head injury was negligible. Conversely the absence of etiologic factors by history or examination does not rule out a small discrete structural lesion, especially in one temporal lobe. Thus inferences as to etiology are at times hazardous, and instead of the simple dichotomy of idiopathic versus symptomatic a clinical classification of 'uncomplicated' epilepsy, to use the term introduced by Rutter, Graham, and Yule (1970), versus epilepsy associated with other central nervous system handicaps appears to be preferable. It is independent of assumptions about etiology, and the severity of the mental handicap lends itself to a gradation by the clinician which can subsequently be verified through specific neuropsychologic measurements.

The prognosis as to educational achievements and resultant life performance will obviously be influenced by the presence or absence of coexisting brain damage. It is also quite apparent from test results that the earlier the insult to

Childhood Epilepsies: Neuropsychological, Psychosocial and Intervention Aspects
Edited by B. Hermann and M. Seidenberg

the central nervous system occurs, the more severe is the mental deficit (Collins and Lennox, 1947; Rodin, 1968; Dikmen, Matthews, and Harley, 1977). There are, however, exceptions because some patients with spastic diplegia due to perinatal injury have measured intelligence quotients which still fall into the average range. While motor handicap is usually associated with lowered intellectual functions, as Sillanpää has pointed out (1973), the diffuseness of the insult—for instance as a result of an anoxic or encephalitic process—may be more important. In patients who have overt cerebral lesions prognostication is relatively simple, because they tend to remain at various levels of retardation although fluctuations can, of course, occur as a result of increased seizure frequency, the consequences of status epilepticus or excessive medication regimens. The question in regard to prognosis for intellectual functions in the 'uncomplicated' epilepsy population is, however, more difficult to answer.

LITERATURE REVIEW UP TO 1968

When I reviewed the literature on this topic during the mid-1960s I was surprised by the paucity of actual follow-up studies of children with epilepsy where the IQ had been measured at regular intervals (Rodin, 1968). The world literature contained at that time only six studies dealing with children, and four where children and adults had not been separated. The test instrument had for the most part been the Stanford-Binet in various translations, and the duration of follow-up was usually less than 2 years. This encompasses a period of time which is clearly too short to allow an accurate prognosis for future life performance. Furthermore, in most instances only one follow-up comparison was available against which improvement or deterioration had been measured. Thus it is not surprising that different authors arrived in part at different conclusions. There were only three studies where a relatively small number of patients had been re-examined at least twice within the mentioned time frame. Since the original review in 1968, only four additional reports seem to have been published. Table 3.1 lists all the studies which could be retrieved through the various national library data banks as well as those which were available in the reprint library at the Epilepsy Center of Michigan. It is apparent that during the past 50 years the subject has clearly not received the attention it deserves.

The investigations shown in Table 3.1 which had been performed prior to 1968 have been discussed previously (Rodin, 1968) and only the conclusions need to be summarized here. These can be listed as follows:

1. The uncomplicated epilepsy group has normal intelligence quotients, but there is a persistent suggestion that they tend to be shifted towards the low end of the normal range rather than being situated at the center.
2. Deterioration from a higher level appears to occur at times, but precise figures about the frequency of this phenomenon are not available due to the paucity of long-term longitudinal studies.

Table 3.1

Year	Author	Source	Number of patients followed	Duration of follow-up	Test instrument
1924	Fox	Colony school	130	1 year (one retest)	Binet
1928	Patterson and Fonner	Colony school	98	1–3 years 10 months (one or two retests)	Binet
1929	Denison and Conn	Children's hospital	21	8 months–4 years 8 months (one retest)	Binet
1934	Fetterman and Barnes	Community hospital clinic	46	1–2 years (one to six retests)	Stanford–Binet
1935	Sullivan and Gahagan	Children's hospital	44	1 month–4 years 11 months (one retest)	Stanford–Binet
1938	Kugelmass *et al.*	Institutionalized private practice and special schools	129 91	3 months–3 years (one retest)	Weighted average of 'appropriate measures'
1942	Yacorzynski and Arieff	Outpatients 'idiopathic'	63	1–3 years (one to three retests)	Stanford–Binet
1942	Arieff and Yacorzynski	Outpatients 'symptomatic'	27	1–10 years (1–4 retests)	Stanford–Binet
1943	Ziskind	Outpatients		1 year (one retest)	Stanford–Binet
1955	Tenny	Special school for epilepsy children	284	?	?
1974	Schlack	Specialized neurologic center	78	10–15 months (one retest)	Various
1976	Steinhäuser *et al.*	University hospital	44	2 years (two retests)	Kramer
1983	Bourgeois *et al.*	Children's hospital	72	Average 4 years, severe 6 years (one to six retests)	Binet WISC
1986	Rodin *et al.*	Outpatient epilepsy center	64	5–33 years, severe 9.6 years (one to five retests)	WISC WAIS

3. Follow-up studies which have been performed tend to show greater variability on test–retest measures than what would be expected from normal control groups.
4. The general trend for a group of patients tends to be in the downward direction, but the overall decrease in IQ points is usually not marked.
5. In the individual patient one may observe either a decrease or an increase in IQ on follow-up examination. A decrease of the IQ on one retest cannot be taken as evidence for permanent deterioration, because it can be offset by an equally large gain in IQ points on subsequent re-evaluations.
6. The most common causes for lowered intellect, even in 'uncomplicated' epilepsy, are early age of onset of the seizure disorder and frequency of major seizures.
7. Increase in IQ tends to be related to remission of seizures. Our own follow-up study of 56 adult patients who had been tested with the Wechsler instrument confirmed these findings, and noted in addition that the Performance rather than the Verbal portion of the test appeared to be more affected in presence of continued seizures.

The subsequent data to be reviewed here will deal only with those studies where follow-up investigations are available. The reader interested in prognostic aspects of specific seizure syndromes may wish to consult the recent review on this topic which updates the 1968 publication (Rodin, 1987).

REVIEW OF STUDIES SINCE 1968

Table 3.1 contains only those studies where measured IQs were available on at least one occasion following an initial baseline IQ assessment, and thus omits the important long-term follow-up studies by Harrison and Taylor (1976) as well as by Britten, Morgan, Fenwick, and Britten (1986), which will be commented upon in the appropriate context.

In Sillanpää's (1973) investigation, which covered a mean follow-up period of 10 years, all children with epilepsy (*N*=245) of the TUCH region of Finland were investigated. Of the 135 whose IQ was measured rather than clinically estimated, only 24 (17 percent) had an IQ of 86 or higher. The author noted this was due to case selection because psychological tests were obtained mainly in cases of suspected mental retardation or behavioral disturbances instead of having been a routine measure. The intellectual level of the other 108 patients was estimated clinically and 90 (83 percent) had a 'normal IQ' as defined above. In my personal experience, clinical estimates correlate reasonably well with measured results at the lower levels, but they can be misleading when one is confronted with a quiet, well-behaved child who cooperates with the neurological examination. In these instances a 'halo' effect may be generated and the significantly poorer performance on psychometric assessment may come as a surprise.

In the 71 children who were followed with psychological tests by Sillanpää, an increase in scores (magnitude not defined) was noted in two (2.8 percent). A decrease of five to nine points had occurred in four (5.6 percent), more than nine points in 39 (55 percent), while 26 (36.6 percent) remained unchanged. The test instrument was not mentioned in the publication, nor was the interval between tests. Several variables were found to be indicators of poor prognosis for intellect: early age at onset of seizures, organic cause, occurrence of seizures in both waking and sleeping state, occurrence of status epilepticus, complete loss of consciousness during the seizures, and a family history of mental retardation. An early good result of therapy correlated with good intellectual functions later on.

A 20-year follow-up on 203 of the original patients was subsequently presented in 1983 by Sillanpää. An IQ of more than 85 was reported in 49.7 percent, mild abnormality in 13 percent (IQ 85–68) and mild to profound retardation was present in 37 percent. The test instrument was not mentioned, nor was the course of individual patients. Concerning educational level, if one excludes from the author's data those patients whose education was either incomplete or who were in training schools for the retarded, one is left with 148 individuals with a completed education. Of these, 55 percent had received only primary schooling, 27 percent lower secondary, 15 percent upper secondary and 2 percent undergraduate or graduate university training. It is apparent that the curve is shifted to lower educational achievements, and this is likely to reflect itself in occupational status. The latter point was especially clearly demonstrated by the 25-year follow-up of childhood seizure patients conducted by Harrison and Taylor (1976). Two hundred of an initial cohort of 628 children who had had at least one seizure were available. Clear differences were obtained between the patients whose seizures had remitted as against those who either still had seizures or were on anticonvulsant medication. When employed they were overrepresented in the lower occupational categories, which corresponds to our previously published findings (Rodin, Rennick, Dennerll, and Lin, 1972; Rodin, Shapiro, and Lennox, 1977).

The studies mentioned above did not differentiate between patients who had epilepsy as a single handicap and those with 'complicated' epilepsy. The most recent publication by Britten, *et al.* (1986) deserves to be noted, although it does not contain IQ measures. Fifty-eight individuals who were born during the first week of March 1946, and formed part of the longitudinal program of the National Survey of Health and Development in the United Kingdom, were re-examined in terms of survival and continued dependence on anticonvulsant medications up to the age of 36. The assessments were compared between ages 26 and 36 to ensure stability of the results. The patients were subdivided into the complicated and uncomplicated groups, but only the results from the uncomplicated group will be mentioned here. Cohort members whose epilepsy had continued were significantly less likely than controls to be in paid work, and more likely to have had previous experience of unemployment. They were also less likely to think that 'life had been good to them.' An important aspect of the study was that at age 26 there had been no significant differences in regard to work between uncomplicated epilepsy patients and controls. This emerged only during the subsequent decade, but the authors had to leave the question open as to whether this was due to lay-offs of patients with seizures during times of economic slow-down or an inherent problem in the patients which manifests itself only later in life. We will return to this important question after we have reviewed the rest of the studies where IQ measurements have been carried out.

From a cohort of 276 children reported by Schlack in 1974, 78 had repeat IQ evaluations over a span of 10–15 months. The test instrument was not specified, nor were the mean IQ and educational levels (EQ). The group was divided into IQ and EQ of less than and more than 50. The fact that 55 children (70 percent) had IQs of less than 50 indicates that one was dealing mainly with a brain-damaged patient population. At follow-up a decrease in IQ (degree unspecified) was observed in 38 children (48.7 percent). The IQ had remained stationary, or had increased to an unspecified extent in the rest. A relationship to seizure freedom was noted. In the 38 patients who were in remission an increased or stationary IQ was observed in 27 (71 percent), but a decrease in IQ was found in 27 of 40 children (67.5 percent) who had continued seizures (p <0.001). Marked increase in IQ (not further defined) was noted in eight children. The probable causes of this increase were listed as: discontinuation of medications after several years of seizure freedom (N=4), reduction of total anticonvulsant dose (N=2), and seizure cessation (N=2). In the six patients whose IQ had markedly deteriorated, an increase in anticonvulsant dosages due to refractory seizures had occurred in four; in the other two there was an additional encephalitic process.

The paper by Steinhäuser, Wagner, and Kulz (1976) is of interest because it deals with a 3-year follow-up of a relatively homogeneous sample of pre-schoolers seen at the Pediatric University Clinic of Rostock. The age at initial evaluation was between 3 and 4 years. There was no selection other than a specified year of birth, and 44 children with seizure disorders formed the sample. These were compared with healthy children of the same age group attending Kindergarten classes. The Kramer test (Buhler and Hetzer, 1953), where the mean for normal individuals is 100, was used to assess intelligence. The patients at initial evaluation had an IQ of 98, which is clearly in the average range. Levels above 110 were found in 16 (36.6 percent); lower than 90 in 25 percent. The extent to which the sample contained patients with simple febrile convulsions or isolated nonfebrile seizures cannot be ascertained from the published data since a description of seizure characteristics was not provided.

At final follow-up when the children were between 5 and 6 years old the mean IQ had decreased to 93 and the number of children with values above 110 had dropped by 50 percent, which was 18.1 percent of the total. The major reduction had occurred at the first-year retest where the mean had dropped to 91. The third and final test showed a slight increase leading to the previously mentioned 93 level. The decrease was most pronounced in children who had initially higher IQs. In 23 children with a mean value of 112 the first-year follow-up showed a level of 103, which rose to 105 by the time of the second evaluation. Patients who improved clinically also showed the first-year decrement from 113 to 103, and ended up with a level of 105 subsequently. The initial IQ drop was independent of EEG findings, because it was also noted in those children whose records had remained normal throughout the observation period. The finding that patients with initially higher IQs are more susceptible to decrease in intellectual functions as a result of seizures thus confirms our findings in adults (Rodin, 1968). The implications will be discussed later in the context of our more recent work.

In contrast to the previous two papers the work by Bourgeois *et al.* (1983) was published in the English language and has enjoyed a wider circulation. It also had the advantage of being a prospective study. Psychological testing was carried out initially within 2 weeks after the diagnosis had been established at the University Children's Hospital in St Louis and anticonvulsant blood levels had been determined. Seventy-two children were followed for an average of 4 years and either the Stanford-Binet or the WISC were used. The children were re-evaluated annually and four groups were initially formed:

1. No change in IQ, i.e. less than a ten point change in either direction between the highest and lowest score was found in 32 percent of the sample. The mean scores were initially 100 versus 101 at final follow-up.
2. Fluctuating course, i.e., differences of ten or more points at times, but no permanent increase or decrease was noted in 40 percent; mean scores 99 versus 100.
3. Permanent increase of ten or more points over initial value in 17 percent; mean scores 93 versus 108.
4. Permanent decrease of ten or more points from initial value in 11 percent; mean scores 108 versus 88.

Since no differences in regard to clinical variables was found between groups 1 and 2, they were subsequently combined for further statistical analyses. The initial IQ was 99.7 and rose to 101 at final evaluation, a nonsignificant difference. The demographic data show that three children had had simple febrile convulsions, but it is not clear how many patients had had only one or two afebrile seizures rather than chronic epilepsy prior to or during the observation period. The 57 children with 'idiopathic epilepsy' had initially, as

Table 3.2
Demographics and seizure characteristics

	N	%				
Sex						
Male	33	51.6				
Female	31	48.4				
Race						
White	57	89.1				
Black	7	10.9				
Seizure type						
Tonic–clonic	43	67.1				
Petit mal absence	14	21.8				
Partial simple	4	6.2				
Partial complex	8	12.5				
Myoclonic	4	6.2				
Other*	5	7.8				
One type only	50	78.1				
Two types	13	20.3				
Three types	1	1.5				
History of status epilepticus	1	1.5				
Family history of epilepsy or febrile convulsions	20	31.2				
Neurological examination						
Normal	45	70.3				
'Soft signs'	16	25.0				
Abnormal	3	4.6				
EEG background						
Normal	46	71.9				
Slight slowing	11	17.2				
Definite slowing	7	10.9				
EEG seizure pattern						
None	12	18.8				
Questionable	7	10.9				
Definite	45	70.3				
School performance						
Below average	33	58.9				
Average	22	39.3				
Above average	1	1.8				
Seizures in remission	8	12.5				
	None		Questionable		Definite	
	N	%	*N*	%	*N*	%
Etiology						
Pre/perinatal injury	41	64.0	19	29.6	4	12.5
Postnatal head injury	56	87.5	8	12.5	–	
Cerebral infection	60	93.7	4	6.2	–	
Other external causes	–		1	1.5	–	

* Ill-defined or poorly described episodic symptoms in addition to at least one of the above

Table 3.3
Epilepsy children, follow-up descriptive data

	Initial evaluation	Last evaluation
Mean age	10.0 years	19.6 years
Mean grade level	3.8	9.9
Seizures in remission	12.3%	50.0%
EEG seizure discharges		
None	18.8%	40.0%
Suggestive	10.9%	14.3%
Definite	70.3%	31.4%
Behaviour problems	31.7%	29.6%

Anticonvulsant regimens

	Initial			Follow-up		
	N	Mean*	Range	*N*	Mean	Range
Phenytoin						
dose	47	205	(32–500)	40	266	(64–575)
level	20	13.5	(3.7–29.8)	19	13.0	(3.6–26.8)
Phenobarbital						
dose	41	63	(15–120)	25	88	(30–200)
level	17	19.7	(5.6–49.3)	17	11.8	(6.7–49.3)
Primadone						
dose	14	612	(125–1000)	8	768	(150–1000)
level	6	10.4	(2.8–14.7)	6	10.1	(2.8–14.7)
Carbamazepine						
dosc	5	560	(200–800)	3	866	(600–1200)
level	4	1.4	(3.3–6.8)	2	3.8	(3.3–4.4)
Valproate						
dose	10	1050	(500–2500)	9	1388	(500–2500)
level	10	43.9	(16.2–78.9)	8	40.1	(11.2–78.9)
Ethosuximide						
dose	17	741	(100–1250)	12	841	(100–1500)
level	7	47.8	(56–120)	6	48.8	(5.6–81.0)
Other (dose)	17			11		
Not on anticonvulsants	8	2.8 years	(<1 year–6 years)	6	3.1 years	(<1 year–7 years)
Number of anticonvulsants per patient		2.3			1.6	

* Doses in mg; levels in μg/ml

slightly increased, as had Color Naming and the recall of the Bender figures. The findings were mild and not statistically significant.

The best indication as to what happened to these children academically was revealed by the WRAT (Wide Range Achievement Test). Although the reading, spelling and arithmetic grade level achievements had increased, the percentile and standard scores had decreased to a statistically significant

In conformity with the data presented by Bourgeois *et al.* (1983) we then divided the sample into patients who had shown a consistent 10-point gain or loss from the initial evaluation for Verbal or Performance IQ. Verbal change did not show definite relationships to clinical findings, but the change in PIQ did. Of the 23 patients who gained or lost at least 10 PIQ points, 13 were in remission and nine of these manifested a gain in IQ. Of the ten patients who continued to have seizures, nine had suffered the mentioned degree of loss ($p < 0.02$). It is thus highly uncommon for the PIQ to rise significantly as long as the patient still has seizures, but remission does not guarantee a substantial rise. Of potential importance is the observation concerning four patients who were in remission but still showed an IQ loss of 10 or more points from their initial values. It would seem that in these patients the epileptogenic process might actually still be active, the remission temporary, and seizures may re-emerge again later in life. We also noted, in concordance with Steinhäuser *et al.* (1976), that when an IQ drop had occurred, it was most marked between first and second evaluation.

In Bourgeois *et al.*'s (1983) sample only 11 percent had shown a persistent 10-point decrease in Full Scale IQ, while this was the case in 28 percent of our sample. The most likely reasons are differences in case selection criteria and length of follow-up. We had excluded all patients with single seizures, febrile convulsions or those who had only two attacks in their lifetime. This was done in order to concentrate on those individuals who have demonstrated the tendency to spontaneously recurring seizures which is the hallmark of clinical epilepsy. We also stayed with the Wechsler scale because the Binet may at times yield higher estimates than the Wechsler and could thus cloud the picture. Furthermore, our follow-up was on the average 5 years longer, which may have provided more time for potential negative changes to take place. Our initial IQs were lower than those reported by Bourgeois *et al.* and are in all probability a result of the first two factors. For the follow-up differences it is probably of importance that in the St Louis sample only 18 percent of patients were regarded as 'difficult to control', while in our group 40 percent still had seizures within the year of the last evaluation.

EFFECTS OF MEDICATIONS

As mentioned earlier, Bourgeois *et al.* had noted that toxic anticonvulsant levels were associated with IQ decline. Our own data on the relationship of anticonvulsant levels to IQ scores are still incomplete, and further data are being collected. Ideally one would want to have the level measured on the day the tests are given, but this can only be done prospectively. In a retrospective study like the one reported here we had to limit ourselves to those patients where anticonvulsant levels had been obtained within a week of psychological testing. The data to be discussed now were collected from the entire case

Table 3.6
Significant correlations of phenobarbital level with IQ measures ($N = 290$)

	r	p
Performance IQ	−0.46	<0.01
Full Scale IQ	−0.38	<0.03
Similarities	−0.39	<0.03
Block Design	−0.37	<0.04
Digit Symbol	−0.45	<0.01

material and are by-and-large single rather than serial determinations. Because of small sample sizes, IQ relationships were investigated only for phenytoin (N=31) and phenobarbital (N=29). No relationships to IQ levels were found for phenytoin, but some were noted for phenobarbital. These findings are in agreement with the results reported by Bourgeois *et al.* (1983).

The different effects of phenytoin versus phenobarbital may be due to the fact that phenytoin levels which are regarded as falling into the 'toxic range' had occurred only twice (26.8 and 29.8 μg/ml respectively) and, since phenytoin has a relatively short half-life, the levels at time of testing may have differed from the day when they were obtained. Phenobarbital, on the other hand, has a long half-life and the literature regards levels of up to 40 μg/ml as being within the therapeutic range rather than the 25 μg/ml for phenytoin. The mean phenobarbital level of 20.5 μg/ml was therefore significantly higher than the mean phenytoin level of 12.3 μg/ml. Table 3.6 shows the significant correlations between phenobarbital levels and IQ measures. The Performance measures are more affected, which is understandable when one considers that these are tests where speed is an important aspect. When the patients were divided above and below the mean of 20 μg/ml phenobarbital levels, the PIQs were 78.7 versus 90.7 respectively (p <0.02). The findings were not statistically significant for the VIQ and FSIQ. It should be re-emphasized, however, that the relationship is not necessarily causal because the physician tends to strive for higher levels when patients are uncontrolled and, as has been shown, seizure persistence is an important contributor to IQ drop.

CONCLUSIONS

From the entire material presented here several conclusions can be drawn. The most apparent is that the topic has so far not received the degree of interdisciplinary scientific attention it deserves. Nevertheless, it can be stated that if epilepsy is 'uncomplicated' and there is only one seizure type which responds promptly to a simple anticonvulsant regimen without leading to toxic levels, the prognosis for intellectual functions is good, especially when seizures started in late childhood or adolescence. The prognosis is somewhat more uncertain with early-onset childhood seizures which have remitted because not enough longitudinal data are available. When seizures persist for several years in spite of adequate treatment, the child is likely to have some educational problems and in spite of an initially higher IQ, the patient may not be adequately prepared to pursue a college career effectively. Nevertheless, the overall life performance is likely to be adequate and satisfactory. Patients whose seizures remain refractory to treatment are in all likelihood going to experience considerable difficulties throughout their life span. Education is likely to be impaired and vocational choices apt to be limited to the lower socio-economic brackets. Furthermore, when these patients reach the age of about 35–40 years they may develop additional mental changes of which viscosity and memory difficulties are the most consistent feature. These patients may then conform in various degrees to the stereotype of the 'chronic epileptic' as found in the older textbooks. In this connection Steinsiek's (1950) autopsy findings are of potential importance. Although he dealt with an institutionalized sample, patients with overt cerebral disease had been excluded. Of special interest are the 140 patients, 27.9 percent of the total sample, which he called 'Lebensinsuffizienz bei Epilepsie'. He meant to indicate by this term that all the internal organs were intact at autopsy but there was a premature 'wearing out' (Verbrauchstein) of the brain. He felt that it could be compared to the debility of old age which occurred in these patients years or decades earlier, and was limited to the brain. This concept of premature aging of certain brain areas is potentially important because it could explain why many of our long-standing epilepsy patients start complaining of memory difficulties when they are in their early 40s. To my knowledge there has so far not been a systematic evaluation of the similarities and differences on psychometric examinations between a group of healthy individuals in their 70s against a group of 'uncomplicated' epilepsy patients who are in their 40s. The reason why this is not entirely irrelevant comes from three of our own studies in a patient population which ranges in age from about 20 to 50 years. Viscosity, the major characteristic of chronic epilepsy patients, is more common in the older individuals (Rodin *et al.*, 1984) and there is a tendency for the auditory cognitive evoked potential to increase in latencies comparable to what is seen in normal individuals in their 60s or 70s (Khabbazeh *et al.*, 1988). Furthermore, measurement of testosterone levels in males showed not only an overall decrease to the low end of the normal range, but also a statistically significant age effect. In the normal person testosterone levels begin to decrease by age 65. In our epileptic patients the phenomenon was apparent at age 33 (Rodin *et al.*, 1987). When one considers that testosterone effects are not limited to the sexual sphere, but involve overall anabolic and energizing functions, the finding does assume relevance in this context.

It is therefore apparent that even 'uncomplicated' epilepsy tends to be more than an occasional seizure, and a great deal of interdisciplinary work which relates psychometric data to clinical seizure parameters, EEG and evoked potential recordings, anticonvulsant levels and hormonal assays on a longitudinal rather than strictly cross-sectional basis needs to be undertaken.

REFERENCES

Arieff, A.J., and Yacorzynski, G.K. (1942). Deterioration of patients with organic epilepsy, *Journal Nervous and Mental Disease*, **96**, 49.

Bourgeois, B.F.D., Prensky, A.L., Palkes, H.S., Talent, B.K., and Busch, S.G. (1983). Intelligence in epilepsy: a prospective study in children, *Annals of Neurology*, **14**, 438–444.

Britten, N., Morgan, K., Fenwick, P.B.C., and Britten, H. (1986). Epilepsy and handicap from birth to age 36, *Developmental Medicine and Child Neurology*, **28**, 719–728.

Buhler, Ch., and Hetzer, H. (1953). *Kleinkindertests*, J. Barth, Munchen.

Collins, A.L., and Lennox, W.G. (1947). The intelligence of 300 private epileptic patients, *Proceedings of the Association for Research in Nervous and Mental Disease*, **26**, 586.

Dawson, S., and Conn, J.C.M. (1929). The intelligence of epileptic children, *Archives of Diseases of Children*, **4**, 142–151.

Dikmen, S., Matthews, C.G, and Harley, J.P. (1977). Effect of early versus late onset of major motor epilepsy on cognitive–intellectual performance: further considerations, *Epilepsia*, **18**, 31–36.

Fetterman, J., and Barnes, M.R. (1934). Serial studies of the intelligence of patients with epilepsy, *Archives of Neurology and Psychiatry*, **32**, 797–801.

Fox, J.T. (1924). The response of epileptic children to mental and educational tests, *British Journal of Medical Psychology*, **4**, 235–248.

Harrison, R.M., and Taylor, D.C. (1976). Childhood seizures: a 25-year follow-up, *Lancet*, **1**, 948–951.

Khabbazeh, Z., Rodin, E., Twitty, G., and Schmaltz, S. (1988). Cognitive evoked potential in epilepsy patients. *Neurology*, **38** (Supp.) 1, p. 320.

Kugelmass, I.N., Poull, L.E., and Rudnick, J. (1938). Mental growth of epileptic children, *American Journal of Disease of Children*, **55**, 295–303.

Patterson, H.A., and Fonner, D. (1928). Some observations on the intelligence quotient in epileptics, a preliminary report, *Psychiatric Quarterly*, **31**, 542–548.

Rodin, E. (1968). *The Prognosis of Patients with Epilepsy*, Charles C Thomas, Springfield, Illinois.

Rodin, E. (1978). Psychiatric disorders associated with epilepsy, *Psychiatric Clinics of North America*, **1**, 101–115.

Rodin, E. (1987). Factors which influence the prognosis of epilepsy, in A. Hopkins (ed.), *Epilepsy*, Chapman and Hall, London, pp. 339–371.

Rodin, E., Rennick, P., Dennerll, R., and Lin, Y. (1972). Vocational and educational problems of epileptic patients, *Epilepsia*, **13**, 149–160.

Rodin, E., Shapiro, H.L., and Lennox, C. (1977). Epilepsy and life performance, *Rehabilitation Literature*, **38**, 34–39.

Rodin, E., Schmaltz, S., and Twitty, G. (1984). What does the Bear–Fedio Inventory measure? In R.J. Porter *et al.* (eds), *Advances in Epileptology: XVth Epilepsy International Symposium*, Raven Press, New York, pp. 551–555.

Rodin, E., Schmaltz, S., and Twitty, G. (1986). Intellectual functions of patients with childhood-onset epilepsy, *Developmental Medicine and Child Neurology*, **28**, 25–33.

Rodin, E., Subramanian, M.G., Schmaltz, S., and Gilroy, J. (1987). Testosterone levels in adult male epileptic patients, *Neurology*, **37**, 706–708.

Rutter, M., Graham, P., and Yule, W.A. (1970). *A Neuropsychiatric Study in Childhood*. Clinics in Developmental Medicine, Nos. 35/36. SIMP with Heinemann Medical, London; Lippincott, Philadelphia.

Schlack. H.G. (1974). Zur Prognose der Intelligenz-und Sozialentwicklung anfallskranker Kinder. *Monatsschrift für Kinderheilk*, **122**, 676–678.

Shafer, S. (1984). Epilepsy and intelligence, *Annals of Neurology*, **15**, 506.

Sillanpää, M. (1983). Social functioning and seizure status of young adults with onset of epilepsy in childhood. *Acta Neurologica Scandinavica*, **96**, 68, 1–81.

Sillanpää, M. (1973). Medico-social prognosis of children with epilepsy, *Acta Paediatrica Scandinavica*, **237**, 1–104.

Somerfeld-Ziskind, E., and Ziskind, E. (1940). Effect of phenobarbital on the mentality of epileptic patients, *Archives of Neurology and Psychiatry*, **43**, 70–79.

Steinhäuser, V.A., Wagner, K.D., and Kulz, J. (1976). Longitudinalstudie zur Entwicklung anfallskranker Vorschulkinder, *Kinderarztliche Praxis*, **11**, 494–500.

Steinsiek, H.D. (1950). Ueber Todesursachen und Lebensdauer bei genuiner Epilepsie, *Archiv für Psychiatrie und Nervenkrankheiten*, **183**, 469.

Sullivan, E.B., and Gahagan, L. (1935). On intelligence of epileptic children, *Genetic Psychology Monographs*, **17**, 309–376.

Tenny, J.W. (1955). Epileptic children in Detroit's special school program, a study, *Exceptional Children*, **21**(5), 162–167.

Yacorzynski, G.G., and Arieff, A.J. (1942). Absence of deterioration in patients with non-organic epilepsy with special reference to bromide therapy, *Journal of Nervous and Mental Disease*, **95**, 687.

Chapter 4

Information Processing in Petit Mal Epilepsy

*Allan F. Mirsky**

The primary symptom in petit mal epilepsy consists of brief lapses or interruptions in the patient's ability to maintain contact with the environment. The French term for these lapses, i.e. 'absence,' has led to the modern designation for this disorder, absence epilepsy. Another, less frequently used designation is 'centrencephalic' epilepsy, due to the theory of Penfield and Jasper (1954). I shall use the three terms interchangeably. The interruptions of contact have been described in various ways, including lapses of consciousness, momentary lapses of attention, or temporary reductions in the capacity to process information. Each type of description stems from a different body of literature and, consequently, leads to different ways of thinking about the disorder. To consider the interruptions as effects on 'information processing' (the most recent term), affords certain advantages in terms of techniques for dissecting and understanding the symptom that other, earlier methods do not provide. It is hoped that this will become evident later in this paper.

The material presented here reviews behavioral and electrophysiological studies that have been aimed at understanding the absence phenomenon. The nature of the deficits seen in the ictal and interictal periods is described, and some suggestions are offered for educational techniques which may be of value in children suffering from the disorder.

A BRIEF HISTORY OF EARLY EXPERIMENTAL STUDIES OF THE INFORMATION-PROCESSING DEFICIT IN PETIT MAL EPILEPSY

The first experimental study of the behavioral effects of petit mal was done by Schwab (1939, 1941, 1947), who reported that the characteristic EEG spike-wave (or wave-spike [WS]; see Mirsky, Duncan, and Myslobodsky, 1986) discharge of this disorder was accompanied by delays in responding to simple visual or auditory stimuli (or complete failure to respond) in a reaction time

* Source: National Institute of Mental Health, Bethesda MD, USA

Childhood Epilepsies: Neuropsychological, Psychosocial and Intervention Aspects
Edited by B. Hermann and M. Seidenberg Published 1989 by John Wiley & Sons Ltd

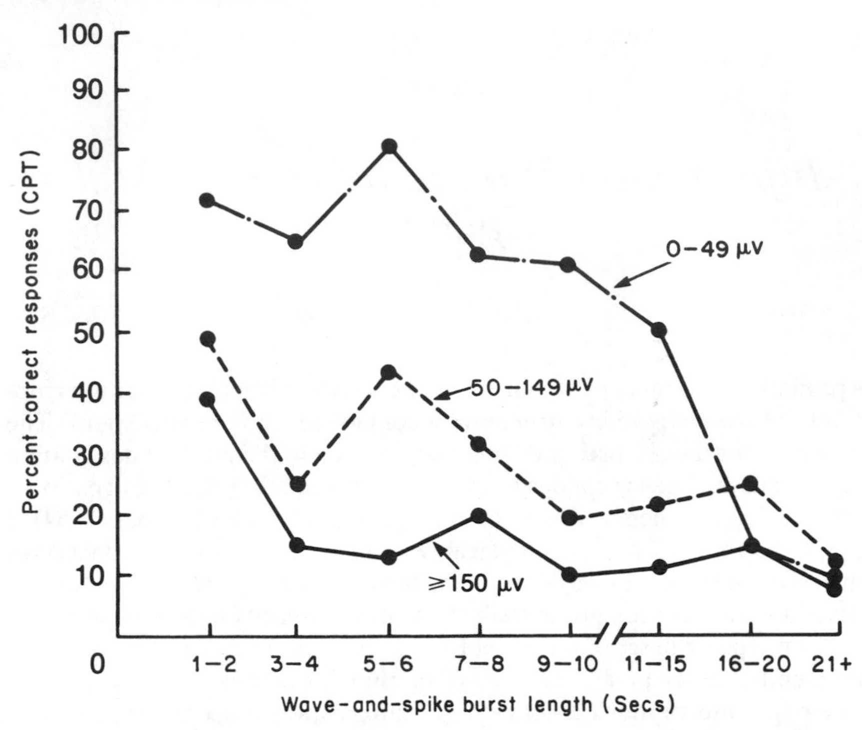

Figure 4.1. Relation between tendency to make correct responses on the CPT during wave-spike burst activity, and amplitude and length of the burst. Long bursts (> 20 sec) and high amplitude bursts (> 150 μ v) are usually accompanied by errors. In other cases, increasing length and amplitude appear to be monitonically related to omission error tendency. (Data from Mirsky and Van Buren, 1965).

task. Schwab was unable to detect the effect of brief WS paroxysms, however. Other workers have reported generally similar effects of WS bursts (Mirsky and Van Buren, 1965; Tizard and Margerison, 1963a,b; Goode, Penry, and Dreifuss, 1970; Orren, 1974; Browne, Penry, Porter, and Dreifuss, 1974). The consensus of these studies is that the likelihood of behavioral interruption by WS bursts is proportional to burst length and to amplitude of the discharge (Figure 4.1). Figure 4.1 demonstrates the relationship between the likelihood of an error of omission on the CPT, amplitude of discharge and length of WS burst. The interpretation of this recruitment-like effect, with more erroneous performance accompanying more robust discharge activity, is debatable. However, it may be argued that the more neural tissue that is brought into the WS paroxysmal process the more likely is the brain system(s) necessary for consciousness/attention/information processing to be rendered temporarily nonfunctional. This also implies, although it may not be immediately evident, that the brain system that generates the WS discharge is not identical with the system that supports the behavior. Van Buren and I advanced this argument some years ago (Mirsky and Van Buren, 1965). We also reported that the

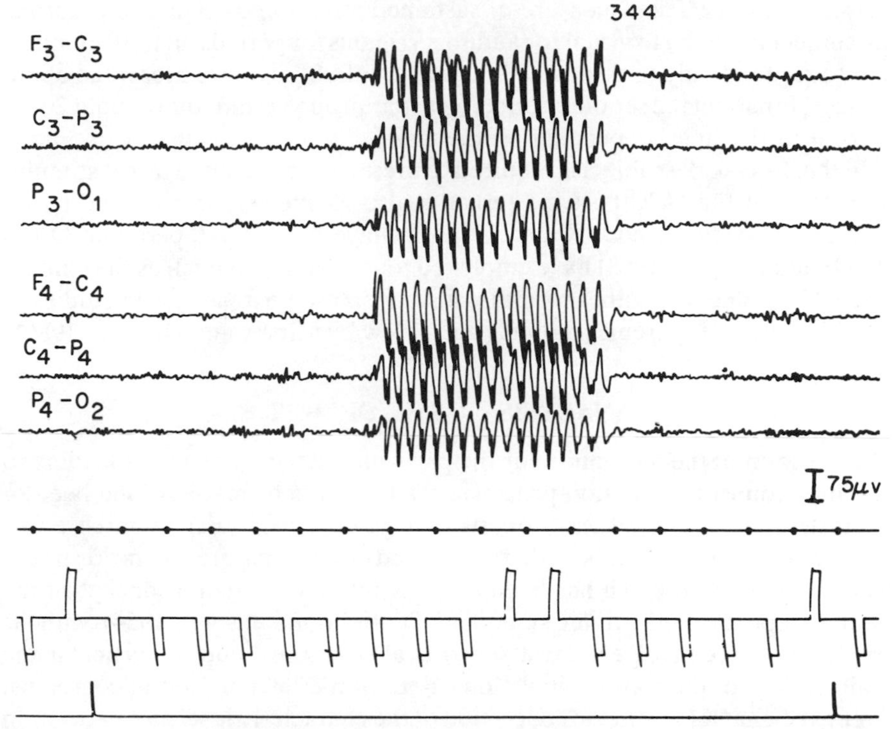

Figure 4.2. The relation between a burst of wave-spike activity and performance in a patient suffering from petit mal epilepsy. The top six channels in the tracing represent a standard anteroposterior EEG run, with electrode placements determined by the '10–20' system (Penfield and Jasper, 1954). The channel below this is a one second time mark. Below this are represented the stimuli (duration = 0.2 second) shown to the patient; those requiring a response (the letter X) are seen as deflections above the baseline; other letter stimuli appear as deflections below the baseline. The patient's response appears on the bottom-most channel as an upward deflection. In this sample, the patient responded correctly to X's presented before and after the wave-spike burst but failed to respond to the two occurring within the burst. (From Mirsky and Tecce, 1968)

following WS burst characteristics are associated with behavioral impairment: bilateral symmetry; organization (i.e. the tendency to generate repetitive, well-organized bursts); and character (i.e. the bursts are comprised of clear WS or W and polyspike complexes). The burst shown in Figure 4.2 would be described as symmetrical, well organized and of clear WS character.

THE CONTINUOUS PERFORMANCE TEST

Figure 4.2 presents an example of an interruption in performance on a visual attention task (the Continuous Performance Test or CPT) occasioned by a WS burst (Rosvold *et al.*, 1956). The CPT has been used extensively in research on the absence phenomenon (see review by Mirsky *et al.*, 1986 and citations in this chapter). The CPT is a measure of sustained attention or vigilance requiring the subject to attend to visual (or auditory) signals for periods up to 10 minutes, and to respond only to designated target stimuli. Stimuli are presented about one/sec, for about 0.2 sec duration; target stimuli appear randomly about 20–25 percent of the time, depending on the task.

In the 'X' task the subject is required to press for a designated target stimulus (e.g. 'X'); in the 'AX' task the target is also X but only if preceded by A. Auditory versions of both X and AX tasks have been developed, and Orren (1974) and Duncan (1988) have employed tones varying in pitch as the stimuli. The CPT in one or another form has also been used extensively in studies of attention in schizophrenic patients (see review by Mirsky and Duncan, 1986).

ANALYSIS OF THE DEFICIT

The question of the mechanism or the particular defect of behavior leading to the attention or information-processing failure in petit mal has long been of interest. The theoretical conceptions that guide a particular research effort may color the interpretation that is offered for the nature of the response failure. My own research has been strongly influenced by the concept of the 'centrencephalic' integrating system of Penfield and Jasper (1954) with its emphasis on the involvement of subcortical structures, and in particular the brain stem, i.e. the 'centrencephalon,' both in the interruption in conscious, attentive behavior and in the generation of the characteristic seizure pattern. In fact, Penfield and Jasper coined the term 'centrencephalic epilepsy' to replace the term petit mal; this label reflected their theoretical conception of the 'focus' of the disorder. The newest label, as noted earlier, is 'absence epilepsy.'

NEUROPHYSIOLOGICAL MECHANISMS

My colleagues and I conducted a series of investigations that involved a variety of manipulations in experimental animals of brain stem reticular nuclei, or other related structures; these were designed to simulate either the electrographic or the behavioral symptoms of absence epilepsy. This follows a long tradition of modeling the electrographic features of the disorder in experimental animals, usually cats, in research conducted by students and colleagues of Jasper (see review by Ajmone-Marson, 1969). Our studies involved such techniques as implantation of epileptogenic substances (i.e. aluminum hydroxide in the thalamus or brain stem (Mirsky and Oshima, 1973)), electrical stimulation of thalamic and reticular formation structures in monkeys trained to perform attention tests (Bakay Pragay *et al.*, 1975), measurement of EEG or event-related potential changes consequent to direct brain stimulation (Mirsky, Bakay Pragay and Harris, 1977), the production of WS complexes by means of steroids (Mirsky *et al.*, 1973), and the search for neurons in the brain stem with a special role in visual attention (Bakay Pragay *et al.*, 1978; Ray, Mirsky, and Bakay Pragay, 1982). Our results indicated that manipulations of brain stem could produce effects which strongly resembled the symptoms seen in petit mal epilepsy (i.e. the arrest in behavior, the errors of omission on attention tests), thus supporting the view of the key role of this brain region in the pathophysiology of this disorder (Mirsky and Bakay Pragay, 1988). Moreover, the behavioral effects of these manipulations could be accounted for as the result of interruption of the activity of the 'attention' cells in the brain stem.

This account does not rule out the possibility, of course, that these cells form part of a larger attention network with widespread rostral anatomical connections (Mirsky, 1987). Our conception is thus consistent with the classical views of Moruzzi, Magoun, Lindsley, and others (Lindsley, 1960) that the brain stem reticular activating system is a major center for the control of the processes of attention and consciousness, and consistent with the views of Penfield and Jasper (1954) concerning the key role of the brain stem in the behavioral manifestations of petit mal seizures. In contrast, the recent views of Gloor (1988), who has led a prolific and sustained research program on the pathophysiology of petit mal, lean toward the notion of the absence as a temporary dementia; this is consequent to the brief, reversible disabling of cortical behavioral systems. This follows from the model Gloor has developed for absence seizures which emphasizes the role of cortical disruption, in conjunction with some disturbance of thalamic function, in the expression of the disorder (Gloor, 1988).

ANALYSIS OF BEHAVIOR

Our attempts to identify the nature of the deficit in WS bursts began with the use of a measure of visual attention—the CPT—which was found to be impaired in absence patients; patients with focal epilepsy, on the other hand, were unimpaired on this test (Mirsky *et al.*, 1960; Lansdell and Mirsky, 1964; Fedio and Mirsky, 1969).

Some years ago Van Buren and I published the results of an intensive behavioral and psychophysiological investigation in a group of 18 patients with absence seizures (Mirsky and Van Buren, 1965). Part of this study included some experiments designed to identify the nature of the behavioral deficit during WS bursts. We created some tests aimed at maximizing sensory, motor, or mnemonic requirements, so as to be able to better characterize the nature of the absence. We then compared the effects of WS bursts on the different tests in the same group of patients. To maximize the sensory and minimize the motor demands on the subjects we developed the delayed identification (DId) task. We asked subjects to attend to various stimuli, visual or auditory, but not to report them until asked to do so by the examiner. Some of these stimuli fell within a WS burst; others came at some interval preceding the bursts; and in other instances no burst was involved. The latter condition served to check on the effects of the passage of time on the ability of these patients to recall simple stimuli.

To maximize the motor demands and to minimize sensory and other information processing requirements, we asked the subjects to perform a simple repetitive motor response (SMR) test—by pressing a response key (of the CPT) at a comfortable rate—and observed the effects of burst activity. We compared the effects of WS activity within patients across the three conditions (i.e. CPT, DId and SMR) and found in general that the CPT was most impaired, followed by the DId and then by the SMR. The data are summarized in Table 4.1. The fact that greater effects of WS bursts were found on the CPT than on the DId or SMR tests indicates that the WS-induced impairment on the CPT cannot be interpreted solely on the basis of a temporary sensory or motor loss; some higher-order processing must be affected as well. By the same token, these contributions to response failure on the CPT may not be ignored. The variability from patient to patient was striking. As can be seen from the range in scores in Table 4.1, some patients were able to achieve high levels of performance during WS bursts; others were totally impaired. A proportion of this variability is due to burst factors such as voltage and duration, represented in Figure 4.2. However, as Mirsky and Van Buren (1965) showed, a considerable amount of performance variability between patients remains, even after all such electrographic factors are controlled. I shall discuss this briefly, later in this chapter.

The analysis presented thus far suggests that sensory and motor—or, more precisely, response-execution factors—are implicated in the impairment seen on the CPT, although they are apparently not sufficient to account entirely for the deficit. A higher-order processing deficit is presumably also involved. Analysis of some of the data gathered in the DId experiment suggests that there may also be a loss of short-term memory. It will be recalled that there were

Table 4.1
Comparison of correct responses made by eight patients on CPT, DId, and SMR tests during WS bursts (adapted from Mirsky and Van Buren, 1965)

Test		Mean percentage correct responses		Range
CPT		17.2[a]	$p<0.02$	0–61.0
DId ('Sensory')	$p<0.01$	42.04[b]	$p<0.20$	0–87.0
SMR ('Motor')		52.9[c]		0–100.0

[a] Correct responses to target stimuli, i.e. correct commissions during WS bursts.
[b] Correct recall of stimuli presented during WS bursts.
[c] Instances when patient continues to press response key at preburst rate during WS bursts (percentage of actual key presses).

Table 4.2
The DId Test as a function of burst activity: percentage errors under various conditions; eight patients (after Mirsky and Van Buren, 1965)

Condition	Mean percentage errors		Range percentage errors	Mean no. stimuli
(A) S–R[a]	2.3	$p<0.01$	0–5.5	204.9
(B) S–B–R[b]	25.6	$p<0.05$	5.0–55.5	26.9
(C) SB/R[c]	58.0		12.5–100.0	46.4

[a] No bursts supervened between presentation of stimulus and request for recall.
[b] Burst occurred between stimulus and request for recall.
[c] Stimuli presented during WS burst; recall requested later.

three conditions in that experiment, in which stimuli were presented either (A) in no immediate relation to bursts, (B) prior to bursts, or (C) during bursts. As Table 4.2 shows, there are striking differences in error rates in recall as a function of the condition: in condition (A) the patients were virtually error-free; in condition (C) are nearly 60 percent of stimuli cannot be recalled. The evidence for a retrograde amnesic effect of the bursts is provided in condition (B): one-quarter of the stimuli presented before bursts could not be recalled. Encoding as well as registration difficulties may be involved in the impaired performance seen in condition (C). The available data suggest that both may be implicated in the WS burst effect. It should be noted that condition (A) controlled for length of time between stimulus and recall.

We can summarize the material presented to this point as follows: much of the neurophysiological studies done in human subjects, and in animal models of petit mal, has supported Penfield and Jasper's centrencephalic hypothesis of brain stem dysfunction. Pathophysiological processes in the brain region are thought to generate both the behavioral and electrographic disturbances in absence epilepsy. Other research (Gloor, 1988) has tended to emphasize the role of cortical factors in the expression and behavioral symptoms of the disorder. A consensus exists, however, that WS bursts can impair sensory, mnemonic-encoding and response-execution capacities, and therefore that no simple description of the disturbance produced by WS bursts is possible.

OCULOMOTOR FACTORS IN ABSENCE SEIZURES

While recognizing that loss of sensory capacity (temporary blindness?) may not account for all of the response failures on tasks such as the CPT, such loss may indeed be a necessary if not sufficient condition for CPT errors of omission in WS bursts.

The possibility also exists that the response failures on a visual task during WS bursts may be a simple result of movement of the subject's eyes away from the target stimulus—an involuntary oculomotor accompaniment of the seizure.

Orren and I provided some data relevant to that possibility in a group of four patients with absence seizures (Orren and Mirsky, 1975). We sought also to examine the latency of the burst-related eye movements in relation to the onset of the burst; this study arose (in part) from a finding reported by Mirsky and Van Buren (1965) that CPT errors *preceded* WS burst onset by 0.5 sec, on the average. We found, however, that if oculomotor changes occurred, they *followed* rather than *preceded* the WS burst. Moreover, two of the patients showed no WS-related eye movements, although they were clearly impaired on the CPT during the bursts (Orren and Mirsky, 1975; Orren, 1974). The results thus suggest that the oculomotor changes which may accompany WS bursts are not sufficient to account for the subject's neglect of visual stimuli.

EFFECTS OF WS BURSTS ON ERPS

Orren also conducted a series of studies of the effects of WS bursts on visual event related potentials (ERP) (Orren, 1974, 1978). The use of the ERP presumably provides a totally response-free measure of information processing. She reported that partial to complete degradation of visual ERPs could be found in absence patients (Figure 4.3) (Orren, 1974); see also discussion of these results in Mirsky *et al.*, 1987, Mirsky and Orren, 1977, and Mirsky and Bakay Pragay, 1988). This finding is consistent with the effects of reticular formation stimulation reported by Mirsky, Bakay Pragay and Harris (1977): reduced amplitude visual ERPs. Moreover, Orren reported that diminution of early (presumably sensory) components of the ERP could be found in the 1-sec. period *prior* to the onset of WS bursts (Figure 4.4) (Orren, 1978). This latter finding is consistent with the occurrence of CPT errors preceding WS bursts reported by Mirsky and Van Buren (1965). The effects of WS bursts on other sensory modalities have not been investigated intensively. There is, however, a report that WS bursts may alter brain stem auditory evoked responses (BAERs) both in animal models of the WS discharge produced by pharmacological methods, and in a patient suffering from absence seizures. Figure 4.5 illustrates WS effects on BAERs in a cat and monkey model of WS discharges and in a patient that Skoff and I studied. The WS activity disrupted the BAER in all three instances; the data from the patient show a delay in component IV, which is compatible with a disturbance at the level of the midbrain, and possibly at the auditory way station, the inferior colliculus (Starr, Sohmer, and Celesia, 1978). These data suggest that disruption of sensory transmission in the auditory modality may also occur in WS bursts, implying that this generalized paroxysm does not preferentially impair vision, but that it probably signals a global impairment of all (or many) sensory modalities. This in turn suggests that the pathophysiological source of the response failure is some generalized disturbance, such as one originating in the structures comprising the reticular activating system.

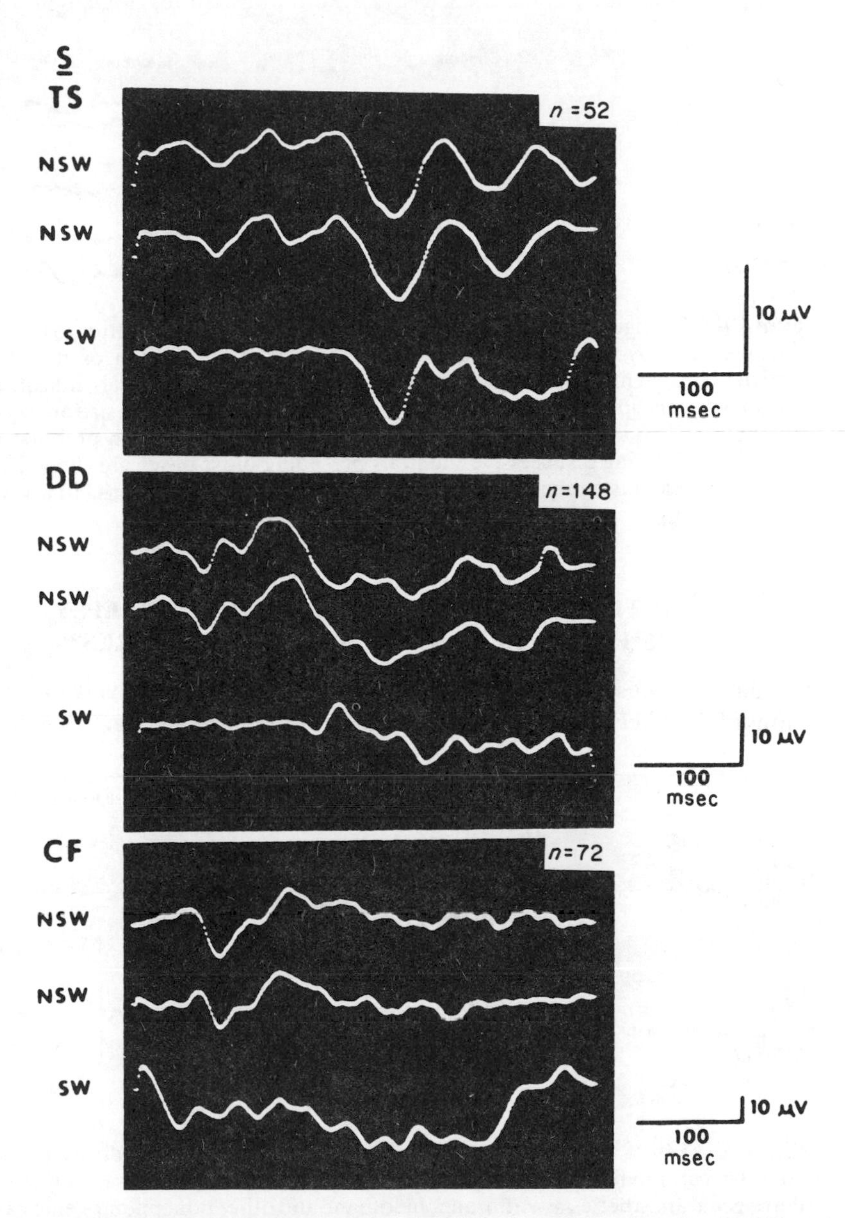

Figure 4.3. Visual event-related potentials (ERPs) during non-wave-spike (NSW) and wave-spike (SW) EEG activity in three absence patients, T.S., D.D., and C.F. The wave forms were obtained from parietal-occipital recordings (P3–10 or P4–02). An upward deflection indicates positivity at the occipital relative to the parietal electrode. Note that sensory components of the ERP, within the first 100–200 msec, were absent during bursts of wave-spike activity. (From Mirsky and Orren, 1977)

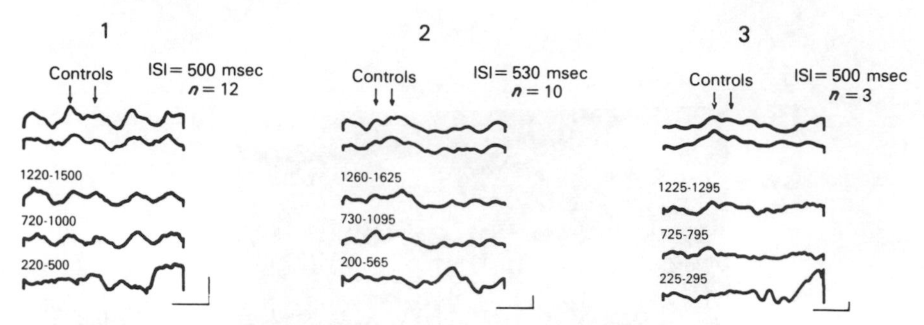

Figure 4.4. Changes in the average flash-evoked ERP of 3 subjects prior to the onset of wave-spike bursts. Single responses were averaged as a function of flash-to-burst interval, indicated in the msec above each curve. Interstimulus interval, indicated in the msec above each curve. Interstimulus interval (ISI) and ERP sample size are shown for each subject. The average ERPs (P–O recording) during the fourth preburst second (controls) and during 3 successive intervals preceding burst onset are shown. Arrows point to components common to both control responses. Calibrations: 10 μ v and 100 msec (From Orren, 1978)

THE INTERICTAL PERIOD IN PETIT MAL EPILEPSY—ARE PATIENTS NORMAL BETWEEN SEIZURES?

The material presented thus far has focused almost exclusively on investigations of the effects of the burst WS on information processing. While it is true

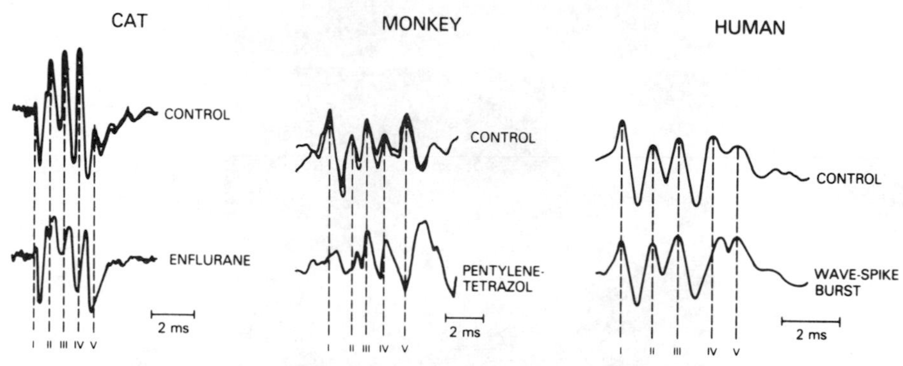

Figure 4.5. Effect of wave-spike bursts of BAER (Brainstem auditory evoked responses) in cat, monkey, and human. The seizure activity in the cat was induced by the epileptogenic anesthetic gas enflurane; halothane and other nonepileptogenic gases are ineffective. Pentylenetetrazol was used to induce generalized seizure activity in the monkey. A change in morphology as well as an increase in brainstem transmission time (interpeak I-V latency) was seen during the seizure period. The averages in the monkey are based on N = 1000 clicks at 20 Hz. In the human, the wave-spike activity was due to spontaneously occurring paroxysmal bursts in a patient with petit mal epilepsy. The average BAER in the patient was based on N = 640 clicks at 20 Hz (From Mirsky, 1988)

Table 4.3
Mean CPT scores (percentage correct responses) in seizure-free intervals: petit mal and focal epileptic patients[a]

		Petit mal patients — *no* WS bursts	Focal epileptic[b] patients
X task	Mean	76.5	94.4
	N	18	122
	Range	17.1–100	35.0–100[c]
AX task	Mean	79.4	83.6
	N	15	122
	Range	20.5–99.2	13.3–100

[a] From Mirsky and Van Buren (1965).
[b] While the EEG was not monitored in these patients during their examination, the nature of their seizure disorder would make it relatively easy to detect the occurrence of convulsive episodes.
[c] The low CPT scores obtained by some focal epileptic patients may reflect concurrent subcortical ('centrencephalic') pathology in such patients.

that behavioral effects are variable from patient to patient, it is clear that for most patients the WS paroxysm signals a global sensory disturbance coupled with reduced motor-executive capacity and higher-order deficits in attention and memory as well. Young untreated patients, who may experience several hundred such episodes daily, are at an enormous disadvantage in any learning setting. Fortunately, effective antiabsence medications such as ethosuximide and valproic acid exist which, for many patients, reduce the seizure frequency to a very low level (Mirsky *et al.*, 1986). However, the interictal period in such patients may not be free of behavioral impairment. The results of several early studies (Mirsky *et al.*, 1960; Lansdell and Mirsky, 1964; Fedio and Mirsky, 1969) pointed to the poor attentive performance in patients with petit mal and, although EEG was not monitored in these reports, the deficit was not clearly linked to obvious absence attacks. Mirsky and Van Buren (1965) provided evidence that even when WS bursts were not present in the EEG, patients with petit mal tended to perform more poorly on the CPT than patients with other 'focal' epileptic diagnoses. These data are summarized in Table 4.3.*

* Although significant differences between groups were seen on the CPT X task ($p < 0.01$), they were not seen on the AX task. Moreover, the wide range of CPT scores emphasizes that some patients with petit mal epilepsy may show little impairment on the task, and that some patients with focal seizures may perform as poorly as patients with petit mal. The poor CPT scores of some focal patients may reflect the presence of some concurrent generalized ('centrencephalic') pathology in such cases; the good CPT scores of some cases of petit mal speaks to the heterogeneity of this disorder and to the possible range of underlying pathophysiological processes (Myslobodsky and Mirsky, 1988; Berkovic *et al.*, 1987).

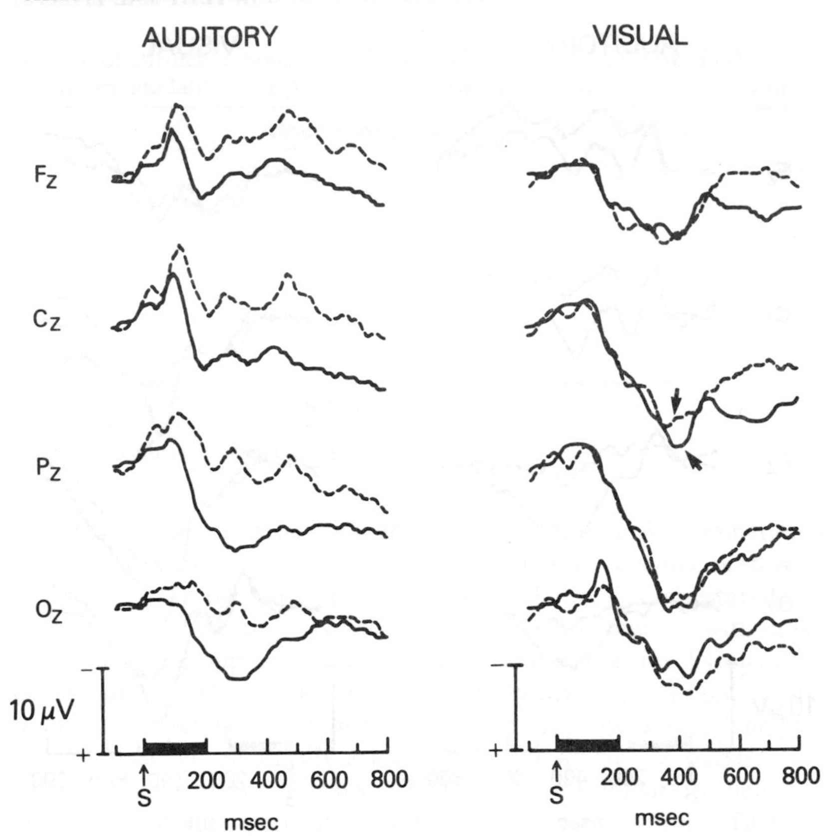

Figure 4.7. Event-related potentials (ERPs) elicited by target ($p = .20$) stimuli in the auditory and visual CPT-AX tasks. The data collected from the two groups were averaged over subjects: the grand-mean ERPs for the normal controls (solid line) and patients with absence epilepsy (dashed lines) are superimposed at four midline scalp sites. Positive peak of visual P300 is indicated by arrow at Cz. It is apparent that the ERPs to visual targets did not differentiate the groups, whereas the ERPs to auditory targets were strikingly different. It is in fact difficult to discern a P300 to auditory AX targets in the ERPs of the absence patients (Adapted from Duncan, 1988)

response processing is not due to the use a more cautious response strategy. Rather, it appears that the execution of the response itself is delayed' (Duncan, 1988). Duncan concludes 'the patients failed to summon and/or sustain sufficient attentional resources to the auditory stimuli . . . [they] do not have attentional capacity sufficient to cope with the additional demands of the auditory CPT task' (Duncan, 1988).

INTERICTAL EVENTS—ANTECEDENTS OF WS BURSTS

Some light may be shed on the impaired information processing between bursts in absence epilepsy from the results of studies done by Siegel, Grady, and Mirsky (1982) and Mirsky and Grady (1988). In this work (e.g. Mirsky and Grady, 1988), frequency analysis of the EEG immediately preceding WS bursts was performed, and such epochs were contrasted with control epochs, remote from the occurrence of WS bursts. Generally, it was found that a significant increase in EEG power in the WS frequency band itself (i.e. 3–4 cps) or in harmonics of this frequency (e.g. 5.5 cps, 12.5 cps) precedes WS bursts; moreover, a monotonic buildup in EEG power in such frequencies may be detected in the 20 sec period preceding bursts. Figure 4.8 presents an example of a progressive buildup of power in the 3.5 and 5.5 cps frequencies preceding bursts in one subject, T.M. The total preburst epoch represented here is 20 sec and epoch 8 is the 2.56 sec period immediately prior to burst onset. The result emphasizes that events can be detected in the scalp EEG reflecting an ongoing process which leads to its most dramatic expression as a WS burst. Thus, the burst does not appear *de novo* without some prodromal antecedent. Presumably these prodromal events are generated by the same pathophysiological process that produces the burst itself. And they would likely be accompanied by behavioral manifestations, however much they may be attenuated, similar to those occurring in the ictal period. 'More and more neurons may be participating in a common activity that, generally speaking, results in (grossly) abnormal behavior only when enough neurons are involved to produce the WS burst itself. Those subjects who show such a progressive reorganization of EEG activity might also be expected to show progressive alterations of behavior or evoked potentials as the burst approaches' (Mirsky and Grady, 1988).

It is also conceivable that events which do not culminate in an obvious WS burst, but remain truly subclinical (without even a manifestation of a short WS burst in the EEG) could have the deleterious effect on information processing seen in Duncan's (1988) study. At the least this appears to be a feasible explanation for the interictally altered ERPs and behavior seen in patients with absence epilepsy.

THE PATHOPHYSIOLOGY OF ABSENCE EPILEPSY IN RELATION TO BEHAVIOR

In recent publications summarizing the current state of knowledge of absence epilepsy (Mirsky *et al.*, 1986; Myslobodsky and Mirsky, 1988) we concluded that the disorder remains largely enigmatic as to its etiology and prognosis, and that no completely satisfactory physiological or neurochemical explanation

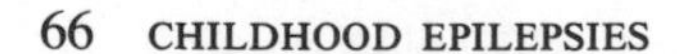

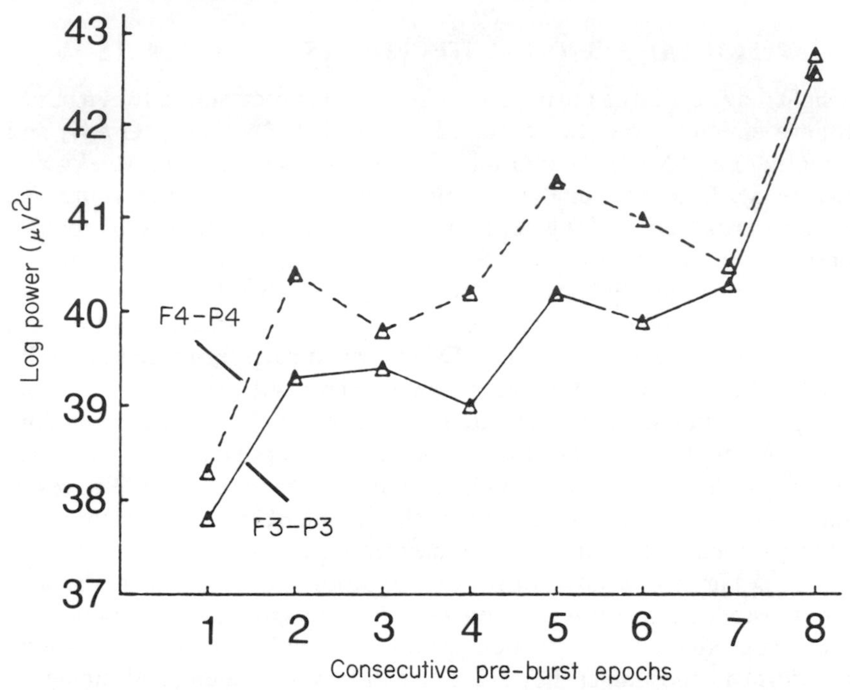

Figure 4.8. Mean total power in the low discriminating frequencies (3.5 and 5.5 cps) plotted against preburst value for 8 successive 2.56-sec epochs for subject T.M. Epoch 8 is closest to burst (From Mirsky and Grady, 1988)

exists which would account for its basic manifestations. Nevertheless, as summarized in these publications, and briefly in this chapter, we do possess at a descriptive level considerable information about the behavioral disturbances present in this form of generalized seizures. Although I have emphasized the distinction between ictal and interictal disturbances, the data suggest that the ictal phenomena are a *crescendo* of what is present in attenuated form, probably at most other times. The capacity to focus, mobilize, and sustain attentional resources waxes and wanes in these patients with absence epilepsy, more or less correlated with the occurrence of WS bursts; however, these functions are rarely unimpaired. These facts are best understood, perhaps, in terms of disturbance in a cerebral attention and/or information-processing support system which is composed of a number of structures ranging from the reticular formation of the brain stem, thalamus, basal ganglia, and hippocampus through prefrontal, temporal and parietal cortices (Mirsky, 1987).

As the disturbance intensifies, more of these structures are recruited into a convulsive process, and the behavioral deficits are intensified. It seems unlikely that all of the behavioral and psychophysiological manifestations (e.g. reduced ERPs, altered attention, disturbed memory, reduced visual and auditory

P300s) could be attributed to a perturbation within a single cerebral region. Although there is considerable variation between patients, it is not clear whether this represents simply degrees of disturbance or different forms of a generalized disorder (Bercovic *et al.*, 1987; Myslobodsky and Mirsky, 1988). Future research will shed light on this issue.

INFORMATION PROCESSING IN ABSENCE EPILEPSY–ICTAL AND INTERICTAL PERIODS COMPARED: SOME TENTATIVE EDUCATIONAL IMPLICATIONS

The data presented indicate that patients with absence epilepsy have difficulty in processing visual and auditory information in both ictal *and* nonictal periods. Whereas the analysis of the ictal and immediate preictal events have focused on the temporary loss of sensory information (i.e. a brief, functional blindness and deafness), the interictal period (as evaluated most recently by Duncan (1988) in a group of high-functioning adult cases) is also characterized by significantly poorer attentional capacity than is seen in control subjects, especially with respect to that aspect of attention related to response execution. Data have been presented which also point to effects of WS bursts on short-term memory consolidation.

One implication of the findings presented in this chapter, with particular relevance to the interictal period, is that the suppression, or non-occurrence, of WS bursts in a person suffering from petit mal epilepsy does not guarantee freedom from cognitive impairment. Parenthetically, the existence of memory impairment in absence patients does not necessarily implicate brain areas concerned with memory (i.e. amygdala, hippocampus) in the disorder; rather, it could represent the sequela of an earlier failure of attention.

The data also suggest that the processing of auditory information may hold special difficulties for patients with absence epilepsy and that *executing responses* is the place in the information-processing chain where the problem may lie.

Two other studies of subjects with petit mal epilepsy are relevant in this context. Kimura (1964) contrasted the performance of several subgroups of epileptic patients and reported that 'centrencephalic' patients (especially those without myoclonic bursts) performed significantly more poorly that groups with focal disorders on a task requiring attention to letters appearing in a visual display. The deficit was apparent when the subjects were asked to order the letters alphabetically before reporting them. Kimura noted, in discussing the nature of the deficit on this test, that 'apart from the degree of concentration . . . the subject must [also] keep in mind more than one event at a time and respond to these events in a sequential way' (Kimura, 1964, p. 294). These results are consistent with the results discussed above, suggesting that both attentive and some types of mnemonic ability may be impaired in patients with absence seizures. Some additional support for this view is provided in a study by Fedio and Mirsky (1969). We reported that, in addition to their poor performance on the CPT AX task, children (mean age 10.8, range 6–14) with centrencephalic epilepsy (as compared with epileptic and normal controls) had difficulty with the *recall* of complex visual material and, among other subtests of the Wechsler Intelligence Scale for Children (WISC–Wechsler, 1949), difficulty on the digit span and arithmetic subtests. Both of the latter tests require the ability to keep numerical material in memory.

Recommending educational enhancements for children with absence epilepsy is beyond my area of expertise; nevertheless, it seems appropriate to suggest that promoting and emphasizing *visual* rather than auditory material might be an effective strategy in teaching new subject-matter to such children. Possibly, combining visual and concurrent auditory inputs would provide special benefits to the child with absence epilepsy. Any memory problems related to WS-burst occurrence might be ameliorated by increased repetitions of material (particularly if it were presented in the auditory modality).

The means or method by which the capacity for *response execution* could be improved by practice or exercise is difficult to conceptualize. Attention training of some specialized variety may be helpful, but a discussion of what this might entail goes beyond the limits of this chapter.

SUMMARY

A series of investigations of attention and/or consciousness, and most recently information processing in patients with petit mal epilepsy, is described. The results of behavioral and electrophysiological experiments designed to elucidate the nature of the absence are discussed, in addition to studies aimed at characterizing the cognitive capacities of such patients in the interictal period. It may be concluded that, although the degree of impairment varies from patient to patient, persons with this disorder have a range of cognitive difficulties involving auditory and visual information processing (possibly related to difficulty in response execution) and in some tasks dependent upon memory. The deficits are most striking in conjunction with the WS burst itself, in which evidence exists for a temporary loss of signals in the visual, and possibly auditory, modality. However, similar deficits also exist in the interictal period, presumably reflecting an ongoing pathophysiological process related to the one that generates the WS burst itself. Some suggestions are offered about educational maneuvers of possible value for children with absence epilepsy.

REFERENCES

Ajmone-Marsan, C. (1969). Pathophysiology of the EEG pattern characteristic of petit mal epilepsy, a critical review of some of the experimental data. In H. Gastaut, H.

Jasper, J. Bancaud, and A. Waltregny (eds), *The Physiopathogenesis of the Epilepsies*. Thomas, Springfield, Il, pp. 237–49.

Bakay Pragay, E., Mirsky, A.F., Fullerton, B.C., Oshima, H., and Arnold, S.W. (1975). Effect of electrical stimulation of the brain on visually controlled (attentive) behavior in *Macaca mulatta*. *Exp. Neurol.*, 49:203–220, 1975.

Bakay Pragay, E., Mirsky, A.F., Ray, C.L., Turner, D.F., and Mirsky, C.V. (1978). Neuronal activity in the brainstem reticular formation during performance of a 'go/no-go' attention task in the monkey. *Experimental Neurology*, **60**, 83–95.

Berkovic, S.F., Andermann, F., Andermann, E., and Gloor, P. (1987). Concepts of absence epilepsy; discrete syndrome or biological continuum? *Neurology*, **37**, 993–1000.

Browne, T.R., Penry, J.K., Porter, R.J., and Dreifuss, F.E. (1974). Responsiveness before, during, and after spike-wave paroxysms. *Neurology*, **24**, 659–665.

Duncan, C.C. (1988). Application of event-related brain potentials to the analysis of interictal attention in absence epilepsy. In M.S. Myslobodsky and A.F. Mirsky, (eds), *Elements of Petit Mal Epilepsy*, Peter Lang, New York, 341–364.

Duncan-Johnson, C.C., and Donchin, E. (1977). On quantifying surprise: the variation of event-related potentials with subjective probability. *Psychophysiology*, **14**, 456–467.

Fedio, P., and Mirsky, A.F. (1969). Selective intellectual deficits in children with temporal lobe or centrencephalic epilepsy. *Neuropsychologia*, **7**, 287–300.

Gloor, P. (1988). Neurophysiological mechanism of generalized spike and wave discharge and its implication for understanding absence seizures. In M.S. Myslobodsky and A.F. Mirsky (eds), *Elements of Petit Mal Epilepsy*, Peter Lang, New York.

Goode, D.J., Penry, J.K., and Dreifuss, F.S. (1970). Effects of paroxysmal spike-wave on continuous visual-motor performance. *Epilepsia*, **11**, 241–254.

Kimura, D. (1964). Cognitive deficit related to seizure pattern in centrencephalic epilepsy. *Journal of Neurology, Neurosurgery and Psychiatry*, **27**, 291–295.

Lansdell, H., and Mirsky, A.F. (1964). Attention in focal and centrencephalic epilepsy. *Experimental Neurology*, **9**, 463–469.

Lindsley, D.B. (1960). Attention, consciousness, sleep and wakefulness. In J. Field (ed.-in-chief), *Neurophysiology*, Vol. III, American Physiological Society, Washington, DC, pp. 1553–1593.

Mirsky, A.F. (1987). Behavioral and psychophysiological markers of disordered attention. *Environmental Health Perspectives*, **72**, 191–199.

Mirsky, A.F,. and Bakay Pragay, E. (1988). Brain stem mechanisms in the processing of sensory information: clinical symptoms, animal models, and unit analysis. In D.E. Sheer and K.H. Pribram (eds), *Attention: Theory, Brain Functions and Clinical Applications*, Erlbaum, Hillsdale, NJ (In press).

Mirsky, A.F., and Duncan, C.C. (1986). Etiology and expression of schizophrenia: Neurobiological and psychosocial factors. *Annual Review of Psychology*, 291–319.

Mirsky, A.F., and Grady, C.L. (1988). Toward the development of alternative treatments in absence epilepsy. In M.S. Myslobodsky and A.F. Mirsky (eds), *Elements of Petit Mal Epilepsy*, Peter Lang, New York, 285–310.

Mirsky, A.F., and Oshima, H.J. (1973). Effects of subcortical aluminum cream lesions on attentive behavior and the electroencephalogram in monkeys. *Experimental Neurology*, **39**, 1–18.

Mirsky, A.F., and Van Buren, J.M. (1965). On the nature of the 'absence' in centrencephalic epilepsy: a study of some behavioral, electroencephalographic and autonomic factors. *Electroencephalography and Clinical Neurophysiology*, **18**, 334–348.

Mirsky, A.F., Bakay Pragay, E., and Harris, D. (1977). Evoked potential correlates of stimulation-induced impairment of attention in *Macaca mulatta. Experimental Neurology*, **57**, 242–256.

Mirsky, A.F., Bloch-Rojas, S., Tecce, J.J., Lessell, D., and Marcus, E. (1973). Visual evoked potentials during experimentally induced spike-wave activity in monkeys. *Electroencephalography and Clinical Neurophysiology*, **35**, 25–37.

Mirsky, A.F., Duncan, C.C., and Myslobodsky, M.S. (1986). Petit mal epilepsy: a review and integration of recent information. *Journal of Clinical Neurophysiology*, **3**, 179–208.

Mirsky, A.F., and Orren, M.M. (1977). Attention. In L.H. Miller, A.J. Kastin and C.A. Sandman (eds), *Neuropeptide Influences on the Brain and Behavior*, Raven Press, New York, 233–267.

Mirsky, A.F., Primac, D.W., Ajmone Marsan, C., Rosvold, H.E., and Stevens, J.A. (1960). A comparison of the psychological test performance of patients with focal and nonfocal epilepsy. *Experimental Neurology*, **2**, 75–89.

Myslobodsky, M.S., and Mirsky, A.F. (eds) (1988). *Elements of Petit Mal Epilepsy*, Peter Lang, New York.

Orren, M.M. (1974). Visuomotor behavior and visual evoked potentials during petit mal seizures. Unpublished Ph.D. dissertation, Boston University.

Orren, M.M. (1978). Evoked potential studies in petit mal epilepsy: visual information processing in relation to spike-and-wave discharges. In W.A. Cobb and H.V. Duijn (eds), *Contemporary Clinical Neurophysiology (EEG Suppl. 34)*, Elsevier, Amsterdam, pp. 251–257.

Orren, M.M., and Mirsky, A.F. (1975). Relation between ocular manifestations and onset of spike-and-wave discharges in petit mal epilepsy. *Epilepsia*, **16**, 771–779.

Penfield, W., and Jasper, M. (1954). *Epilepsy and the Functional Anatomy of the Human Brain*, Little, Brown, Boston.

Ray, C.L., Mirsky, A.F., and Bakay Pragay, E. (1982). Functional analysis of attentional-related unit activity in the reticular formation of the monkey. *Experimental Neurology*, **77**, 544–562.

Rosvold, H.E., Mirsky, A.F., Sarason, I., Bransome, E.D., Jr., and Beck, L.H. (1956). A continuous performance test of brain damage. *Journal of Consulting Psychology*, **20**, 343–350.

Schwab, R.S. (1939). A method of measuring consciousness in petit mal epilepsy. *Journal of Nervous and Mental Disease*, **89**, 690–691.

Schwab, R.S. (1941). The influence of visual and auditory stimuli on the electroencephalographic tracing of petit mal. *American Journal of Psychiatry*, **97**, 1301–1312.

Schwab, R.S. (1947). Reaction time in petit mal epilepsy. *Res. Publ. Association for Research into Nervous and Mental Disease*, **26**, 339.

Siegel, A., Grady, C.L., and Mirsky, A.F. (1982). Prediction of spike-wave bursts in absence epilepsy by EEG spectrum signals. *Epilepsia*, **23**, 47–60.

Starr, A., Sohmer, H., and Celesia, C.D. (1978). Some applications of evoked potentials to patients with neurological and sensory impairment. In E. Calloway, D. Tueting and S.H. Koslow (eds), *Event-Related Potentials in Man*, Academic Press, New York, pp. 155–121.

Tizard, B., and Margerison, J.M. (1963a). The relationship between generalized paroxysmal E.E.G. discharges and various test situations in two epileptic patients. *Journal of Neurology, Neurosurgery and Psychiatry*, **26**, 308–313.

Tizard, B., and Margerison, J.M. (1963b). Psychological functions during spike-and-wave discharge. *British Journal of Social and Clinical Psychology*, **3**, 6–15.

Wechsler, D. (1949). *Wechsler Intelligence Scale for Children*. Psychological Corporation, New York.

Chapter 5

Neuropsychological Functioning of Children with Epilepsy

Michael Seidenberg

Investigation of the neuropsychological correlates of the epilepsies has provided useful information in the treatment and management of adults with epilepsy (Dodrill, 1981; Klove and Matthews, 1974). Knowledge of the nature, degree, and determinants of cognitive dysfunction among *children* with epilepsy is perhaps even more crucial, as they are in the process of acquiring skills which will be necessary for further academic achievement and subsequent psychosocial adjustment. Impairment in the development of these skills because of compromise in basic underlying cognitive processes could clearly have far-reaching effects. Identification of the factors responsible for neuropsychological impairment in children with epilepsy holds forth the promise of early identification of those children at most risk, with subsequent provision of appropriate remediation services at a time when these services are likely to have their greatest impact.

Surprisingly, there has been only a modest amount of investigation into the neuropsychological characteristics of children with epilepsy. This is noteworthy, particularly when it is considered that epilepsy is one of the most prevalent of the neurological disorders, that a majority of the epilepsies have their onset in childhood and adolescence, and that neurological compromise is a known etiological factor for cognitive learning and achievement problems.

Much of the previous work in this field, particularly prior to 1970, focused on the assessment of intellectual abilities with standardized instruments such as the Wechsler Tests (WISC and WISC-R) or the Stanford-Binet. These measures provide useful indicants of some broad domains of cognitive functioning, but lack the comprehensiveness afforded by a neuropsychological investigation of adaptive and behavioral abilities (Boll, 1981). A second major limitation of earlier research in this area relates to the use of institutionalized samples of children with epilepsy which represent a very selective and unrepresentative sample. Several review articles have shown, not surprisingly, that when

Childhood Epilepsies: Neuropsychological, Psychosocial and Intervention Aspects
Edited by B. Hermann and M. Seidenberg

noninstitutionalized epilepsy patients are studied, the degree of intellectual deficits and deterioration is markely diminished (Keating, 1960; Tarter, 1972). More recent investigations of cognitive functioning in children have examined specific domains such as attention (Mirsky, this volume) and memory (Schefner and Weber, 1981; Stores, 1981) in relation to various aspects of epilepsy, and these investigations have the potential to shed light on specific brain–behavior relationships.

It is apparent from the published literature, as well as from clinical experience, that there is considerable variability among children with epilepsy in the adequacy of their cognitive functioning. Knowing that a child has epilepsy provides one with little predictive information about the level or nature of cognitive ability to anticipate for the child. A myriad of neurological, psychosocial, and medication factors impinge on the child with epilepsy, and may affect the adequacy of the child's development and neuropsychological functioning. Research in this area has therefore been primarily aimed at detecting which variables, primarily seizure-related variables, are particularly important determinants of cognitive functioning.

This chapter will review the data available concerning several epilepsy-related factors and the neuropsychological performance of children with epilepsy, including age of seizure onset, seizure type, and seizure frequency. The focus of the review will be on studies which have used standardized neuropsychological test batteries and which therefore represent a broad and comprehensive evaluation of cognitive function. The chapter will also discuss, albeit briefly, the relevance of neuropsychological assessment and functioning for psychosocial functioning. Specifically, it will review investigations of the relationship between adequacy of neuropsychological functioning and psychopathology.

EFFECTS OF SEIZURE-RELATED VARIABLES ON NEUROPSYCHOLOGICAL FUNCTIONING

Age of onset

Several investigations have examined the potential significance of the age at which seizures begin for cognitive sequelae. Most studies have found that persons with an early onset of seizures perform more poorly than do people with a later seizure onset. There are, however, several methodological issues to consider in relation to these findings. For example, few studies make a distinction between age of onset and duration of epilepsy. Since these are typically highly correlated (i.e. the earlier the onset the longer the duration), it becomes difficult to disentangle the effects of one from the other.

Two studies reported by Dikman, Matthews, and Harley (1975, 1977) exemplify the difficulties of controlling all relevant variables when studying persons with epilepsy. In their initial study they found that persons with major motor seizures of early onset were impaired relative to individuals with later onset on a variety of measures from the Halstead Neuropsychological Test Battery. In a second subsequent study, which matched the two onset groups for both seizure duration and seizure frequency, most of the group differences were no longer evident. Hence, factors other than age of onset may be critical for determining neuropsychological performance.

A few studies have examined age of onset effects in children with epilepsy instead of adults. Since the majority of persons with epilepsy begin having their seizures early in life, it would seem important to determine the effects of age of onset during childhood. O'Leary, Seidenberg, Berent, and Boll (1981) examined the test performance of 48 children, aged 9–14, who had been classified by a neurologist as having tonic–clonic seizures as their primary seizure type. Children were tested with the Halstead Neuropsychological Test Battery for Children and Allied Procedures (see Boll, 1981, for a detailed description of these tests). Analysis of covariance procedures were used in order to control for the effects of seizure duration. The findings supported the conclusion that children who began to have tonic–clonic seizures at an early age (prior to age 5 years) were more impaired than children with a later onset of tonic–clonic seizures. The early-onset children performed significantly worse on eight of the 14 test measures. Deficits were observed on tasks of motor speed, attention and concentration, memory, and complex problem-solving.

Is the effect of age of onset similar for other seizure types? O'Leary *et al.* (1983) examined this question by studying the neuropsychological test performance of children with partial seizures of early (N=27) and late onset (N=22), and comparing their performance with that of children with early (N=33) or later onset (N=24) with generalized seizures. All children were between the age of 9 and 14, and had obtained a score of 70 or greater on at least one of the summary WISC-R IQ scales (i.e. Verbal IQ, Performance IQ, Full Scale IQ). Early-onset groups had their initial seizure before the age of 5 years, and later-onset groups had their initial seizure dated to after 5 years of age. All children were administered the Halstead Neuropsychological Test Battery for Children and Allied Procedures.

The results indicated that children with an early onset of seizures performed more poorly than the late-onset group, regardless of whether the seizures are partial or generalized. Statistically significant differences were observed for the effects of age of onset (summed over seizure type) on four measures: Verbal IQ, Performance IQ, Trails A and Trails B. None of the interaction effects for onset by seizure type reached statistical significance.

Hermann *et al.* (1988) examined the effects of age of onset of epilepsy in a sample of 64 children with epilepsy, aged 6–11, using the Luria Nebraska Neuropsychological Battery–Children (LNNB-C) (Golden, 1981). The sample consisted of 34 children with primary generalized epilepsies (GE) and 30 children with complex partial seizures of temporal lobe origin (CPS). The effects of age of onset were investigated in the total group of children as well as in each of the seizure-type subgroups.

For the total sample of children statistically significant inverse correlations were noted (i.e. the earlier the onset of seizures the poorer the performance) on eight of the 11 scales of the LNNB-C including Receptive Speech, Expressive Speech, Writing, Reading, Mathematics, Memory, Intelligence, and Rhythm. When the effects of age of onset were examined within seizure subgroups, it was found that earlier onset in the CPS group was associated with significantly poorer performance on the Memory, Expressive Speech, and Reading Scales. For the GE group, earlier age of onset was associated with significantly poorer performance on the Receptive Speech, Writing, Mathematics, and Intelligence Scales.

In summary, similar to results using the Halstead Battery (O'Leary *et al.*, 1981, 1983), age of onset of epilepsy was found to be inversely correlated with neuropsychological performance on the LNNB-C. The effect of age of onset was observed for the total sample as well as in the individual seizure subgroups. It is of interest that the Hermann *et al.* study found different scales to be significantly correlated with age of onset for the two seizure subgroups. Future research will need to determine the significance of these findings and their potential implications for the neuropsychological functioning of children with epilepsy.

In reviewing the data available on the effects of age of onset for neuropsychological functioning of children with epilepsy, several summary points are worth emphasis. First, the data seem to indicate that the potential deleterious effects associated with earlier age of onset can be observed (at least for some children) at a relatively young age and across a diversity of neuropsychological tests and batteries. Given the significance of neuropsychological deficits for educational attainment (see Seidenberg, Chapter 7 in this volume) and more general vocational outcome (see Fraser and Clemmons, Chapter 13 in this volume), the potential role of neuropsychological evaluation in children with epilepsy should be evident.

It remains unclear whether there is a broad-based generalized impairment associated with age of onset or whether more specific domains are more vulnerable at different points in development or within different seizure-type subgroups. Further research may help to determine if there are corresponding critical periods of behavioral development and impairment associated with onset age of different times in childhood.

It should be noted that there are inherent limitations to the assessment of age of seizure onset which might be expected to minimize its association with cognitive functioning. First, it may be quite difficult to determine with any degree of accuracy when the first seizure episode occurred, particularly for some seizure types (e.g. absence seizures). Also, the occurrence of a seizure is, for some children, the initial symptomatic manifestation of some underlying brain dysfunction which actually occurred at an earlier point in time. Factors such as these can serve to mitigate against strong associations between onset age and behavioral functioning.

Seizure type

Much of the research examining seizure type has focused on the study of the relationship between specific domains of neuropsychological dysfunction and the brain regions or focus of the epileptiform activity. In this context the study of attention and memory abilities in those with temporal lobe seizure involvement or centrencephalic seizures has received the greatest amount of investigation. Memory deficits have been associated with children with temporal lobe epilepsy (Fedio and Mirsky, 1969) while those with centrencephalic epilepsy are more impaired on measures of sustained attentional abilities.

There has been a very limited number of investigations to date comparing children of different seizure type across a broad base of neuropsychological abilities. The O'Leary *et al.* (1983) study, described earlier, provides some data relevant to this issue. They examined 106 children between the ages of 9 and 15 years of age who had been diagnosed as having generalized seizures (N=57) or partial seizures (N=49). These children were compared on the WISC-R as well as the Halstead Neuropsychological Test Battery for Children. For the 13 measures examined, only one showed significant group differences between seizure type, with the Partial group being better than the Generalized group on Tactual Performance Test–Total Time.

The authors suggest that one of the factors which may have limited the observation of greater group differences had to do with the lumping together of children with partial seizures of varying types (i.e. simple partial, complex partial, and partial secondarily generalized seizures) into a single category They carried out a second analysis to compare the test performance between these three partial seizure groups. There were no group differences on age, duration, or onset. Although significant group differences emerged for only one of the 13 measures (TPT–Localization), a consistent pattern of poorer performance for the partial secondarily generalized group was evident on 11 of the 13 test measures. A chi-square analysis indicated that such a distribution would be highly unlikely to result by chance (chi square=15.4, p <0.001). This pattern of results is similar to that reported by Giordani *et al.* (1985) in their comparison of the WAIS performance of 350 adult patients with epilepsy.

A similar point could be made for the composition of the generalized group which in the O'Leary *et al.* study (1983) included 47 children with tonic–clonic seizures only, and 10 children with both tonic–clonic and absence seizures. Children with mixed seizures tend to perform more poorly than those with a single seizure type (Seidenberg *et al.*, 1986) on measures of intellectual ability and academic achievement, and it is likely then that they would also perform more poorly on a set of broader measures of neuropsychological functioning. If that were the case, the results from the O'Leary *et al.* (1983) study may not have provided an accurate characterization of the level of neuropsychological functioning for the tonic–clonic seizure group.

Similar patterns of results emerged when Hermann *et al.* (1988) examined seizure-type differences in neuropsychological functioning as assessed by the LNNB-C. Comparing a group of children with complex partial seizures of temporal lobe origin (N=30) to those with primary generalized epilepsies (N=34) on the 11 scales of the LNNB-C, the generalized epilepsy group was found to perform significantly worse on three of the scales (Writing, Mathematics, Intelligence). Thus, similar to O'Leary *et al.* (1983), the significant differences between the partial epilepsy and generalized epilepsy groups were small in number, but when significant the generalized epilepsy group performed in a more impaired fashion.

Further, interesting differences appeared when the generalized epilepsy and partial epilepsy groups were further subdivided into clinically meaningful groups. For instance, when children who experience *only* absence seizures (N=13) were compared to children who experience *only* primary generalized tonic–clonic seizures (N=8), the latter performed in a more impaired fashion on 10 of the 11 scales of the LNNB-C with the absence group performing more poorly only on the Motor scale.

In summary, it appears as if more informative statements regarding the effects of seizure type on neuropsychological function will depend on sophisticated subgrouping of seizure types. Perhaps when seizure type is covaried with other variables, like etiology or seizure frequency, clearer distinctions will be possible. Such research will require large numbers of very carefully diagnosed children, but the findings should yield substantial benefits and aid in efforts aimed at prevention of associated psychosocial problems.

Seizure frequency

It would seem reasonable to expect that increased seizure frequency would be related to greater cognitive impairment. However, studies in both the adult and child literature have not consistently found such a relationship. Dodrill (1981) suggested several methodological reasons which might underlie the differences reported in the literature. These include: the use of a variety of seizure types grouped together which may obscure effects for some types of seizures (presumably the more serious seizure types such as tonic–clonic seizures), and the use of seizure frequency indices which reflect only a single point in time (seizures in the last month or year) rather than the lifelong history of seizure episodes.

Some recent findings provide support for Dodrill's suggestions. Aschkenase

(1979) studied the neuropsychological test performance of 73 children with seizures between the ages of 9 and 15 years. Children from three seizure groups were included: major motor (N=46), psychomotor (N=19), and petit-mal (N=8). Tests administered included the WISC and measures from the Halstead Neuropsychological Test Battery for Children—Category Test, Tactual Performance Test, Trail Making Test, and Tapping Test. Results indicated that as seizure frequency increased, test scores on several measures of neuropsychological functioning also significantly declined: WISC Full Scale IQ, Performance IQ, Verbal IQ, Tactual Performance Test, and Trails A. Further analyses broken down by seizure type, and using an estimate of total lifetime number of seizures (i.e. seizure duration multiplied by seizure frequency), yielded significant correlations with cognitive performance only for the major motor seizure group, and not for the psychomotor seizure group.

Dean (1983) in a study of 61 children (aged 10–14 years) with tonic–clonic seizures also found significant correlations between lifetime total of seizures and several measures of neuropsychological functioning—Full Scale IQ, Performance IQ, Trails B, Category Test, and Finger Tapping Test.

Both these studies found significant correlations with test performance when employing an estimate of seizure frequency based on lifetime total rather than one based upon a single point in time. Of interest too, both these positive findings were observed for children with tonic–clonic seizures. Indeed, in the Aschkenase study there was no significant correlation between seizure total and test performance in the psychomotor seizure group. Hermann *et al.* (1988) also found a consistent inverse relationship between seizure control and cognitive functioning (more seizures correlated with poorer performance) for children with generalized seizures but not for children with temporal lobe seizures. For the group with generalized epilepsies, those with poor seizure control (N=7) performed more poorly than those children with good control (N=15) on all 11 scales of the LNNB-C. When children with partial seizures were similarly subdivided, no such trend was seen.

These findings raise questions concerning the possible differences for the effect of seizure frequency depending on seizure type. That is, perhaps the effect is most evident for the more 'serious' seizure types. Alternatively, we may simply be observing a measurement problem, as tonic–clonic seizures may be more reliably reported and counted than other seizure types. Future studies examining different indices of seizure frequency (e.g. time since last seizure, seizures within the last month and year, lifetime seizure total, frequency of subclinical EEG discharges) within seizure type categories, would be of considerable use in disentangling this issue but need to attend to the issue of establishing reliable frequency estimates. Furthermore, there is the issue of severity of the seizure episode itself, which could be of some importance beyond the sheer number of seizure episodes.

Neuropsychological performance and psychopathology

The relationship between epilepsy and behavioral–psychosocial problems remains far from clear (see Chapter 9), yet it does appear that children with epilepsy are more likely to be perceived as having psychological adjustment and behavioral problems than are children who do not have a seizure disorder (Graham and Rutter, 1968; Mellor, Lowit, and Hall, 1974). No doubt multiple factors operate and interact to influence behavioral functioning and adjustment in epilepsy (Hermann and Whitman, 1984).

Several investigators have suggested that there may be a link between behavioral and psychosocial adjustment in children with epilepsy and the adequacy of neuropsychological functioning (Hermann, 1982; Stores, 1971). A similar viewpoint has recently been extended in the examination of the behavioral and adjustment problems often observed with learning-disabled children (Porter and Rourke, 1985). According to this viewpoint, cognitive deficits may serve to underlie some of the problems in social learning abilities, thereby promoting the occurrence of behavioral and adjustment difficulties.

Hermann (1982) divided 50 children with epilepsy (aged 8–12) into two groups (good versus poor) based on their performance on the Luria–Nebraska Neuropsychological Battery—Children's Version. The two groups were then compared on the behavioral measures derived from the Child Behavior Checklist (CBCL) (Achenbach, 1978). There were no group differences in gender, age, age of seizure onset, or seizure types represented. Significant differences did emerge between groups on the behavioral checklist on all dimensions examined (i.e. Total Behavioral Problems, Total Social Competence, and Aggression), with the poor neuropsychological functioning group obtaining scores indicative of greater problems in these areas.

A recent study by Camfield *et al.* (1984) also reported that social maladjustment in children with epilepsy was related to cognitive deficits. They studied a group of 27 children (aged 6–17) with unilateral temporal lobe epilepsy (13 had a left-sided focus and 14 had a right-sided focus). There were no significant behavioral or cognitive differences between those with a left- and those with a right-sided focus. A group of 10 'maladjusted' children were selected based upon their score on the Personality Inventory for Children (Lachar and Gdowski, 1979). This group was compared with the remaining 17 children who obtained normal adjustment scores. Significant group differences were found for 12 of the 25 measures from the neuropsychological test battery, and in every instance the 'maladjusted' group performed more poorly than the 'well-adjusted' group.

The hypothesis that neuropsychological deficits may be an important factor in the occurrence of behavioral adjustment difficulties of children with epilepsy is an intriguing one, and one that, if additional studies demonstrate to be valid, would have potential remedial and intervention implications. Future research directions could include determining whether specific cognitive deficits are linked to behavioral adjustment problems or simply global neuropsychological deficits are the key factor. Studies investigating the development and efficacy of intervention strategies are also necessary.

The contribution of neuropsychological assessment

The current review has focused on the examination of the significance of some epilepsy-specific variables for neuropsychological functioning in childhood epilepsy. The review has been limited in scope, as many other variables which are of potential significance (e.g. etiology of seizures, laterality of seizure focus, anticonvulsant effects) have not been discussed. Nevertheless, it should be apparent that none of these factors, either alone and probably in combination, is likely to provide a full account of the variability observed in the test performance among children with epilepsy.

The unique contribution of neuropsychological assessment to patient care is by providing a comprehensive evaluation of adaptive abilities, in terms of strenghts and deficits, and in a manner which can be of some utility for treatment planning. There is no epilepsy-specific pattern of neuropsychological dysfunction; however, the nature and level of neuropsychological abilities and deficits can be of considerable utility for understanding and treating educational problems, vocational planning, and psychosocial adjustment. Other important areas of application in childhood epilepsy include monitoring of treatment effects with anticonvulsants. Neuropsychological evaluation pre- and post-initiation of treatment, and at points of major changes in drug regimen, can provide an important objective set of data by which to evaluate the efficacy of such treatment. We refer the interested reader to Chapter 6 in this volume, by Cull and Trimble, for a comprehensive review of this area, and some of their recent work aimed at examining this question.

REFERENCES

Achenbach, T.M. (1978). The child behavior profile: I. Boys aged 6–11. *Journal of Consulting and Clinical Psychology*, **46**, 478–488.

Aschkenase, L.F. (1979). Neuropsychological sequelae of childhood epilepsy. Unpublished dissertation.

Boll, T.J. (1981). The Halstead–Reitan Neuropsychology Battery. In S.B. Filskov and T.J. Boll (eds), *Handbook of Clinical Neuropsychology*, John Wiley & Sons, New York, pp. 577–607.

Camfield, P.R., Gates, R., Ronen, G., Camfield, C., Fergueson, A., and MacDonald, G.W. (1984). Comparison of cognitive ability, personality profile, and school success in epileptic children with pure right versus left temporal lobe EEG foci. *Annals of Neurology*, **15**, 122–126.

Dean, R.S. (1983). Neuropsychological correlates of total seizures with major motor epileptic children. *Clinical Neuropsychology*, **5**, 1–3.

Dikman, S., Matthews, C.G., and Harley, J.P. (1975). Effects of early versus late onset of major motor epilepsy on cognitive-intellectual performance. *Epilepsia*, **16**, 31–36.

Dikman, S., Matthews, C.G., and Harley, J.P. (1977). Effects of early versus late onset of major motor epilepsy on cognitive-intellectual functions in adults: further considerations. *Epilepsia*, **18**, 31–36.

Dodrill, C.B. (1981). Neuropsychology of epilepsy. In S.B. Filskov and T.J. Boll (eds), *Handbook of Clinical Neuropsychology*, John Wiley & Sons, New York, pp. 366–398.

Fedio, P., and Mirsky, A.F. (1967). Selective intellectual deficits in children with temporal lobe or centrencephalic epilepsy. *Neuropsychologica*, **7**, 287–300.

Giordani, B., Berent, S., Sackellares, J.C., Rourke, D., Seidenberg, M., O'Leary, D.S., Dreifuss, F.E., and Boll, T.J. (1985). Intelligence test performance of patients with partial and generalized seizures. *Epilepsia*, **26**, 37–42.

Golden, C.J. (1981). The Luria–Nebraska children's battery: Theory and initial formulation. In G. Hynd and J. Obrzut (eds), *Neuropsychological Assessment and the School-Age Child: Issues and Procedures*, Grune & Stratton, New York, pp. 277–302.

Graham, P., and Rutter, M. (1968). Organic brain dysfunction and child psychiatric disorder. *British Medical Journal*, **2**, 695–700.

Hermann, B.P. (1982). Neuropsychological functioning and psychopathology in children with epilepsy. *Epilepsia*, **23**, 545–554.

Hermann, B.P., Desai, B., and Whitman, S. (1988). Epilepsy. In V. Van Hasselt, P. Strain, M. Hersen (eds), *Handbook of Developmental and Physical Disabilities*, Pergamon Press, New York, pp. 247–270.

Hermann, B.P., and Whitman, S. (1984). Behavioral and personality correlates of epilepsy: A review, methodological critique, and conceptual model. *Psychological Bulletin*, **95**, 451–497.

Keating, L.E. (1960). A review of the literature on the relationship of epilepsy and intelligence in school children. *Journal of Mental Science*, **106**, 1042–1059.

Klove, H., and Matthews, C.G. (1974). Neuropsychological studies of patients with epilepsy. In R.M. Reitan and L.A. Davison (eds), *Clinical Neuropsychology: Current Status and Applications*, Winston and Sons, Washington, DC, pp. 237–265.

Lachar, D., and Gdowski, C.L. (1979). *Actuarial Assessment of Child and Adolescent Personality*, Western Psychological Services, Los Angeles.

Mellor, D.H., Lowit, I., and Hall, D.J. (1974). Are epileptic children behaviorally different from other children? In P. Harris and C. Maudsley (eds), *Epilepsy: Proceedings of the Hans Berger Centenary Symposium*, Churchill Livingstone, Edinburgh, pp. 313–316.

O'Leary, D.S., Seidenberg, M., Berent, S., and Boll, T.J. (1981). The effects of age of onset of tonic–clonic seizures on neuropsychological performance of children. *Epilepsia*, **22**, 197–203.

O'Leary, D.S., Lovell, M.R., Sackellaras, J.C., Berent, S., Giordani, B., Seidenberg, M., and Boll, T.J. (1983). Effects of age of onset of partial and generalized seizure on neuropsychological performance in children. *Journal of Nervous and Mental Disease*, **171**, 624–629.

Porter, J.E., and Rourke, B.P. (1985). Socioemotional functioning of learning disabled children: a subtypal analysis of personality patterns. In B.P. Rourke (ed.), *Neuropsychology of Learning Disabilities*, Guilford Press, New York, pp. 257–280.

Schefner, D., and Weber, R. (1981). Review on epilepsy and memory in children. *Acta Neurologica Scandinavica*, **64**, 157–164.

Seidenberg, M., Beck, N., Geisser, M., Giordani, B., Sackellaras, J.C., Berent, S., Dreifuss, F.E., and Boll, T.J. (1986). Academic achievement of children with epilepsy. *Epilepsia*, **27**, 753–759.

Stores, G. (1971). Cognitive function in children with epilepsy. *Developmental Medicine and Child Neurology*, **13**, 390–393.

Stores, G. (1981). Memory impairment in children with epilepsy. *Acta Neurologica Scandinavica*, **64**, 21–27.

Tarter, R.E. (1972). Intellectual and adaptive functioning in epilepsy. *Diseases of the Nervous System*, **33**, 763–770.

Chapter 6

Effects of Anticonvulsant Medications on Cognitive Functioning in Children with Epilepsy

Christine A. Cull and Michael R. Trimble

It has been estimated that, in the UK, there are 90,000 children on antiepileptic medication, of whom 54,000 have active epilepsy (Hopkins, 1981). The majority of these children are able to lead relatively normal lives, but many children are further handicapped by learning and behaviour problems. A number of factors have been suggested to be related to these difficulties, such as epilepsy variables, EEG abnormalities, brain damage, parental attitudes and adverse environmental factors. Investigations in this area have often yielded inconclusive and conflicting findings. It is probable that the causation in many cases is multifactorial.

One factor that is common to all children with epilepsy is the ingestion of antiepileptic medication, which has been mentioned by a number of authors as having a potentially important role in their psychosocial functioning (Keating, 1960; Ounsted, Lindsay, and Norman, 1966; Holdsworth and Whitmore, 1974; Knaven, 1978). There is a growing body of literature on the relationship of these drugs to cognitive performance in adults with epilepsy (see Trimble, 1979). By comparison, relatively little in the way of systematic research has been undertaken in children.

In this chapter we will review previous studies reporting on the effects of anticonvulsant drugs on cognitive function in school-age children with epilepsy. We have chosen to exclude studies which have investigated the prophylactic use of these drugs for febrile convulsions because of the young age of the subjects, and the different problems posed by the assessment of preschool children. Following the review of the previous literature we present data from our laboratory which explore further the relationship between antiepileptic medications and cognitive function.

Childhood Epilepsies: Neuropsychological, Psychosocial and Intervention Aspects
Edited by B. Hermann and M. Seidenberg

ANTIEPILEPTIC DRUGS AND COGNITIVE FUNCTIONING

Phenobarbitone

Holdsworth and Whitmore (1974) found no difference in school performance attributable to drugs. In their sample 73.7 per cent of 20 children doing well at school were taking phenobarbitone, as were 69.2 per cent of those failing at school (*N*=44). Additionally, 9 per cent of the latter group were not taking any medication.

Wapner, Thurston, and Holowach (1962) investigated changes in learning, behaviour and intellect in children with epilepsy following the introduction of phenobarbitone. Thirty-six children (aged 8–12 years) were tested prior to the introduction of phenobarbitone, at an average dose of 1.8 mg/kg/day, only one child having received any medication previously. A control group matched for race, sex, age and approximate IQ on initial testing, was selected from regular schools. Both groups were retested after an interval of 6 weeks. Measures used were the Stanford-Binet Intelligence Test, the Full Range Picture Vocabulary Test, and a multiple-T-stylus maze. All types of seizures were represented in the group with epilepsy, and although the number of seizures following administration of phenobarbitone was significantly less than prior to its use, complete control was not achieved. There was no significant change in any of the measures for the phenobarbitone group, and they did not differ significantly from the control group, either in respect of the initial assessment or the degree of change over time.

Phenytoin

Investigating reading attainment in children with epilepsy, Stores and Hart (1976) found that children who had been prescribed phenytoin continuously for at least 2 years had significantly lower accuracy and comprehension scores than children on other drugs. Utilizing measures of attentiveness, Stores, Hart and Piran (1978) found no significant differences between children on different anticonvulsant drugs, although there was a tendency for children taking phenytoin to perform less well on some measures.

Ethosuximide

Guey *et al.* (1967) studied 25 children with epilepsy (6–17 years of age), half of whom were suffering from absence seizures, while the remainder also had tonic–clonic seizures. Fifteen children were mentally retarded, while the remainder were of average intelligence. Ethosuximide in a dose of 750–1500 mg/day was added to their existing treatment. Test–retest evaluations ($\bar{x}$=7 months; range 1–30 months) included the WISC, the Bender Visual Motor

Test, the Benton Visual Retention Test, and additional drawing tests. On the WISC, all scores at retest were lower than those at initial testing. Significant differences were found only for the Full Scale IQ, Verbal IQ, and four subtests (Comprehension, Digit Span, Information and Vocabulary). For those children who were retested within the first 6 months of treatment the results were similar, with a significant drop in Full Scale IQ, Verbal IQ, and two subtest scores (Comprehension and Digit Span). However, for those retested after 6 months, although the second scores were lower there was no significant difference between pre- and post-treatment tests. Sixty per cent of the children had lower retest scores on the Benton Visual Retention Test, and the Bender Visual Motor Test. Given the overall pattern of results, the authors concluded that ethosuximide exerts a negative influence on intellectual efficiency.

Roger, Grangeon, Guey, and Lob (1968) studied a random sample of 100 young children (median age 8 years 7 months), with absence seizures (alone or in combination with grand mal seizures) being treated with ethosuximide (500–2500 mg/day). It was not clear whether this was used alone or in combination with other drugs. Cessation of seizures was seen in 57 per cent, a lessening in 29 per cent, and no change in 14 per cent of subjects. In 41 per cent there was reported to be a fall in school performance, and a significant drop in FSIQ (initial mean value 78.0; retest value 69.6) was reported for a group of 34 children who were assessed on the WISC. Deterioration was also seen on the Benton Visual Retention Test for 13 out of 20 subjects who received this test; the Bender Gestalt Test for 10/13 subjects and the Goodenough drawing test for 8/11 subjects. The effects were more pronounced for those children on higher dosage levels of at least 750 mg/day.

A group of 37 children (aged 5–15 years) with previously untreated absence seizures treated with ethosuximide (750–1500 mg/day) were studied by Browne *et al.* (1975). Of the total group, 32 per cent were already receiving medication for other seizure types. Subjects were initially given placebo capsules for 1 week, followed by ethosuximide for 8 weeks, and tested on the WISC and a modified Halstead–Reitan Battery (which assessed language, sensory-perceptual functions, motor functions, and intelligence) at both these times. A control group of 36 healthy children matched for age, sex, race, and socio-economic status was assessed over the same time period. For both groups the results of the retest were evaluated by a blind rater as being much worse, worse, unchanged, improved, or much improved relative to the first evaluation. None of the children were rated in the first (much worse) category, one was worse, 19 were unchanged, 15 were improved, and two were much improved. There was no change between first and second tests for any of the control subjects. The difference between the distribution of the retest scores for the control group and the ethosuximide group was significant. Thus the results indicate that there was no significant deterioration in performance after 8 weeks of treatment with ethosuximide. On the contrary, the performance of 17 patients was rated as having improved significantly. However, it must also be noted that there was a significant improvement in seizure control in the epilepsy group. Thus it is not clear whether the observed improvement in cognitive functioning was attributable to improved seizure control or the drug effect.

In a recent investigation of the clinical efficacy of ethosuximide, Blomquist and Zetterlund (1985) treated 11 newly diagnosed cases of typical absence seizures (aged 4–14 years) with ethosuximide monotherapy (10–20 mg/kg/day). The children were reported to be normal in all other respects. A reduced frequency of seizures was observed for all children, and improved school performance was reported in four. No adverse reactions were noted.

The results of these studies are clearly conflicting. Two studies show deterioration in performance in the short term (Guey *et al.*, 1967; Roger *et al.*, 1968), while the other two studies report improvement in similar areas of cognitive function at similar dose levels (Browne *et al.*, 1975; Blomquist and Zetterlund, 1985). In the latter studies this improvement could also be attributed to improved seizure control. The only obvious difference is a greater proportion of retarded children in those studies showing decline, and a greater use of concomitant medications. A control group comparison was not used in these studies either, which were conducted over much longer periods of time than that of Browne *et al.* (1975). As yet, the effect of ethosuximide on the cognitive functioning of children with epilepsy remains unclear, but it may be suggested that less able children are more at risk for cognitive disturbance, as also might be those where it is used in combination with other medications.

Carbamazepine

Martin, Movarrekhi, and Gisiger (1965) studied 12 children with epilepsy (aged 6–13 years) who were attending a special boarding school. They were assessed prior to the addition of carbamazepine (600 mg/day) to their existing drug regimen, and followed up 4–5 months later. The children were tested on the Terman or Borel-Maisonny IQ tests; the Goodenough Draw-A-Man test; Raven's Progressive Matrices; Rey's Incomplete Figures, Disks, Rings, Tapping, Dotting, and Rolls; and the Rey-Osterreith Figure—copy and memory versions. The majority of the children were described as being mentally handicapped. Overall there was an average rate of improvement of 34.4 per cent, 52.3 per cent of scores were unchanged, and a deterioration was seen in 13.3 per cent. Marked improvements were seen on the Progressive Matrices (66 per cent), and Rey's Dotting Test (58 per cent), which assesses speed and visuomotor coordination. The scores of nearly half the subjects improved on Rey's incomplete figures, rings, and tapping (measures of overall functioning and visuomotor coordination). In 33 per cent of subjects there was an improvement of at least 5 points with respect to IQ, and no change in 67 per cent. In contrast, 42 per cent showed a decrease in score on the Goodenough Test, 50 per cent were unchanged, and only 8 per cent showed an improvement. The authors concluded that the addition of carbamazepine had a beneficial effect in the areas of perceptual organization, practical intelligence, manual motor skills and visuomotor coordination. However, there was also some considerable decline in the skills necessary to complete the Goodenough test, suggesting that carbamazepine is not without some detrimental effect. Further, the authors fail to comment on the statistical significance of these findings. With respect to seizure frequency, there was a marked improvement in five children, no change in 11, and a deterioration in four, but it is not clear how this relates to change in cognitive performance.

Schain, Ward and Guthrie (1977) investigated 45 children (aged 5½–15 years) with major motor or psychomotor seizure disorders who were treated with carbamazepine (at a maximum dose of 30 mg/kg/day). Barbiturate anticonvulsants were concurrently withdrawn over a 4-week period; non-barbiturates were maintained in 28 children. A battery of tests including the WISC, the Matched Familiar Figures Test, the Children's Embedded Figures Test, and the Porteus Maze (the latter three being used as a measure of problem-solving abilities, attentiveness, and impulse control) were administered before and 4–6 months after the initiation of carbamazepine. Statistically significant improvements on all measures were found at retest. In addition, parents and teachers reported improved attentiveness and alertness. The authors suggest that these changes are due to a drug effect rather than a practice effect, although it is not clear whether this is attributable to the introduction of carbamazepine *per se* or the withdrawal of other anticonvulsants. The final mean carbamazepine dose was 19.1 mg/kg/day and the serum level was 7.8 μg/ml. No relationship was found between improvement in test performance and epilepsy variables (seizure type, seizure frequency at onset and follow-up), dose or plasma levels of anticonvulsants (carbamazepine, phenytoin, and phenobarbitone). A very large range of intellectual ability was represented in this study (WISC FSIQ values ranged from 52 to 130, with a mean of 87), and it would have been helpful to examine whether this improvement was found for all children, or whether there was any difference depending on ability level.

Rett (1976) studied three groups of children with grand mal seizures. Group I consisted of 10 children who were being changed to carbamazepine monotherapy, and were tested before and 11–12 months later. In Group II there were nine patients who were receiving carbamazepine monotherapy as their first treatment, and Group III consisted of 10 children who were taking other anticonvulsants. Psychological examination consisted of the WISC (mean IQ values: Group I, 99.8; Group II, 77.9; Group III, 95.0) and the Walther Test (a measure of motor function). No changes between pre- and post-test were seen in Group I. For Group II there was a significant improvement on the Walther Test, and no statistically significant changes were noticeable in Group III. From these results the author concluded that there was no evidence of a psychotropic effect of carbamazepine. However, he fails to comment on the initial comparability of the groups, and it is clear from the data they present that the groups were not equivalent, which may have had some influence on the outcome.

Jacobides (1978) studied 46 children (aged 6½–16 years) attending a neurology outpatient clinic, before and 1 year after treatment with carbamazepine. A variety of seizure types were represented in the sample (focal temporal in 19 patients, grand mal in 16, and a mixed type in 12 cases). Nineteen patients were treated with carbamazepine only at a dose of 15–25 mg/kg/day, and 27 were on polytherapy and a carbamazepine dose of 10–15 mg/kg/day. Assessments consisted of psychological assessments, scholastic ratings, and teachers' reports. Intellectual ability was assessed by means of the WISC; the revised Binet; or the Georgas test which included Raven's Progressive Matrices, vocabulary tests, and a measure of visuomotor integration. The IQ of the whole group was 65–110 and above; 17 children had a FSIQ of less than 80. There was no change in seizure control. The arithmetic mean of school marks rose by an average of 22 per cent, this was most marked for those children whose intellectual ability was average and above. The IQ scores increased from an average of 87.0 to 100.3. Alertness was reported to be generally improved in most patients. These results indicate a very positive effect of carbamazepine on cognitive function, but statistical comparisons are not presented. In addition, it is not clear how comparable the different IQ measures are, so caution is required in interpreting these results.

In summary, an improvement in different areas of cognitive functioning has been found in three studies (Martin *et al.*, 1965; Schain *et al.*, 1977; Jacobides, 1978), no change in two studies (Martin *et al.*, 1965; Rett, 1976) and deterioration in some aspects in one study (Martin *et al.*, 1965). The evidence thus far remains inconclusive but suggests that, if there is a beneficial effect of carbamazepine, it is specific to some aspects of functioning such as problem solving, visuomotor coordination and alertness, and is not a global effect. The least effect seems to be found in children of below average ability (Jacobides, 1978). It may thus be that difficulties in evaluating these studies are due, in part, to the different ability levels of the subjects.

Sodium valproate

Barnes and Bower (1975) investigated the clinical efficacy of sodium valproate in the treatment of 24 children with intractable epilepsy. Sodium valproate, at a dose of 20–80 mg/kg/day, was added to the existing drug regimen. Changes in school performance and alertness were noted over a follow-up period of at least 4 months, and information concerning school performance was available for 18 of these 24 children. There was no change in nine children, a definite improvement in six, and a marked improvement in three. Alertness was noted to be improved in 17/23 cases, and there was no change in the remaining six. No deterioration with respect to either aspect was reported.

Harding, Pullan, and Drasdo (1980) tested 35 children (aged 3–20 years) with generalized photosensitive epilepsy prior to receiving sodium valproate and again when they had attained the dosage of the drug which provided an elimination or maximum reduction of photosensitivity. An additional eight patients were tested when they had remained symptom-free for a minimum of 2 years, and once again after the drug had been successfully withdrawn for at least a month. The measures used were the Contingent Negative Variation (CNV) as an indicator of arousal or attention, and a simple reaction time task. The results were conflicting. The amplitude of the CNV was clearly reduced during treatment with sodium valproate, which the authors thought to be indicative of a sedative effect. The mean reaction time was significantly shorter when patients were on the drug, which was not dose-related, indicative of an alerting effect. Both of these changes occurred irrespective of the direction of change in medication.

Thus, in terms of objective measures of performance, sodium valproate would appear to have little in the way of sedative effects. But no reports are available as to the range of ability levels of these groups, so it is not clear whether these findings are applicable to children of normal, or below average, ability, or both.

Comparisons of antiepileptic drugs

Ozdirim, Renda, and Epir (1978) randomly assigned 63 newly diagnosed children with epilepsy (aged 5–12 years) attending a neurological outpatient clinic, to monotherapy treatment with phenobarbitone, phenytoin, or placebo (dosage not specified). The children were tested, before and 3 months after the initiation of treatment, on the Goodenough–Harris Drawing Test, the Peabody Picture Vocabulary Test (PPVT), and the Bender–Gestalt Visual Motor Test. There were no significant differences between the groups on initial testing; none of the groups showed any changes in perceptuomotor functioning as measured by the Bender–Gestalt test, and all groups improved significantly on the PPVT. The phenytoin and placebo groups showed improvement in performance on the Goodenough–Harris Drawing test, but this was significant only for the placebo group; no change was evident for the phenobarbitone group. On the basis of this, the authors suggest that phenobarbitone exerts a negative influence on cognitive function relative to other treatment conditions. From the reviewers' point of view, this conclusion is unwarranted, given the little differences that were apparent. No relationship was found between serum levels of antiepileptic drugs and scores on the psychological tests.

Nolte, Wetzel, Brugmann, and Brintzinger (1980) investigated two different therapeutic regimens. First, they assessed children before and 6 months after starting treatment with phenytoin. Children were randomly assigned to a high (Group I: N=4) or low (Group II: N=4) plasma level group. A second sample of children was tested before and 6 months after ending long-term therapy with either phenytoin (Group III: N=8) or primidone (Group IV: N=4). A group of six healthy children in the same age range served as a control group. All children were tested twice with the WISC or WPPSI, the 'd2 Concentration Test', the Benton Visual Retention Test, and a test of motor performance. The IQs obtained were found to be within the average range. Improvement on the WISC was found on second testing for all groups with the exception of Group I, with a high phenytoin plasma level (22.0 mg/L), where there was a reduction of mean scores. In Group IV (plasma level: 14.1 mg/L of phenobarbitone, 7.1 mg/L of primidone) there was a marked increase in Performance IQ, which was not so for Group III (plasma level: 13.7 mg/L). Similarly, scores on the motor performance tests deteriorated in Group I, were equivalent to the control group for Group II (plasma level: 5.9 mg/L), and higher than the control group for Groups III and IV, indicating improvement. Children in the phenytoin-treated groups were seizure-free over the 6-month period. Thus phenytoin would seem to impair some aspects of performance but only at high serum levels, whereas primidone, even with low plasma concentrations, seems to have a pronounced negative effect, particularly on motor performance.

Schain, Shields, and Dreisbach (1981) compared the efficacy of carbamazepine and phenobarbitone in the single-drug treatment of childhood seizure disorders. A group of 24 children (aged 6–16 years) of normal intellectual ability were assessed before and 6 weeks after the initiation of medication on the WISC, a paired-associate test, Matched Familiar Figures Test, a children's checking task, and a single-digit modality task. Carbamazepine (10–20 mg/kg/day) was given to 12 children, and the remaining 12 children received phenobarbitone (4–5 mg/kg/day), with mean serum levels of 6.8 μg/ml and 323.8 μg/ml respectively. A statistically significant change was found on only one test, the children's checking task (a test of sustained attention), in which there was a significant increase in the number of omission errors, following treatment with both carbamazepine and phenobarbitone. Thus both drugs were found to interfere with the children's ability to sustain attention. Six children who were initially on phenobarbitone were later crossed over to carbamazepine, because of poor seizure control or behaviour disturbance, and in the long term there was reported to be a pattern of improved performance on the Matched Familiar Figures Test and the paired-associate test. However, it is difficult to determine whether this was due to improved seizure control, improved behaviour, or a drug effect, or a combination of these.

Harding *et al.* (1980) investigated seven children who were changed from phenobarbitone to sodium valproate, and tested while on each drug by means of the CNV, and a simple reaction time task. The CNV amplitude did not change, but the reaction time was significantly shorter on sodium valproate than on phenobarbitone. They also investigated seven children with absence epilepsy who were transferred from ethosuximide to sodium valproate or vice-versa, and tested using the same measures as above, on each drug. There was no significant change with respect to CNV amplitude or reaction time. These studies suggest that phenobarbitone has more of a detrimental effect than sodium valproate, and that the effects of the latter drug and ethosuximide are equivalent. However, the authors do not comment on the ability level of the subjects, or whether they were comparable for each group.

In a study of teachers' questionnaire ratings of cognitive dysfunction, Bennett-Levy and Stores (1984) made comparisons among 39 children with respect to their type of antiepileptic medication. Those having any form of antiepileptic drug treatment (N=25) had significantly worse ratings on concentration, processing ability, and alertness, as well as having poorer attainments, than other children with epilepsy who had not taken any antiepileptic medication for at least 2 months (N=14). Those taking either sodium valproate or a combination of drugs (N=12) showed the same pattern of deficits as the total group taking drugs, whereas children on carbamazepine alone (N=13) only showed differences from the no-treatment group in having lower attainment ratings. When the very small group on valproate alone (N=5) were considered, they similarly appeared to be no different from the no-treatment group, except for having lower attainments. Children with epilepsy no longer on treatment were the same as their normal controls in all respects except for being significantly less alert, suggesting that this was not related to type of drug treatment. The authors fail to address the issue of seizure frequency, and it is not clear how this may be related to their findings.

Matched groups of individuals (including some children) whose epilepsy was well controlled by carbamazepine (N=21) or phenytoin (N=21), in a monotherapy regimen, were investigated with respect to their performance on a number of cognitive tasks by Andrewes *et al.* (1986). Significant differences between the groups were found on learning and memory tasks (both short-term and delayed), the better performance being shown by the carbamazepine group.

Trimble and Corbett (1980), in a study of 312 children with epilepsy, found a group of 31 who had a fall in IQ of at least 10 points (mean=21.3 points), over a period of at least a year. Sodium valproate, sulthiame, primidone, and phenytoin were the drugs most associated with this fall in IQ, and phenobarbitone and carbamazepine were the least associated. However, this information is difficult to evaluate because most of the children were taking more than one drug concurrently. The children with deterioration were found to have signifi-

Table 6.1
Summary of the main longitudinal studies — Anticonvulsants and cognitive function

Author	Year	Anticonvulsant	Dose/day (mg)	*N*	Age (years)	IQ	Design	Retest (months)	Seizure frequency	Effect	Notes
Wapner *et al.*	1962	Phenobarbitone	1–4 mg/kg	36	8–12	n/k	O–PHB	1½	+	=	1,3
				36			O–O				
Guey *et al.*	1967	Ethosuximide	750–1500	25	6–17	15 LD	AED+ETH	1–30	n/k	=–	3
Roger *et al.*	1968	Ethosuximide	500–2500	100	8:7	LD normal	AED+ETH	7	+=	–	3
Browne *et al.*	1975	Ethosuximide	750–1500	37	5–15	n/k	AED+ETH	2	+	17+ 1–	1,2,3
Blomquist and Zetterlund	1985	Ethosuximide	10–20 mg/kg	11	4–14	normal	O–ETH	n/k	+	4+	
Martin *et al.*	1965	Carbamazepine	600	12	6–13	LD	AED+CBZ	4–5	+=–	+=–	3
Schain *et al.*	1977	Carbamazepine	10–30 mg/kg	45	5–15	LD	PHB–CBZ	4–6	+=	+	2,3
Rett	1976	Carbamazepine	n/k	10	12–16	normal	CBZ	11–12	n/k	=	1,3
				9		LD	O–CBZ			+=	
Jacobides	1978	Carbamazepine	15–25 mg/kg	19	6–16	17 LD	O–CBZ	12	=	+=	3
		Carbamazepine	10–15 mg/kg	27			AED+CBZ				

Harding *et al.*	1980	Sodium valproate	n/k	35	3–20	n/k	AED–VPA	n/k	n/k	+−	
				8			VPA–O	1	=	+−	
Ozdirim *et al.*	1978	Various	n/k	63	5–12	n/k	O–PHB	3	n/k	=+	1,2,3
							O–PHT			=+	
							O–PBO			=+	
Nolte *et al.*	1980	Various	n/k	4	n/k	normal	O–PHT	6	+	−	1,2,3
				4			O–PHT		+	=	
				8			PHT–O			+	
				4			PRIM–O			+	
Schain *et al.*	1981	Carbamazepine	10–20 mg/kg	12	6–16	normal	O–CBZ	1½	n/k	=−	2,3
		Phenobarbitone	4–5 mg/kg	12			O–PHB			=−	
Harding *et al.*	1980	Various	n/k	7	n/k	n/k	PHB–VPA	n/k	n/k	+	3
				7			ETH–VPA			=	

1: Control group used; 2: blood level assessed; 3: standardized measures used; +: improvement, =: no change, −: deterioration; LD: learning disability; n/k = not known.

cantly higher mean serum levels of phenytoin and primidone than children who did not show such intellectual deterioration. This association remained true for phenytoin when children having less than 10 seizures a month were considered. For those children within the normal ability range there was a negative correlation between phenobarbitone and phenytoin levels and Performance IQ, and a trend in this direction for primidone. Thus blood levels of anti-epileptic medication may be an important factor with respect to intellectual deterioration.

Number, dose, and blood level of anticonvulsants

A number of authors have commented on the role of dose and duration of therapy. Glaser (1967) reported that dose of medication was important, insofar as a low IQ tended to be present in those children who were on the highest doses of medication. Children in special education were found to be particularly likely to receive heavy and multiple medication with anticonvulsants. Thus Ross and Peckham (1983) suggested that withdrawal of antiepileptic medications may have a beneficial effect on educational outcome.

Rodin, Schmaltz, and Twitty (1986), in a retrospective investigation of intellectual ability in children with epilepsy (aged 5–16 years at their initial contact), found no relationship between phenytoin level and IQ measures. However, for phenobarbitone level a significant inverse relationship was found for Peformance IQ, Full Scale IQ, and three subtests. Further, when two subgroups of patients who had phenobarbitone levels of less, or more, than 20 μg/ml were compared, there was a significant difference in Performance IQ, in favour of the group with the lower blood level.

Similarly, children with subtherapeutic drug levels were found to perform significantly better on a test of attention than children with therapeutic levels, by Niemann, Boenick, Schmidt, and Ettlinger (1985). There was also a nonsignificant trend for an inverse association between the level of medication and motor speed. Nineteen of these children were classified as being 'backward' and 18 were retarded. It is difficult to put these findings in perspective because the authors fail to inform about the range of medications employed, or the number taken by each child.

In a longitudinal study of IQ in 72 children with epilepsy, over periods of up to 6 years, Bourgeois *et al.* (1983) found eight children who showed a persistent decrease in IQ. The mean initial value was 108.1, and that of the last assessment was 88.0. These children were found to have a significantly higher incidence of drug levels in the toxic range. They were also significantly more likely to have had toxic drug levels of more than one drug at different times during the study.

A summary of the main studies is shown in Table 6.1.

SUMMARY

The little available evidence suggests that phenobarbitone does not exert a significant effect on cognitive function (Wapner *et al.*, 1962; Holdsworth and Whitmore, 1974; Ozdirim *et al.*, 1978; Trimble and Corbett, 1980; Schain *et al.*, 1981) but may be more detrimental than sodium valproate (Harding *et al.*, 1980). Primidone has been reported to have a detrimental effect (Nolte *et al.*, 1980), as has phenytoin (Stores and Hart, 1976) particularly at high blood levels (Nolte *et al.*, 1980), but the studies are few.

Ethosuximide has been found to both impair (Guey *et al.*, 1967; Roger *et al.*, 1968) and improve (Browne *et al.*, 1975; Blomquist and Zetterlund, 1985) efficient cognitive processing. Beneficial effects have also been reported for sodium valproate (Barnes and Bower, 1975; Harding *et al.*, 1980), and carbamazepine (Martin *et al.*, 1965; Schain *et al.*, 1977; Jacobides, 1978) which has less of an effect on cognitive function than phenytoin (Andrewes *et al.*, 1986) but is not without some detrimental effect (Martin *et al.*, 1965; Schain *et al.*, 1981).

Thus, for many of the compounds reviewed, beneficial, detrimental, and no effects have been reported, making it difficult to arrive at any firm conclusions. What is clear is that no anticonvulsant is free of potentially disruptive effects on cognitive functions in some individuals. The evidence would seem to suggest that this is more likely to occur with primidone and phenytoin, and least likely with phenobarbitone, carbamazepine, and sodium valproate. This conclusion is based on a limited number of studies and more information is obviously needed.

These studies do demonstrate, however, that the question of whether a particular anticonvulsant is likely to have adverse effects is somewhat simplistic. It is becoming more and more evident that, before arriving at an answer in the individual case, a number of other factors must be taken into account.

First, the status of the individual child must be considered. Thus no significant effect, or even beneficial effects, may be more likely to be apparent in children who do not have learning difficulties (Browne *et al.*, 1975; Jacobides, 1978). This may be due to the limitations of testing such patients, or may reflect real differences in the effect of drugs in this population.

Secondly, the clinical effect of the drug on seizure frequency may be important. In two studies improved cognitive function was reported as well as improved seizure control (Browne *et al.*, 1975; Schain *et al.*, 1981). Thirdly, the occurrence of high and toxic blood levels may be an important factor in any deterioration of cognitive ability (Nolte *et al.*, 1980; Trimble and Corbett, 1980; Bourgeois *et al.*, 1983; Niemann *et al.*, 1985; Rodin *et al.*, 1986). The use of drugs in a polytherapy regimen can also impede cognitive development (Ross and Peckham, 1983; Bennett-Levy and Stores, 1984).

CRITICISM OF THE STUDIES REVIEWED

Many of these studies are subject to methodological limitations which complicate the interpretation of the results. For example, the use of target drugs concomitantly with other medications, and the potential subsequent anticonvulsant drug interactions, makes it difficult to determine what any observed effect should be attributed to. For this reason the use of serum level monitoring in these kinds of studies is invaluable. It is not always clear whether any observed changes occur dependently, or independently, of any effect on seizure frequency. Many studies failed to incorporate a placebo control comparison in order to determine the degree to which practice effects, for example, might be operating. This is an important consideration in view of the fact that these investigations are often conducted over relatively short periods of time, typically 6 months or less.

The nature of the measures employed must also be considered. To assess cognitive functioning, investigators have frequently used measures of global ability such as IQ tests, developmental tests, and neuropsychological measures, which were not designed for repeated use in the short term and may not be sensitive enough to detect more subtle drug effects.

NATIONAL HOSPITAL AND GREAT ORMOND STREET HOSPITAL STUDY

In the foregoing literature review the impact of the pharmacological treatment of epilepsy on cognitive variables in children with this disorder has been presented. It is clear that relatively few studies have been done in this field, the results of which are inconclusive. As mentioned previously, one major stumbling block has been the inadequacy of assessment procedures. In our studies we have chosen to explore the value of microcomputer-delivered tests in the assessment of cognitive function in children with epilepsy in an attempt to rectify some of these inadequacies, and to examine further the relationship between anticonvulsant drugs and cognitive function. This work was carried out in association with Dr John Wilson (consultant paediatric neurologist) and his colleagues at Great Ormond Street Hospital.

Automated assessment offers a number of advantages over traditional face-to-face testing, including: standardized presentation of stimuli (Miller, 1968); and accurate and controlled time intervals of stimulus presentation, exposure and delay (Flowers, 1968; Gedye and Miller, 1969). All of these factors facilitate test reliability, minimize the influence of experimenter bias, and would thus seem an eminently suitable tool for psychopharmacological investigations (for review see Cull and Trimble, 1987). For this purpose a Research Machines Ltd 380Z microcomputer was programmed to deliver a battery of tests of cognitive function (see Figures 6.1 and 6.2), looking broadly at perceptuomotor performance, attention and sensory processing, central cognitive processing and memory.

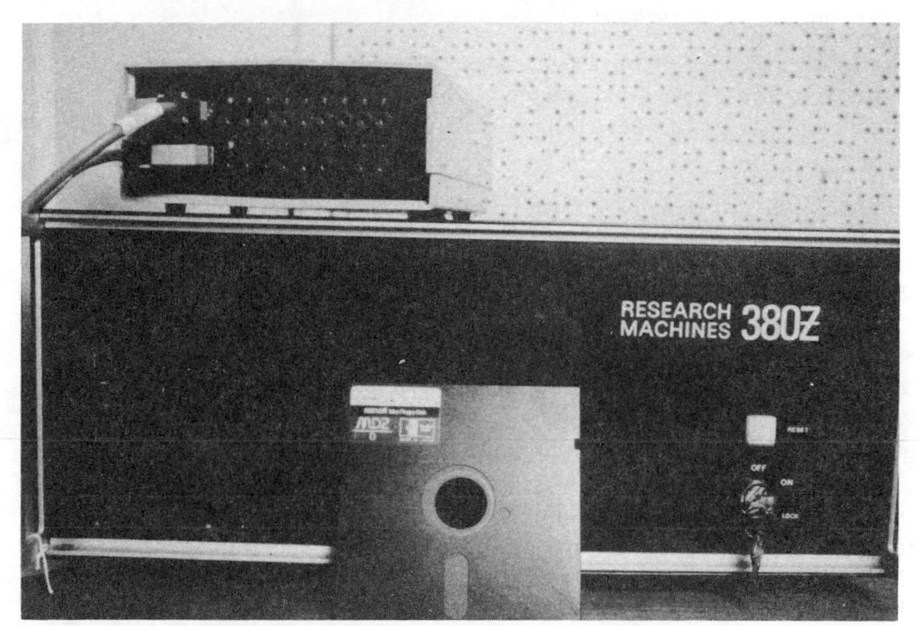

Figure 6.1: 380Z Microcomputer and floppy disc

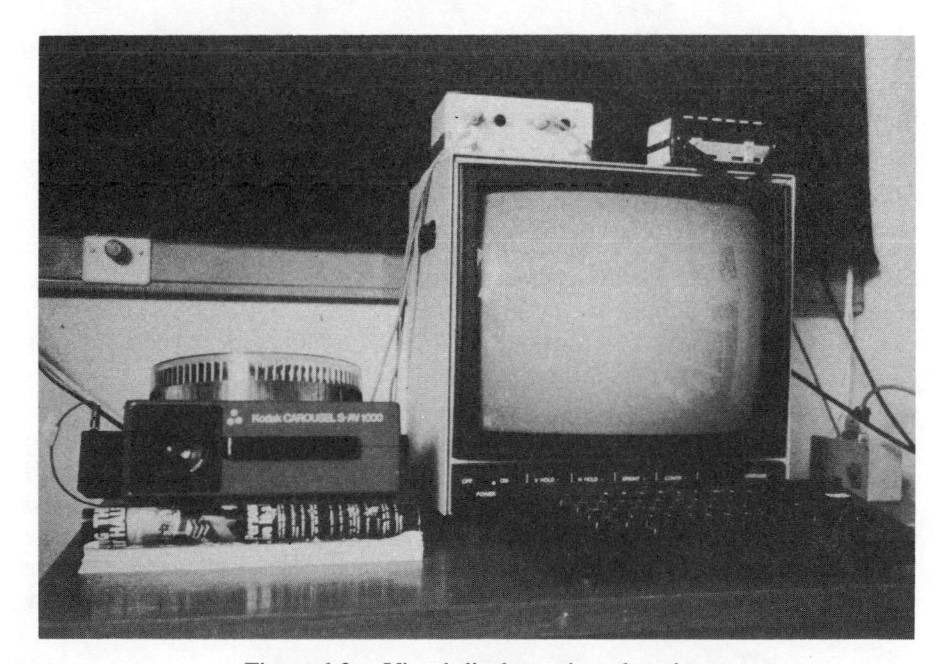

Figure 6.2: Visual display unit and projector

Perceptuomotor performance

Three simple reaction time tasks were used to assess the perceptuomotor element of the response sequence required in the remaining tasks. These involved pressing a predetermined key in response to a specified stimulus.

Attention and sensory processing

Four tasks were designed to assess attention to specific stimuli, maintaining performance on a long task, and the ability to explore complex stimuli in a planned and efficient way. In the first of these, 'Three-target Scanning Task', subjects were presented with 100 single digits consecutively, in random order. To each of these they had to indicate the recognition of the stimulus by responding YES/NO as to whether it was the same as any of three target digits also present on the visual display unit continuously throughout the task. The second task, 'One-target Scanning Task', was similar to the first, but had only one target digit on the screen and 300 items to be responded to. The third task in this series was a modification of the Digit Symbol Substitution Task found in the Wechsler intelligence scales (Wechsler, 1955). In our automated version the subjects had to match a number with a symbol and respond by pressing the appropriate key. The fourth task involved responding YES/NO to a simple perceptual identification task, answering the question 'Is it a picture?' in response to a visual display of either a word or a picture.

Central cognitive processing ability

To assess the ability of subjects to handle and process numerical information, they were required to complete 25 simple mental arithmetic (addition) tasks.

Memory

Tests of memory included recognition memory for words (presented via a tape cassette recorder) and pictures of faces (projected onto a screen). The ability to access information already stored in memory was also assessed by means of a task where subjects were required to make a YES/NO response to questions ('Is it living?', 'Is it bigger than you?') about pictures of familiar objects (projected onto a screen).

With the exception of the memory tasks, test items were presented on the visual display unit. Subjects responded by pressing keys either on the standard typewriter keyboard (which was used with a shield so that only those keys to be used were available to the subject), or a specially designed YES/NO response box (see Figure 6.3). Response latencies were recorded for all tasks, with the exception of the verbal recognition memory task for which error scores only were recorded.

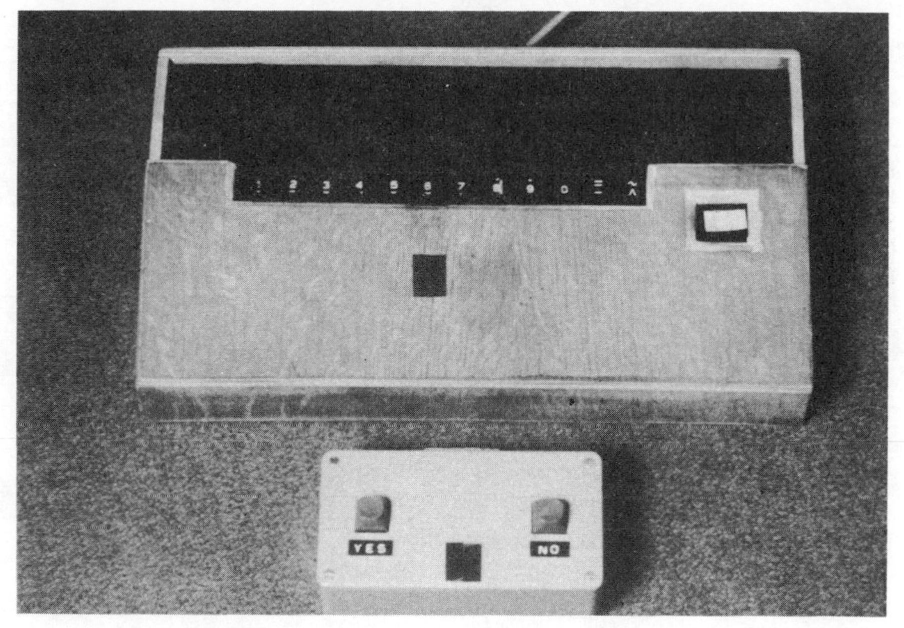

Figure 6.3: Keyboards

Sample studied

Forty-four children with epilepsy (aged 7–17 years) and 21 healthy children (aged 7–12 years) were compared with respect to their performance on the automated test battery. All children were assessed three times over a period of 6 months, at 3-monthly intervals.

The control group was compared with three subgroups of children with epilepsy: (1) those who remained on the *same* antiepileptic drug regimen throughout the period of study (N=18); (2) those who underwent a *decrease* in dose or number of drugs (N=16); and (3) children who had an *increase* in the dose or number of drugs (N=10). The initial drug regimens are shown in Table 6.2. The epilepsy groups were comparable with respect to age, and Full Scale IQ which was within the average range. The normal control group had a significantly lower age and higher Full Scale IQ, but this was taken into account in the statistical analyses. The epilepsy groups did not differ with respect to the age of onset and duration of the seizure disorder, neither was there any significant change in seizure frequency for any of the groups over time.

There was little in the way of change in error scores, so analysis concentrated on response latencies. Clear differences between the *increase* and *decrease* groups were apparent on a number of the cognitive tests, in favour of the latter group. Thus, an *increase* in antiepileptic drug load appeared to have a

Table 6.2
Initial drug regimens of children with epilepsy

	Groups		
	Epilepsy control	Decrease	Increase
Ethosuximude	1	1	—
Phenytoin	1	3	—
Sodium valproate	6	6	1
Carbamazepine	7	3	5
Polytherapy	3	3	4

Table 6.3
Summary of significant findings — cognitive measures

	Groups			
	Normal control	Epilepsy control	Decrease	Increase
DSST	S1 vs S2 S1 vs S3	S1 vs S2 S1 vs S3	S2 vs S3 S1 vs S3	S1 vs S3
Is it a picture?	S1 vs S2	S1 vs S2 S1 vs S3	S1 vs S2	ns
Is it living?	S1 vs S3	S1 vs S2 S1 vs S3	S1 vs S3	ns
Recognition memory for faces — immediate	ns	ns	S1 vs S2 S1 vs S3	ns

S1 : Session 1; S2 : Session 2; S3 : Session 3; ns = not significant

detrimental effect on the simple perceptual identification of stimuli (Is it a picture?), and the time taken to access previously stored information (Is it living?), which was not apparent for the *decrease* group. This latter group further showed improved performance on a face-recognition task not exhibited by the other groups, and a greater degree of improvement on a coding task than the other groups. A summary of these results is shown in Table 6.3.

SUMMARY AND CLINICAL IMPLICATIONS

A decrease in anticonvulsant drug load was found to be beneficial, whereas an increase was, by comparison, detrimental, with respect to response latency. Interestingly, this was apparent only on certain tasks which did not appear to be solely related to simple perceptuomotor responses which were unaffected; that is, the resulting effect was a slowing in the speed of cognitive processing. These data on children are complementary to the more extensive information now available on adults. This has been reviewed elsewhere (Trimble and Reynolds, 1976; Trimble and Thompson, 1986), and the problems of polytherapy, and differences between phenytoin and carbamazepine, especially with regards to cognitive function, noted.

From a practical point of view the influences of anticonvulsant drugs on cognition are important. Educational and vocational problems of children and adolescents with epilepsy are common, and any contribution of medication needs to be carefully considered. Children take anticonvulsants for many years, and through the more formative times of their lives. We believe that adverse cognitive effects of antiepileptic drugs can be minimized by taking into account the child's pretreatment intellectual status, and by prescribing the minimal anticonvulsant load necessary for adequate seizure control. Regular assessment of cognitive status should form part of the evaluation of children with epilepsy. However, this should not be restricted to traditional IQ measures, but should be sensitive to the clinical problems of the child with epilepsy. As with adults, the newer drugs are to be preferred over the older hydantoins and primidone, and polytherapy should always be a cause for concern.

REFERENCES

Andrewes, D.G., Bullen, J.G., Tomlinson, L., Elwes, R.D.C., and Reynolds, E.H. (1986). A comparative study of the cognitive effects of phenytoin and carbamazepine in new referrals with epilepsy. *Epilepsia*, **27**, 128–134.

Barnes, S.E., and Bower, B.D. (1975). Sodium valproate in the treatment of intractable childhood epilepsy. *Developmental Medicine and Child Neurology*, **17**, 175–181.

Bennett-Levy, J., and Stores, G. (1984). The nature of cognitive dysfunction in school-children with epilepsy. *Acta Neurologica Scandinavica*, **69**, Suppl. 99, 79–82.

Blomquist, H.K., and Zetterlund, B. (1985). Evaluation of treatment in typical absence seizures: the roles of long-term EEG monitoring and ethosuximide. *Acta Paediatrica Scandinavica*, **74**, 409–415.

Bourgeois, B.F.D., Prensky, A.L., Palkes, H.S., Talent, B.K., and Busch, S.G. (1983). Intelligence in epilepsy: a prospective study in children. *Annals of Neurology*, **14**, 438–444.

Browne, T.R., Dreifuss, F.E., Dyken, P.R., Goode, D.J., Penry, J.K., Porter, R.J., White, B.G., and White, P.T. (1975). Ethosuximide in the treatment of absence (petit mal) seizures. *Neurology*, **25**, 515–524.

Cull, C.A., and Trimble, M.R. (1987). Automated testing and psychopharmacology. In I. Hindmarch and P.D. Stonier (eds), *Human Psychopharmacology, vol. 1*, John Wiley & Sons, Chichester, pp. 113–153.

Flowers, K. (1968). An automated short-term visual memory test. *Bulletin of the British Psychological Society*, **21**, 102.

Gedye, J.L., and Miller, E. (1969). The automation of psychological assessment. *International Journal of Man–Machine Studies*, **1**, 237–262.

Glaser, G.H. (1967). Limbic epilepsy in childhood. *Journal of Nervous and Mental Disease*, **144**, 391–397.

Guey, J., Charles, C., Coquery, C., Roger, J. and Soulayrol, R. (1967). Study of psychological effects of ethosuximide (Zarontin) on 25 children suffering from petit mal epilepsy. *Epilepsia*, **8**, 129–141.

Harding, G.F.A., Pullan, J.J., and Drasdo, N. (1980). The effect of sodium valproate and other anticonvulsants on performance in children and adolescents. In M.J. Parsonage and A.D.S. Caldwell (eds), *The Place of Sodium Valproate in the Treatment of Epilepsy: The Royal Society of Medicine International Congress and Symposium Series, Number 30*, Royal Society of Medicine, Academic Press, Grune & Stratton, London, pp. 61–71.

Holdsworth, L., and Whitmore, K. (1974). A study of children with epilepsy attending ordinary schools. I: Their seizure patterns, prognosis and behaviour in school. *Developmental Medicine and Child Neurology*, **16**, 746–758.

Hopkins, A. (1981). *Epilepsy. The Facts*. Oxford University Press, Oxford.

Jacobides, G.M. (1978). Alertness and scholastic achievement in young epileptics treated with carbamazepine (Tegretol). In H. Meinardi & A.J. Rowan (eds), *Advances in Epileptology—1977*, Swets & Zeitlinger, Amsterdam, pp. 114–119.

Keating, L.E. (1960). A review of the literature on the relationship of epilepsy and intelligence in school children. *Journal of Mental Science*, **106**, 1042–1059.

Knaven, F.H.J. (1978). A keynote on cognition in children with epilepsy. In H. Meinardi and A.J. Rowan (eds), *Advances in Epileptology—1977*, Swets & Zeitlinger, Amsterdam, pp. 28–33.

Martin, F., Movarrekhi, M., and Gisiger, M.G. (1965). Etude de quelques effets du tegretol sur une population d'enfants epileptiques. *Schweizerische Medizinische Wochenschrift*, **95**, 982–989.

Miller, E. (1968). A case for automated clinical testing. *Bulletin of the British Psychological Society*, **21**, 75–78.

Niemann, H., Boenick, H.E., Schmidt, R.C., and Ettlinger, G. (1985). Cognitive development in epilepsy: the relative influence of epileptic activity and of brain damage. *European Archives of Psychiatry and Neurological Sciences*, **234**, 399–403.

Nolte, R., Wetzel, B., Brugmann, G., and Brintzinger, I. (1980). Effects of phenytoin and primidone monotherapy on mental performance in children. In S.I. Johannessen, P.L. Morselli, C.E. Pippenger, A. Richens, D. Schmidt & H. Meinardi (eds), *Antiepileptic Therapy: Advances in Drug Monitoring*, Raven Press, New York, pp. 81–86.

Ounsted, C., Lindsay, J., and Norman, R. (1966). Biological factors in temporal lobe epilepsy. *Clinics in Developmental Medicine*, No. 22. Spastics Society Medical Education and Information Unit, Heinemann Medical Books, London.

Ozdirim, E., Renda, Y., and Epir, S. (1978). Effects of phenobarbital and phenytoin on the behaviour of epileptic children. In H. Meinardi & A.J. Rowan (eds), *Advances in Epileptology—1977*, Swets & Zeitlinger, Amsterdam, pp. 120–123.

Rett, A. (1976). The so-called psychotropic effect of Tegretol in the treatment of convulsions of cerebral origin in children. In W. Birkmayer (ed.), *Epileptic Seizures–Behaviour–Pain*, Hans Huber, Bern, pp. 194–204.

Rodin, E.A., Schmaltz, S., and Twitty, G. (1986). Intellectual functions of patients with childhood-onset epilepsy. *Developmental Medicine and Child Neurology*, **28**, 25–33.

Roger, J., Grangeon, H., Guey, J., and Lob, H. (1968). Incidences psychiatriques et psychologiques du traitement par l'ethosuccimide chez les epileptiques. *L'Encephale*, **57**, 407–438.

Ross, E.M., and Peckham, C.S. (1983). Schoolchildren with epilepsy. In M. Parsonage, R.H.E. Grant, A.G. Craig & A.A. Ward Jr (eds), *Advances in Epileptology: XIVth Epilepsy International Symposium*, Raven Press, New York, pp. 215–220.

Schain, R.J., Ward, J.W., and Guthrie, D. (1977). Carbamazepine as an anticonvulsant in children. *Neurology*, **27**, 476–480.

Schain, R.J., Shields, W.D., and Dreisbach, M. (1981). Comparison of carbamazepine and phenobarbital in treatment of children with epilepsy. Paper presented at the XIIIth Epilepsy International Symposium, Kyoto, Japan.

Stores, G., and Hart, J. (1976). Reading skills of children with generalised or focal epilepsy attending ordinary school. *Developmental Medicine and Child Neurology*, **18**, 705–716.

Stores, G., Hart, J., and Piran, N. (1978). Inattentiveness in school children with epilepsy. *Epilepsia*, **19**, 169–175.

Trimble, M. (1979). The effect of anti-convulsant drugs on cognitive abilities. *Pharmacological Therapy*, **4**, 677–685.

Trimble, M.R., and Corbett, J.A. (1980). Behavioural and cognitive disturbances in epileptic children. *Irish Medical Journal*, **73**, Suppl. 10, 21–28.

Trimble, M.R, and Reynolds, E.H. (1976). Anticonvulsant drugs and mental symptoms: A review. *Psychological Medicine*, **6**, 169–178.

Trimble, M.R., and Thompson, P.J. (1986). Neuropsychological and behavioral sequelae of spontaneous seizures. *Annals of the New York Academy of Sciences*, **462**, 284–291.

Wapner, I., Thurston, D.L., and Holowach, J. (1962). Phenobarbital, its effect on learning in epileptic children. *Journal of the American Medical Association*, **182**, 139.

Wechsler, D. (1955). *Wechsler Adult Intelligence Scale—Manual*, Psychological Corporation, New York.

Chapter 7

Academic Achievement and School Performance of Children with Epilepsy

Michael Seidenberg

The development of basic academic competencies in reading, writing, and computational abilities is of considerable importance for future educational, social, and occupational adjustment and functioning. It is a well-established finding that children with epilepsy frequently have difficulties in the acquisition and development of these academic skills. Numerous studies have reached the conclusion that children with epilepsy are frequently significantly behind their similar-aged peers in academic achievement levels. In a recent review of the literature, Yule (1980) concluded that, as a group, children with uncomplicated epilepsy were about 1 year behind expectations based on chronological age in reading ability, and that about 20 percent of these children experienced severe specific deficits in reading. We have recently reported that significant impairments in academic ability in children with epilepsy extend to include spelling and arithmetic abilities as well as reading (Seidenberg *et al.*, 1986).

Although the occurrence of educational underachievement in children with epilepsy is well documented, the factors underlying this academic vulnerability have not yet been clearly identified. Identification of these factors is important in order to determine appropriate evaluation and treatment programs. The determinants of academic achievement are multivariate and one can anticipate that a variety of factors are critical to establishing a complete account of the academic and learning problems observed in children with seizures. Hermann and Whitman (1984) have recently suggested a multivariate framework for the examination of epilepsy and psychopathology which delineates three subsets of variables: neurological variables (e.g. EEG features, clinical epilepsy variables), psychosocial variables (e.g. chronic illness factors, social attitudinal factors specific to epilepsy), and medication variables (e.g. side-effects).

Such a tripartite framework is also appropriate for examining the potential sources of influence for the academic achievement of children with epilepsy.

Childhood Epilepsies: Neuropsychological, Psychosocial and Intervention Aspects
Edited by B. Hermann and M. Seidenberg

Indeed it is useful to utilize this framework as a means of organizing and presenting the findings currently available in the literature on academic achievements and epilepsy in children. Following this review, the results of some recent investigations which I have conducted examining clinical seizure and neuropsychological correlates of academic achievement of children with epilepsy will be presented.

NEUROLOGICAL VARIABLES

Seizures represent a transient paroxysmal disturbance of brain functioning. One might expect that the features and characteristics of this neural disturbance would influence the efficiency and nature of learning and information acquisition. There is a large literature suggesting an association between epileptiform activity and deficits in attention, memory, motor and cognitive functioning in adults (Dodrill, 1981). Several investigators have suggested that attention problems may be a critical feature underlying the educational problems of children with epilepsy (Holdsworth and Whitmore, 1974; Stores, 1973). The potential significance of spike-wave bursts for attention and/or consciousness, and information processing is discussed in detail in Chapter 4 of this volume by Dr Mirsky.

Baird, John, Ahn, and Maisel (1980) evaluated the electrophysiological correlates of school achievement and underachievement in groups of children with and without epilepsy. They divided the children with epilepsy into two groups based on their academic performance; successful performance versus a history of school failure (based on review of school records). The two groups were matched for duration of medication usage and degree of seizure control. All children were of normal intelligence based on scores from the Wechsler Intelligence Scale for Children or the Peabody Picture Vocabulary Test. A group of 'healthy' control children were also divided into two similar academic achievement groups based on their school history and record. Visual examination and quantitative analysis of the EEG and Visual Evoked Potential (VEP) showed many abnormal features for both groups of children with epilepsy. According to the authors, the most salient features characterizing the children with epilepsy with school problems were excessive activity in theta and beta bands, especially in the central and frontotemporal regions, and hyperreactivity of evoked responses in the frontal and frontopolar regions. Baird *et al.* suggest that these findings may be related to the attention problems of children with epilepsy experiencing school problems.

Several studies have attempted to relate seizure history or clinical seizure variables to cognitive and academic development of children with epilepsy. The literature relevant to more general aspects of cognitive functioning is reviewed in Chapter 5 of this book, while the current presentation focuses on studies specific to the adequacy of academic performance in children with epilepsy. The determination of epilepsy-related variables which correlate with academic difficulties would be useful for early identification and screening of those children at greatest risk for academic failure and the greatest need for appropriate educational remediation services.

Holdsworth and Whitmore (1974) reported on a group of 85 children with epilepsy who were attending regular school. Based on teacher report, 50 percent of the children were rated as functioning below grade level and 16 percent were significantly behind in their educational attainment. Children with major motor seizures, as compared to petit-mal seizures, were seen as experiencing the most educational difficulties. Seizure frequency was not related to educational rating, though it was related to behavioral problems.

Stores and Hart (1976) compared the reading ability of children with generalized seizure discharges with the performance of children with focal spike abnormalities, and to a group of control children matched for age and gender. They found that the average reading level of the generalized group was no different from the control group, whereas the group with focal spike abnormalities did perform significantly more poorly than its control comparison group on a measure of reading accuracy. Further examination of the data for the group with focal spike abnormalities indicated that the laterality of the epileptic focus may be relevant. Those children with a left hemisphere focus had poorer reading comprehension scores than those with a right hemisphere focus. This finding would be consistent with the greater propensity for language difficulties with left hemisphere dysfunction in adults, though the findings are less clearcut for children (Boll and Barth, 1981).

A recent study by Camfield *et al.* (1984), however, failed to find a relationship between site of EEG foci and academic performance among children with unilateral temporal lobe epilepsy. Several methodological differences exist between the two studies, which could account for the different findings. The Camfield study included only subjects with spikes restricted to the temporal lobes, while the Stores and Hart study included several subjects with EEG spikes extending beyond the temporal lobe, as well as secondary generalization. Also the academic measures employed in the two studies tapped different aspects of reading ability. Stores and Hart included a measure assessing *both* reading accuracy and reading comprehension in their study. The difference reported between the left and right hemisphere focus groups reached statistical significance for the reading comprehension measure but not for the reading accuracy measure. The Camfield study employed a reading accuracy measure only. It is noteworthy that both studies suffer from small sample sizes and it is clear that additional large-scale studies with well-defined groups are needed to clarify the role and relationship of the nature of the EEG abnormality, both type and laterality, for reading ability.

In summary, the current literature does not provide any clear basis for characterizing the neurological variables which would predict why some children with epilepsy do well in school and others do not. In a subsequent section the results of some recent studies investigating clinical seizure variables ad academic achievement are reported.

PSYCHOSOCIAL FACTORS

Several psychosocial factors, including chronic-illness factors (both general and epilepsy-specific), teacher and parent behavior and attitudes toward the child with epilepsy, as well as misconceptions about the disorder, have been suggested by numerous investigators as having a significant impact on scholastic achievement. Hartlage and Green (1972) studied parental attitudes in relation to the academic achievement of a group of 54 children and adolescents with epilepsy. Statistically significant correlations between measures of parental overprotection and acceptance of lower educational performance and the child's academic achievement were found (*r* values in the 0.25 range).

Long and Moore (1979) studied parental expectations for children in 19 families containing both a child with and without epilepsy. The findings indicated that the parents had lower expectations for school performance for their child with epilepsy, and saw themselves as displaying a more restrictive attitude toward the child with epilepsy. The greater prevalence of such attitudes among parents of children with epilepsy, and the association between these attitudes and poorer achievement in children with epilepsy (Hartlage and Green, 1972), has significant implications for the role these factors may play in the social and cognitive development of children with epilepsy. The chapters by Drs Ferrari (Chapter 10) and Taylor (Chapter 8) in this volume provide some additional discussion and data on the significance of parental expectations and attitudes for the personal and social adjustment of the child with epilepsy.

Teacher attitudes and expectations have also been implicated as a possible negative source of influence on the academic performance of children with epilepsy (Holdsworth and Whitmore, 1974). It seems evident that any complete model (and intervention framework) for identifying and treating the school difficulties of children with epilepsy will have to take into account the potential significance of a set of environmental, familial, and societal factors.

Children with epilepsy are at a greater risk for developing behavioral and emotional problems (Rutter, Graham, and Yule, 1970). Several studies which have reported a relationship between behavioral problems and academic difficulties in children with epilepsy have led some investigators to suggest that the poor academic abilities of children with epilepsy were primarily due to these behavior and emotional problems (Bagley, 1970; Pazzaglia and Frank-Pazzaglia, 1976). Yule (1980) cogently cautions that such arguments fail to appreciate the multiple concurrent sequelae of epilepsy, and confuse correlational results with cause-and-effect findings.

MEDICATION FACTORS

Stores and Hart (1976) reported that children on phenytoin performed more poorly than children on other anticonvulsant medications, but this was based on a very small sample size. Holdsworth and Whitmore (1974) found no difference in educational attainment according to whether phenobarbitone was being taken. However, this study based the assessment of educational attainment on teacher ratings rather than direct assessment of academic achievement. Overall, there have been very few investigations directly examining drug/achievement scores, so at this point there is little definitive data available on this subject.

The potential effect of anticonvulsant medications on learning, memory, attention, and other aspects of cognitive functioning has clearcut and significant implications for school performance. There are many methodological factors involved in the evaluation of anticonvulsant effects for behavioral functioning. A detailed review of these issues, and discussion of the current literature and findings on the effects of anticonvulsant drugs on general intellectual and cognitive functioning in school-aged children with epilepsy is provided in Chapter 6, by Cull and Trimble.

RECENT STUDIES

Studies investigating the factors related to school performance of children with epilepsy have implicated potential factors across the three major domains suggested by Hermann and Whitman (1984); neurological factors, psychosocial factors, and medication factors. In the next section, data are presented from several studies from our research group which have attempted to provide some additional information about the potential significance of clinical seizure and cognitive–neuropsychological correlates for academic performance.

In our initial study of clinical seizure variables (Seidenberg *et al.*, 1986), we attempted to expand on the previous literature in three major ways. First, we studied four separate areas of academic abilities: word recognition, spelling, reading comprehension, and arithmetic. Most previous studies have focused on reading skills and few have examined other academic areas. Second, we examined the predictive significance of several clinical seizure variables simultaneously through multivariate statistical analyses. While many of these variables have been implicated by previous studies, their combined predictive power is unknown, and it is also unclear as to whether the risk factors change across academic areas. Finally, we used an objective basis for defining achievement level that took into account the child's level of intellectual ability, therefore providing a more valid basis to evaluate academic performance.

The children included in this study were seen at the Behavioral Studies Section of the Epilepsy Center of the University of Virginia Hospital. Children who were included in this study were between the ages of 7 and 15 years, had received a confirmed diagnosis of epilepsy from a staff neurologist, and obtained a Wechsler Intelligence Scale for Children–Revised (WISC-R) Full Scale IQ score > 70. One hundred and twenty-two children met these criteria—72 children with generalized seizures (tonic clonic = 46, absence = 16, tonic clonic plus absence = 10), and 50 children with partial seizures (simple partial seizures = 6, complex partial = 25, and partial secondarily generalized = 19). There were 54 males and 68 females in the sample.

The academic achievement scores for the group of 54 boys and 68 girls is provided in Table 7.1. As a group the children made less academic progress than expected for their IQ level (difference scores) and age level (percentile scores). Furthermore, there was a substantial percentage of children who were experiencing significant levels of academic underachievement in the four academic areas; ranging from 10 percent in word recognition to 33 percent in arithmetic. These descriptive data of academic achievement levels are consistent with earlier reports of academic deficiencies for children with epilepsy in reading skills and further extend these findings to include other academic areas. Indeed, the present data suggest that arithmetic and spelling abilities are even more greatly impaired than reading skills. Educational evaluations and remedial programs for children with epilepsy need to recognize the possible widespread academic impairments that can be found among these children.

Several previous studies have reported academic performance differences for male and female children with epilepsy. Holdsworth and Whitmore (1974) found more boys than girls among their epilepsy sample to be experiencing educational difficulties. Stores and Hart (1976) found that the reading skills for boys with epilepsy was poorer than for the girls with epilepsy across both generalized and focal seizure types examined.

Do these findings indicate that gender is a specific risk factor for academic abilities in children with epilepsy? Probably not. At least no more so (and perhaps appreciably less) than it is for learning disability and dyslexia in the non-epilepsy population where males outnumber females about 5 to 1 (Hynd and Cohen, 1983). In this sample of 122 children with epilepsy we found that the females performed significantly better than the males only on measures of word recognition and spelling, but not on measures of reading comprehension and arithmetic. These results indicate that the academic superiority of females over males is evident only for some language-related academic areas rather than academic performance in general.

Academic underachievement was apparent across all seizure types in this sample of children. Within the generalized seizure types there was a consistent non-significant trend for children with tonic–clonic seizures to perform more poorly than those with absence seizures across all academic areas. Children with mixed seizures (absence and tonic–clonic) were significantly more impaired across all academic areas than either of the groups of children with only

Table 7.1
Academic achievement scores of male and female children with epilepsy

Variable	Males (N = 54)			Females (N = 68)		
	Mean of difference scores	Mean of percentile scores	Percentage significantly underachieving[a]	Mean of difference scores	Mean of percentile scores	Percentage significantly underachieving[a]
Word recognition	1.39 (13.44)	38.95 (29.90)	10.5	4.33 (13.34)	39.24 (29.07)	10.1
Spelling	−3.86 (16.34)	33.60 (31.85)	33.3	1.46 (15.19)	35.14 (30.05)	15.9
Arithmetic	−4.78 (12.49)	27.67 (23.81)	28.1	−5.81 (10.97)	22.47 (21.79)	31.9
Reading comprehension	−0.74 (12.62)	33.77 (28.99)	22.8	−0.38 (10.51)	31.33 (25.04)	13.0

[a] Children were classified as significant underachievers of their obtained academic score was 1 SD below (12 points) their expected score based on WISC–R Full Scale IQ level.

a single generalized seizure type. However, the children with mixed seizures also tended to have a more severe seizure disorder as reflected by their higher seizure frequency, earlier age of onset, and higher average number of anticonvulsant medications they are being maintained on, so it is difficult to tease apart the bases for their academic problems. Within the partial seizure groups there were no differences in the level of academic achievement scores between those with partial complex seizures and those with partial secondarily generalized seizures. Both groups were again significantly below norms for their same-aged peers.

Subsequent multiple regression analyses examined the predictive relationship of several clinical seizure factors on academic acheivement (age of seizure onset, seizure type, lifetime seizure frequency, and number of medications). Among these variables, age of seizure onset and lifetime total seizure frequency emerged as the strongest correlates of academic achievement scores. These findings are consistent with previous reports demonstrating the significance of earlier age of onset for cognitive vulnerability in children with epilepsy (O'Leary, Seidenberg, Berent, and Boll, 1981). Lifetime seizure frequency has also been shown to be a significant predictor of neuropsychological functioning in a previous study of children with tonic–clonic seizures (Dean, 1983).

Although statistically significant findings emerged from these analyses on a variety of neuroseizure variables, the overall relationships were modest. The combination of neuroseizure predictor variables accounted for a total of between 6 percent of the variance (for word recognition) and 17 percent of the variance for arithmetic scores. Knowledge about various aspects of the seizure history and characteristics is obviously of great importance for accurate diagnosis and medical treatment; however, it appears to be of only modest value for anticipating the academic achievement levels of these children. Similar findings have been recently reported in relation to behavior problems in children (Hermann, 1982), and the vocational adjustment and independent living of adolescents with epilepsy (Dodrill and Clemmons, 1984). In contrast, both these studies found that measures of cognitive abilities were fairly good predictors and discriminators of adjustment and behavioral functioning. One would anticipate a similar relationship for academic performance since various aspects of cognitive abilities are basic to the acquisition of basic academic skills such as reading and writing. Furthermore, such information can be critical in developing the appropriate educational intervention programs for children experiencing educational difficulties.

Our next study was therefore an attempt to specifically examine the cognitive–neuropsychological correlates of academic functioning of children in epilepsy in more detail. Up to this point there have been few studies directly examining the neuropsychological correlates of academic vulnerability for children with epilepsy. Of particular interest to us was whether observed academic impairments were related to generalized cognitive and intellectual impairment (e.g. overall IQ level) or whether academic progress was tied to more specific cognitive deficiencies (e.g. specific problems in language or visuospatial functions). This issue has important practical implications for the assessment and remediation of the educational difficulties of children with epilepsy.

An initial pool of 147 school-aged children (ages 9 to 14) with a confirmed diagnosis of epilepsy had undergone a complete neuropsychological evaluation as part of their diagnostic workup at the University of Virginia Comprehensive Epilepsy Program. The test battery included the Halstead Neuropsychological Test Battery for Children, the Wechsler Intelligence Scale for Children–Revised, and the Wechsler Memory Scale. These tests provided a total set of 30 measures or cognitive variables which are listed in Table 7.2 by their representation in a six-factor solution derived by a principal-component factor analysis of the entire test battery.

We then selected two groups of children for further analyses and comparisons based on their academic achievement scores. One group was composed of children who were making academic progress commensurate with or above age and IQ level expectations (Successful Achiever Group—SA group) (N=18) and the second group was achieving below age and IQ expectations (Unsuccessful Achiever Group—UA group) (N=30). All children had WISC-R Full Scale IQ scores above 80. Basic clinical seizure data, along with academic achievement and overall IQ scores for the two groups are provided in Table 7.3 and 7.4.

The Unsuccessful Academic group was older than the Successful Academic group (12.8 years versus 11.6 years; $p<0.05$) but there were no differences in the overall IQ scores between the two groups (both groups mean IQ scores are within the average range) despite dramatic differences in their academic achievement levels. There are no significant differences between the two groups in terms of age of seizure onset, seizure control, or seizure type (though there was a trend for children with generalized seizures to be overrepresented in the Unsuccessful group compared to the Successful group).

Examination of the results of the neuropsychological assessment battery provides some data indicative of basic cognitive ability differences between the two groups. These group differences are not, however, apparent across the full range of the six factors of the test battery. Rather, significant group differences emerged only for Factor 1 (Verbal Abilities) and Factor 3 (Attention and Concentration).

These findings are significant in two respects. First, they indicate that academic difficulties within a sample of children with epilepsy of Average to Low Average IQ are not related to generalized cognitive impairment. Second, the areas of verbal abilities and attention/concentration abilities are identified as the areas distinctly impaired in the poor academic achieving group. The importance of language-related verbal abilities (e.g. auditory–visual

Table 7.2
Loadings of cognitive measures with means and standard deviations for the academic groups

Cognitive measures	Unseccussful achievers		Successful achievers		
	M	SD	M	SD	F-value[b]
Factor 1					
WISC–R Information	8.43	2.56	9.61	2.28	2.59
Comprehension	8.90	2.19	9.33	2.06	0.46
Vocabulary	8.00	2.45	9.00	2.25	1.99
Similarities	8.67	2.41	9.22	2.60	0.56
Speech Perception Test[a]	11.03	4.07	6.89	3.69	10.91**
Aphasia Screening Test[a]	11.20	6.44	6.29	3.57	15.90**
Passage Recall	8.26	3.20	9.47	3.33	8.15**
Paired Associate	16.02	2.86	17.25	2.18	3.75
Wechsler Memory Scale					
Information	3.93	0.80	3.94	1.26	0.93
Orientation	4.21	1.29	4.22	0.88	0.46
Factor 2					
WISC–R Picture Completion	9.63	2.88	8.94	2.31	0.74
Picture Arrangement	9.77	2.60	9.33	2.91	0.29
Block Design	8.80	2.61	8.67	2.59	0.03
Object Assembly	10.17	2.77	8.61	2.09	4.22*
Category Test[a]	37.53	16.04	41.72	20.11	0.04
Factor 3					
Rhythm Test	22.47	4.45	25.56	4.91	7.83**
Sensory Total[a]	7.07	6.83	5.93	4.56	1.16
WMS Mental Control	5.93	1.62	6.67	1.33	3.70
WMS Digit Span	8.97	1.86	10.06	1.96	6.55**
WISC–R Arithmetic	9.50	2.60	11.17	2.23	5.13*
Factor 4					
TPT Time[a]	8.00	3.57	8.98	3.73	0.97
TPT Memory	4.63	1.03	4.44	1.25	0.74
TPT Localization	3.60	1.59	2.94	1.83	0.34
Figural Memory	8.31	3.56	9.33	3.07	3.19
Factor 5					
Tapping Speed	38.19	7.79	36.61	7.17	0.02
Grip Strength	23.20	7.66	18.48	6.56	0.92
Spatial Score[a]	3.53	1.20	3.76	1.56	0.09
Factor 6					
Trails A[a]	17.90	6.33	19.90	14.14	0.04
Trails B[a]	35.91	16.88	41.76	35.34	0.08
Coding	6.97	3.12	8.44	2.36	2.99

[a] Higher scores on these measures (e.g. errors or time) indicate poorer performance; on all other measures, higher scores indicate better performance.
[b] *, **, denotes p values at 0.05 and 0.01 level, respectively.

Table 7.3
Clinical seizure characteristics of successful and unsuccessful academic achievers

	Successful achiever		Unsuccessful achiever		
Variables	M	SD	M	SD	F-ratio[a]
Age of seizure onset	64.70	42.83	69.22	32.57	0.13
Duration	67.22	32.57	94.23	38.38	6.22*
Seizure control[b]	1.50	0.73	1.95	0.90	0.86
Number of medications	1.40	0.63	1.79	1.07	1.64
Seizure type					
Generalized	7		19		
Partial	9		9		
Unknown	2		2		

[a] * denotes p values significant at 0.15 level.
[b] Seizure control was rated good, fair, poor as a function of seizure type and seizure frequency using the rating system described by Hermann *et al.* (1980). Higher scores indicate poorer seizure control.

integration, verbal conceptualization, verbal expression and word knowledge, and short-term verbal memory) for academic functioning has been well documented in studies of the neuropsychological correlates of academic success in normal children (Townes, Trupin, Martin, and Goldstein, 1980) as well as with learning-disabled children (Rourke, 1982). A recent study of the social and vocational adjustment of high school-aged children with epilepsy reported

Table 7.4
Academic achievement scores and WISC–R IQ summary scores for the successful academic achievers and unsuccessful academic achievers

	Successful achiever		Unsuccessful achiever		
Measure	M	SD	M	SD	F-value[a]
Difference scores					
Word recognition	13.70	7.45	−10.73	7.55	119.21*
Spelling	14.51	9.95	−15.62	10.32	98.41*
Arithmetic	6.19	4.63	−15.06	9.52	78.41*
Percentile scores					
Word Recognition	71.33	19.10	18.70	15.57	108.39*
Spelling	72.22	20.01	14.43	16.66	116.38*
Arithmetic	55.67	14.13	14.13	14.71	76.41*
WISC–R Full Scale IQ	93.83	9.91	92.00	10.18	0.80 ns
WISC–R Verbal IQ	97.61	9.97	92.00	10.94	2.45 ns
WISC–R Performance IQ	91.28	10.86	93.77	11.92	1.07 ns

[a] Results of one-way analyses of variance between the two groups.
* denotes p-values significant at 0.001 level; ns denotes non-significant p-values >0.05.

that language skill had the strongest predictive relationships with these outcome measures (Dodrill and Clemmons, 1984). It is tempting to speculate that the academically unsuccessful children examined in our study represent a similar group of children tested at an earlier age. If this is the case, the importance of early identification of cognitive deficits and academic performance becomes critical in the development of appropriate comprehensive treatment programs for children with epilepsy.

SUMMARY AND IMPLICATIONS

The determinants of academic achievement of children is multifactorial, and any complete model must include biological and environmental dimensions. For children with epilepsy, the presence of a chronic neurological disorder adds several additional factors (e.g. brain dysfunction, medication effects) and intervening variables (e.g. parent and teacher expectations and attitudes, school absence) which must be considered. There is considerable variability among children with epilepsy as to the presence, degree, and nature of the academic difficulties being experienced. For the individual child being evaluated, one must be prepared to examine the various potential sources of influence and their interaction, so that effective and appropriate educational intervention programs are developed.

Many questions remain unanswered in relation to the area of academic and school functioning among children with epilepsy. There are some important points, however, which clearly come across in considering the data available in the literature. First is the recognition of the problem. It is only recently that some investigations have directly examined the educational attainment of children with epilepsy and differentiated it from more general intellectual or cognitve impairments. These studies indicate that academic underachievement is not uncommon, with perhaps as many as one out of five children with epilepsy experiencing significant problems in reading (Yule, 1980). Corbett and Trimble (1983) suggested that the problem may be even more pronounced among children with complicated epilepsy.

For those working with children with epilepsy a number of other points can be made. It should be evident that not all children with seizures will have problems keeping up at school. However, given the high rates which do seem to occur, specific inquiry into this important area of development is appropriate. In this regard one should be aware that information about grade level, or whether a child has been asked to repeat a grade, is not sufficient to determine academic development. Oftentimes these data are too crude to provide a basis to determine whether a child is achieving at levels commensurate to his/her overall intellectual ability. Similarly, impressions and ratings by either parents or schoolteachers may also not provide accurate estimates of a child's functioning. It would be helpful to examine the data from standardized achievement testing which are typically conducted on a yearly basis in the school system. Attention should be paid to academic areas other than just reading ability, as our data have indicated the presence of academic deficiencies to be widespread, including arithmetic and spelling areas. If questions remain after examining these data, or certainly if there are indications of significant levels of underachievement (e.g. over a year behind actual grade level), then consideration for a referral for a more thorough neuropsychological evaluation is warranted. The results of such an evaluation can be very useful in identifying areas of cognitive and behavioral strengths and deficits which can be critical for developing an intervention and remedial program. Finally, as I have maintained throughout this chapter, the potential sources of academic difficulties for children with epilepsy are often multifactorial, and a thorough functional analysis of the potential influence and contribution of these various factors is necessary for a more complete understanding of the child and the bases for their academic difficulties.

REFERENCES

Bagley, C.R. (1970). The educational performance of children with epilepsy. *British Journal of Educational Psychology*, **40**, 82–83.

Baird, H.W., John, E.R., Ahn, H., and Maisel, E. (1980). Neurometric evaluation of epileptic children who do well and poorly in school. *Electroencephalography and Clinical Neurophysiology*, **48**, 683–693.

Boll, T.J., and Barth, J.T. (1981). Neuropsychology of brain damage in children. In S.B. Filskov and T.J. Boll (eds), *Handbook of Clinical Neuropsychology*, John Wiley & Sons, New York, pp. 418–452.

Camfield, P.E., Gates, R., Rosen, G., Camfield, C., Fergueson, A., and McDonald, G.W. (1984). Comparison of cognitive ability, personality profile, and school success in epileptic children with pure right versus left temporal lobe EEG foci. *Annals of Neurology*, **15**, 122–126.

Corbett, M.B., and Trimble, M.R. (1983). Epilepsy and anticonvulsant medication. In Rutter, M. (ed.), *Developmental Neuropsychiatry*, Guilford Press, New York, pp. 112–129.

Dean, R.S. (1983). Neuropsychological correlates of total seizures with major motor epileptic children. *Clinical Neuropsychology*, **5**, 1–3.

Dodrill, C.B. (1981). Neuropsychology of epilepsy. In S.B. Filskov and T.J. Boll (eds), *Handbook of Clinical Neuropsychology*, John Wiley & Sons, New York, pp. 366–398.

Dodrill, C.B., and Clemmons, D. (1984). Use of neuropsychological tests to identify high school students with epilepsy who later demonstrate inadequate performances in life. *Journal of Consulting and Clinical Psychology*, **52**, 520–527.

Hartlage, L.C., and Green, J.B. (1972). The relation of parental attitudes to academic and social achievement in epileptic children. *Epilepsia*, **13**, 21–26.

Hermann, B.P. (1982). Neuropsychological functioning and psychopathology in children with epilepsy. *Epilepsia*, **23**, 545–554.

Hermann, B.P., Schwartz, M.S., Karnes, W.E., and Vahdet, P. (1980). Psychopathology in epilepsy: relationship of seizure type to age at onset. *Epilepsia*, **21**, 15–23.

Hermann, B.P., and Whitman, S. (1984). Behavioral and personality correlates of epilepsy: A review, methodological critique, and conceptual model. *Psychological Bulletin*, **95**, 451–497.

Holdsworth, L., and Whitmore, K. (1974). A study of children with epilepsy attending ordinary schools. I. Their seizure patterns, progress and behavior in school. *Developmental Medicine and Child Neurology*, **16**, 746–758.

Hynd, G., and Cohen, M. (1983). *Dyslexia: Neuropsychological Theory, Research, and Clinical Differentiation*, Grune & Stratton, Orlando, Florida.

Long, C.G., and Moore, J.R. (1979). Parental expectations for their epileptic children. *Journal of Child Psychology and Psychiatry*, **20**, 299–312.

O'Leary, D.S., Seidenberg, M., Berent, S., and Boll, T.J. (1981). The effects of age of onset of tonic-clonic seizures on neuropsychological performance of children. *Epilepsia*, **22**, 197–203.

Pazzaglia, P., and Frank-Pazzaglia, L. (1976). Record in grade school of pupils with epilepsy: an epidemiological study. *Epilepsia*, **17**, 361–366.

Rourke, B.P. (1982). Central processing deficiencies in children: towards a developmental neuropsychological model. *Journal of Clinical Neuropsychology*, **4**, 1–18.

Rutter, M., Graham, P., and Yule, W. (1970). *A Neuropsychiatric Study in Childhood*, Spastics International Publications, London.

Seidenberg, M., Beck, N., Geisser, M., Giordani, B., Sackellaras, J.C., Berent, S., Dreifuss, F.E., and Boll, T.J. (1986). Academic achievement of children with epilepsy. *Epilepsia*, **27**, 753–759.

Seidenberg, M., Beck, N., Geisser, M., O'Leary, D.S., Giordani, B., Berent, S., Sackellaras, J.C., Dreifuss, F.E., and Boll, T.J. (1987). Neuropsychological correlates of academic achievement of children with epilepsy. *Journal of Epilepsy*, **1**, 23–30.

Stores, G. (1973). Studies of attention and seizure disorders. *Developmental Medicine and Child Neurology*, **15**, 376–382.

Stores, G., and Hart, J. (1976). Reading skills of children with generalized or focal epilepsy attending ordinary school. *Developmental Medicine and Child Neurology*, **18**, 705–716.

Townes, B.D., Trupin, E.W., Martin, D.C., and Goldstein, D. (1980). Neuropsychological correlates of academic success among elementary school children. *Journal of Consulting and Clinical Psychology*, **48**, 675–684.

Yule, W. (1980). Educational achievement. In B.M. Kulig, H. Meinardi, and G. Stores (eds), *Epilepsy and Behavior*. Swets & Zetlinger, Lisse, The Netherlands, pp. 162–168.

Chapter 8

Psychosocial Components of Childhood Epilepsy

David C. Taylor

INTRODUCTION

The medical definition of epilepsy, as a recurrent transient brain dysfunction with altered consciousness associated with abnormal electrical discharges which may be detectable by electroencephalography, has hardly changed since that type of analogy was proposed by Hughlings Jackson when the electrical metaphor was novel. But it allows that epilepsy connotes one variable aspect of brain dysfunction which may also betoken the coexistence of other forms of brain abnormality, damage or dysfunction. When epilepsy is severe and persistent it is not surprising that it will be associated with behavioural and with cognitive disorder, since social behaviours are every bit as dependent upon adequate cerebral functioning as are cognitions. In practice, most of the deficiencies of their performances are overlooked, when ordinary social judgements are made, unless the abnormalities obtrude in social transactions. Thus hyperkinesis, which leads to the discomfiture of normals, has been accorded a relatively greater degree of interest than hypokinesis (ixophrenia) though, as in the case of schizophrenia, the negative symptoms of epilepsy are at least as pervasive and disadvantaging to sufferers. Epilepsy has maintained a negative stereotype throughout recorded history, though the manner of its social expression has changed, with changes in our concepts of causation, from florid demonology to sophisticated social constraints and special categorizations. Thus one contemporary advocate claimed somewhat triumphantly that he had been falsely categorized as 'epileptic' for several years before his preferred category 'having a brain tumour' was conferred by more precise diagnosis. There thus persists, even in the minds of devoted modern advocates, some notion that epilepsy is a stigma *in itself*, a view which illustrates the persistence of pre-Hippocratic demonology. It goes without saying that it is perfectly possible to suffer seizures and yet be demonstrably normal in every other

Childhood Epilepsies: Neuropsychological, Psychosocial and Intervention Aspects
Edited by B. Hermann and M. Seidenberg

respect. The problem of epilepsy is that it is a potentially public declaration of a chronic health problem, and that its appearance *does* recategorize its sufferers into a general class of persons with greater than average risk. Like the word 'cancer', 'epilepsy' only has a general meaning in that sense, in the sense of a social categorization. Some of the reasons for this will be evident in other chapters. This chapter will aim directly to examine the origin and sources of the negative stereotype both within the range of organic, physical possibilities and within the range of reactions of significant others to seizures. It cannot be overstressed that most of the destructive potential attributed to 'epilepsy' is worked out in early childhood and enters the popular belief system from that source. Many of the children whose lives with epilepsy contribute to the popular stereotype do not survive, or do not survive in the public domain, hence the part their fate plays in maintaining popular beliefs becomes obscure. The popular nostrum that 80 per cent of people with epilepsy live out normal and useful lives in the community is an acceptable optimism, as it refers to the bulk of the grown-up population; but it precludes from consideration the attrition of childhood epilepsy, and it anyway nicely circumvents the true import of a one in five chance of an impaired life. Modern epilepsy treatment, notably surgery, has revealed how many individuals who cease to suffer epilepsy make substantial and significant improvements in their mental state, their social performance and their well-being. The sum of these improvements might fairly be adduced to be the prior cost of the burden of their epilepsy (Taylor and Falconer, 1968, Ounsted, Lindsay, and Richards, 1987). But they also change their social category.

CHRONIC ILLNESS

Childhood epilepsy is a chronic illness, and consideration must be given to the constraints derived from suffering any chronic illness before specific links between epilepsy and psychosocial development are pursued. These were considered at length in Taylor (1985), but in brief it needs to be considered whether:

1. People of certain personality make-up may be prone to certain sorts of disease; very little support has been adduced for this in people with epilepsy or with asthma and diabetes where it has often been searched for. However, the concept of vulnerability and invulnerability, to giving expression to illness for which there is an hereditable potential given sufficient life stress (Lockyer, 1981) is of interest since it directly links psychological stress and the illness, in which case associated psychological disorder would become probable.
2. There is no doubt that early-onset epilepsies are more generally of poor prognosis in every sphere (Aicardi, 1986) but there is little evidence to

suggest greater psychosocial impairment to other chronic diseases of early onset unless cerebral development is in some way implicated (as in the treatment of leukaemia including X-irradiation of the head).

3. Any chronic illness may become caught up in personality development and become a mode of living 'as a diabetic' or 'as a leukaemic' or an 'epileptic person' (Taylor, 1969a) where fulfilment is found through sick group membership. This dangerous strategy becomes most evident if a cure is effected and the formerly sick person finds he or she has nothing left to live for (Ferguson and Rayport, 1965).
4. Having a chronically sick child generates extra work, chronic anxiety, unresolved grief, which may produce patterns of parenting which eventually affect personality development.
5. Similarly, the strains on the individual may render him or her increasingly liable to various forms of psychiatric disorder without the family or the environment being particularly disadvantageous. The realization of mortality in adolescents with cystic fibrosis and its associated depression is such an instance. But the realization of limitation which comes to adolescents with epilepsy barred from driving produces a similar effect. Treatment non-adherence in teenagers with diabetes or epilepsy charged with their own management similarly suggests their wish to manipulate at least some part of their health management.
6. Being chronically ill in any way is a minority categorization which can be resisted, or may be clung to obsessionally, or else used to be hidden within. These challenges do not exist for the non-sick, and this may underlie some of the differences in personality development seen in certain chronic illnesses, though not necessarily specific to any one.

However, there are relatively few chronic brain diseases of early onset and long duration. Those that exist are often associated with cognitive impairment and, since epilepsy is also evident, their independent effect is not easy to determine.

THE PREDICAMENT

As a result of several personal research studies on the outcome of epilepsy (Taylor, 1972; Taylor and Falconer, 1968; Taylor and Harrison, 1976; Hackney and Taylor, 1976) it became evident that the overall prognosis, the outcome of a sickness, has to be seen as the resultant of several components of that sickness which, though they interact, are actually very different conceptually. They are in different universes of discourse and there is a danger, if that fact is not understood by physicians and other helpers, of believing that effective change in one universe will produce change in another. This will not necessarily happen. The epilepsy might be known, aetiologically, to be grounded in a structural, tangible, cerebral *disease*, for example tuberous sclerosis, or be the direct or indirect consequence of a known biochemical disorder such as Batten's disease or pyridoxine dependency (see Table 8.1).

Alternatively, epilepsy may have no known structural or biochemical concomitants, and the diagnosis of the *illness* depends entirely upon the subjective or objective aspects of the behaviour with support from electroencephalography. Then people suffering from epilepsy are in a particular *predicament*, and this predicament may contribute substantially to the amount of sickness which is experienced. The 'predicament' was the word chosen by Taylor (1979, 1981, 1982) to cover the complex of an individual's particular and personal psychosocial interconnections, not just their living environment but that particular part of the social nexus occupied by them at that time. How any given predicament is being experienced depends upon the history of that person in the world. This history of a person becomes a crucial aspect of diagnosis which is different from the 'history of the presenting complaint'.

The structural component of sickness, that which is most easily validated by biomedical technology, is referred to as 'disease'. Disease is biomedically attractive and respectable. Several of the major advances in epileptology derive from pursuing that line. But, for the most part, epilepsy in this schema is an 'illness'. From Table 8.1 under 'illnesses' epilepsy can be seen as a declaration specifically about cerebral dysfunction though the underlying 'disease' or structural component may not be known. Epilepsy is a behaviour; it constitutes a social manifestation which will be a limitation (on trustworthiness? on driving?) and which may become a 'role' in Goffman's (1963) sense, either aspired to or attributed by others. These role components may be recast, can change for better (seizure-free periods) or worse, and they will be judged morally. The diagnosis of epilepsy is essentially descriptive and leads to a 'semantic reattribution' that is a biomedical attempt at precision, such as 'atypical petit mal', 'complex partial seizures', 'gelolepsy'. The illness will vary over time and space, and alter with development. Knowledge about epilepsy, as can be seen in other chapters, has much to do with classification and attempts at palliation. There is scope for personal change in lifestyle, attitude, habits, which might be ameliorating.

These aspects of epilepsy, viewed as an interactive function of disease, illness and predicament, are illustrated in a case:

> A.B. was 15 years old when brought to the neuropsychiatric clinic by his community psychiatric nurse. He had lived 5 days a week in a boarding school for children with cerebral palsy since the age of 12. The problem was said to be aggressiveness and simulated seizures. His epilepsy had been diagnosed and treated but it was thought that he 'put on' seizures, and that these were becoming troublesome. The boy's 'disease' was evident enough; he suffered cerebral palsy, spastic diplegia, associated with his preterm birth and low birthweight, 3 lbs 5 oz. His 'illness' consisted of his epilepsy and his

Table 8.1

Diseases	Illnesses	Predicaments
Discernible as physical reality. Not necessarily organ-specific	The declaration of the disease in its specific forms. More probably organ-specific	The complex of psychosocial ramification with immediate bearing on the individual
Specific changes in structure or functional organization of tissue	Essentially a social manifestation, a limitation, a commentary, a role, a behaviour pattern	Diffuse, multifactorial, personal but not necessarily unique
May be trivial	May change for better or worse without reclassifying 'the disease'. Capable of being recast as a role	Very unstable structure
Valid without 'illness'. Does not depend upon its implications	Valid without discoverable disease	Valid without disease or illness
Amoral	Probably judged 'morally'. Psychosocial processes modify	Highly charged with moral implication. Dependent upon social mores
Diagnosis is discovery — specifying structural–functional change	Diagnosis is description and semantic reattribution	Diagnosis is discernment
Space, place, and time irrelevant	Space, place, and time relevant. Developmental process modifies. Significance contracts and expands	Space, place, and time paramount
Knowledge grows with investigation	Knowledge grows with classification	Knowledge grows with 'understanding'
Scope for specific therapy, scope for reconciliation	Scope for palliation, scope for personal change	Scope for social and political remedies

> cognitive deficit which was greater than seemed apparent because of relatively good language and socialization. His seizures were first apparent, but later reappeared in the form of absences. Lately the attacks he was said to dissemble were 'tonic', and often nocturnal.
>
> His predicament was that his father left the family as soon as he became aware of A.B.'s handicap, and that his mother had raised him and his sister despite her own sickness (chronic and incapacitating headaches diagnosed as neurotic) until, some 4 years prior, whilst he was in a double-hip spica, incapaciated after surgery for his spastic legs, she had collapsed and died of a cerebral haemorrhage in his presence. Subsequently, his rearing fell to his maternal grandmother and his aunt, who seemed clearly to have been overtaxed by the unlooked-for task. He described discipline at home as severe, unfair and uncompromising. At school he was slapped (albeit in good conscience) to bring him out of his attacks. Examination of his mental state revealed a piteous unresolved grief reaction and 'smiling' depression of considerable severity combined with suicidal ideas 'What's the worth of living?', he remarked in our interview, 'You're just born, then you die!' He confessed to have last been happy 4 years ago 'Before me mother didn't die.'

He proved to have epilepsy of the Lennox–Gastaut type which was resolving into frontal epilepsy which, because of the retention of awareness, was being misconstrued as 'hysterical'.

He was easy to treat but hard to benefit. Much effort was put into his grief work, not only over his mother, but his absent father too. His educational needs were redescribed more appropriately to his cognitive capacity and his psychological needs. His aggression was shown to be closely related to periods of obtunding by status of minor epilepsy.

Nevertheless, the image of the boy held in his own locality by those who 'had known him well for years', together with negative projections about boarding schools for cerebral palsied boys and the highly defensive images held by his relations, all conspired to preclude a really useful restart. Given this, our own role turned rather sour, and following further aggressiveness in a spate of seizures he was discharged from our unit. However, this created a sharp change in the way he was perceived and managed local to his home, and this was of lasting benefit to him and his family.

The vignette illuminates the use of postulates about Predicaments given in Table 8.1, their complexity, their diffuse and multifactorial but not necessarily unique nature, their being highly morally charged and recruiting powerful fixed attitudes from significant others. Understanding the vignette derives from the reader's discernment as well as that of the treating psychiatrists. Knowledge grows with understanding, what Jaspers (1962) called 'Verstehen'. The vignette reveals the scope for a wide variety of changes of a social and political nature which might facilitate the plight, the predicament, of a youth such as this.

THE PREDICAMENT OF EPILEPSY

Several psychosocial constructs have been described which bear directly upon the predicament of the child with epilepsy and deserve particular attention.

Prejudice

One of the curious aspects of prejudice is encapsulated in the distress caused to a patient neurologically normal and with mild epilepsy, by being given the soubriquet 'Spas'(tic) by his schoolfellows. The inaccuracy is obviously not the source of his distress; indeed it highlights the fact that his distress is caused by any attention whatever, accurate or not, being drawn to his membership of a minority group. Prejudice has come to mean ascribing attributes of such overwhelming significance that they override individual characteristics; it is a limitation upon personal expression imposed from outside. Prejudice seems to this author (Taylor, 1973, 1987) to derive directly from the ordinary cognitive process of categorization. Any minority group will be categorized 'unlike me' by most people. Ignorance of the precise characteristics of the minority group is likely, but probably some component of the negative stereotype will be 'true' though exaggerated. Hence 'Spas' does portray the association between seizures and cerebral palsy, though this is unlikely to be known to my patient with epilepsy or his heckler. The effect of the association between epilepsy and deleterious outcomes being weak and irregular does not necessarily weaken it in the public mind. Only some toadstools need to be poisonous for people to tend to leave them alone altogether. Stigmata is the name given to signs which declare minority status. People with epilepsy can have this declaration forced upon them.

B.C., a charming and gracious girl of good background, had only enrolled in her new senior school for 2 weeks when, whilst standing in the queue for lunch, she found that she had voided urine in such a manner that it was obvious to at least a hundred fellow-pupils. Apart from the trauma of this manner of onset of her teenage epilepsy, the loss of esteem she perceived in the unwonted micturition precipitated severe and lasting school phobia. The events rekindled an earlier attachment problem which had had a psychological basis. The onset of epilepsy and its treatment actually created a physical (disease and illness) basis for a regression which was also, wrongly, attributed to psychological causation.

This girl, B.C., found that her entry into the epileptic role created subsequently such overwhelming expectation of her being in that role that her role as her normal self was not sustainable. The clearest stigmata of epilepsy are the seizures, but there are also the pills and regimens, the constraints and the vigilance, the days absent and unaccounted for, which suddenly or gradually create the climate for modern equivalents of ancient demonology to be exhibited, in this instance relabelling as 'physically handicapped' and separation within a special school.

Pseudo-death

Previously I described (Taylor, 1969a) an epileptic seizure as 'a brief excursion through madness into death'. The seizure is the quintessence of dyscontrol but it leads so often to the pseudo-death. Despite 10 years' experience of children with epilepsy, and despite personally having drawn attention to the phenomenon of pseudo-death, I recently described a frightening personal reminder. The parents of a toddler were giving details of their child's intractable seizures, which were continuing at the rate of six or so per day rather than the previous sixty. I sat with the child in my lap to see if I could palpate the jerks and twitches which accompany some nasty childhood epilepsies. Suddenly the child threw back her head, gazed in terror, stiffened at every joint, turned grey and relaxed, lifeless. With such equanimity as I had left, I took the child to an adjacent clinical room and gathered resuscitation equipment and collected my words to her parents. As I turned back to the child she was sitting composedly on the bench. 'Give you a nasty shock didn't she doctor', said her mother reassuringly as I reappeared with her.

The commonest situation of the occurrence of these pseudo-deaths is in febrile convulsions where about 50 per cent of parents will have experienced this brief but awesome scenario (Baumer *et al.*, 1981). Deaths in seizures *do* occur, and with sufficient frequency to feed the possibility that any seizure may be a child's last.

Being personally privy to the experience of the convulsion can radically alter a physician's perception of a case. The care which is given can be radically altered as a result of the chance involvement of a physician in the drama of the seizure, rather than through the cold composure of the casualty room.

> C.D. suffered a catastrophic seizure with fever in early childhood which continued unabated for at least an hour before it could be stopped. Two years later the parents described what was quite clearly the onset of psychomotor epilepsy. These attacks remained unattended to until finally one occurred in the physician's presence, which led to immediate removal of the child to hospital for investigation.

It is part of the predicament of epilepsy that it generates a sense of menace; it suggests the possibility of catastrophe. However remote that might be it often leads to avoidance. Physicians are not precluded from making those responses.

Hyperpaedophilia

This important but unfortunately named concept was introduced by Ounsted (1955) and Ounsted, Lindsay, and Norman, (1966). It refers to the situation where endless doting, care, and devotion are lavished upon a severely handicapped developmentally retarded child to the detriment of the carers' well-being. It implies treating the child inappropriately to its needs, but to a point more appropriate to its perceived developmental level. In introducing the concept, Ounsted *et al.* (1966) quoted Lord Brougham and Vaux in Paley's *Natural Theology* (1845), which provides the clearest explanation of his aims.

> Birds and Beasts after a certain time banish their offspring, disown their acquaintance and seem to have no knowledge of objects which lately engrossed the attention of their minds and occupied the industry and labour of their bodies. This change in different animals takes place at different distances of time from the birth, but the time always corresponds with the ability of the young animal to maintain itself—never anticipates it. In the sparrow tribe, when it is perceived that the young can fly themselves then the parents forsake them for ever, and, although they continue to live together pay them no more attention than they do other birds in the same flock.

In a footnote Brougham and Vaux adds,

> In the natural and instinctive feelings of a man as contradistinguished from those which have been modified by reason, something of the same kind can be observed. The mutual relation of protection and dependence produced by power and weakness is of this description. A helpless infant excites much stronger sympathy in the mother than a child that can shift for itself. Hence that partiality, accompanied by blindness to defects, which most parents entertain towards children whose natural deficiency, whether bodily or mental, throws them on their care long after the season of infancy.

> D.E. was seen at the age of 10. His parents described a wide variety of unmanageable behaviours giving the initial impression that D.E. was moderately severely mentally retarded. They described tantrums in public which would lead to him laying down in the street or sitting rocking on the footpath. He would easily become very angry. He would use these behaviours to obtain gifts and favours if the family were shopping, but once he had achieved his immediate aims he would produce further tantrums to make his parents take him home. His sleep/waking pattern was made chaotic

by similar manipulations. He was often up and about the house with them until 3 a.m. His parents were dismayed and upset by all this but they readily devoted themselves to meeting his whims.

He was one of four children of mother's previous liaison; no other child was problematic. But he suffered neonatal seizures and was in intensive care for 2 weeks. It is probable that nocturnal seizures and daytime absences started in early childhood but were not 'perceived' by his parents until schoolteachers drew their attention to the absences. Other children disliked D.E. and would avoid him. He currently had problems in dressing and managing his bowel movements. His eating was so messy the family allowed him to eat alone.

The family's formulation of him as a handicapped person was inaccurate and unhelpful, since it actually maintained many of his disagreeable behaviours. Work was done with the family to allow them to let him be admitted for observation to a child psychiatric unit. But they were averse to the process and soon found reasons to remove the child and severely criticize the treatment they had received. This allowed all family members to maintain their uncomfortable but fixed position.

It is not necessary for a child to be mentally retarded to produce high degrees of solicitude. Anxious attachment can be provoked in many ways and to various degrees. Green and Solnit (1964) described a 'vulnerable child syndrome' emerging out of a situation where a child survives what had been thought of as a mortal peril. This may be true for children with epilepsy not once but many times in early childhood. In essence the child's impending death is grieved but, as it does not actually occur, it leaves the child and parents in a psychologically anomalous situation.

Humans make heavy investment in rearing relatively few offspring. There are broadly two main strategies for sexual reproduction labelled *r* and *K* (MacArthur, 1962; Daly and Wilson, 1978). Whereas *r* strategists produce large numbers of young in such quantity that some will survive even if abandoned to their fate; *K* strategists produce few, care for them with great concern and usually form a pair-bond which provides an enduring monogamous relationship. Humans are nowadays extreme *K* strategists and, what is more, their developmentally immature young persist in a helpless state for a long time. This accentuates their devoted attachment and determination to succeed even at considerable self-sacrifice. The reduction in infant mortality and morbidity also increases *K* strategy since it increases the potential value of any given conceptus. All this without consideration of the effects of guilt on parents' reactions to the loss of the 'perfect child'. Thus the frustration or potential frustration of bringing any given conceptus to reproductive capacity is likely to involve very powerful feelings and energies. At times these can seem, superficially, to be misplaced; more often they can be seen as not necessarily serving the best interests of the child.

Paroxysmal displays

It is worth recognizing that seizures, as social events, and probably as biological events too, are one of a class of 'paroxysmal displays'. These include labour, orgasm, defaecation, micturition, vomiting, yawning, laughing, crying, rage, etc. (Ounsted, 1971). All these phenomena are regarded as socially proscribed because they are potentially aversive and are thus undertaken in private or under very controlled conditions or in conditions of intimacy. Biologically they are characterized by a period of forewarning or prodrome followed by a further urgent warning that the system (for example the bowel-voiding response) is about to go 'absolute', out of voluntary control to prevent it. The behaviour then supervenes (for example the irrepressible but inappropriate yawn), and this is followed by a feeling of relaxation during which the system is refractory.

The rage component of these paroxysmal behaviours has been singled out, in the so-called epileptic 'dyscontrol' syndrome, for special attention, and it has been regarded as a component of, or especially associated with, epileptic seizures. It is the modern analogue of the 'epileptic furor' which was often described in the old houses of confinement but seems now to be never reported. The evidence to associate epilepsy with crimes of rage and violence is lacking (Gunn, 1969) and derives largely anecdotally from sporadic association (Walker, 1961). Given the general level of aggressive crime, it will not be surprising that some of it is perpetrated by people with epilepsy. Aggression, especially in children, is usually verbal, disorganized and interactive (Taylor, 1969b; Ounsted, 1971) or derives from interference with the epileptic whilst he or she is in an obtunded state. It is perhaps indicative of the level of institutionalized prejudice that, quite recently under English law, a defence against violence committed in that condition was not accepted except as a plea of insanity (Fenwick and Fenwick, 1985).

Menace

Projective mechanisms allow the potential of people with epilepsy who threaten our capacity to cope in the event of their paroxysmal display, or of their death, or of their creating harm, to be viewed as a sense of menace emanating from them, usually undefined and unspoken, but experienced with a deep sense of unease. These mechanisms tend to provide extensive rationalization, and indeed to create conditions for self-fulfilling prophecy.

> E.F. was the son of ageing parents both previously married, their only child of their reconstituted family. He was socially precocious and assertive. His father was a policeman. In early childhood he suffered a severe and prolonged epileptic seizure following which occasional lapses of attention and arousal were noted. At school he was seen as an overactive, intrusive and 'potentially aggressive' child. Moving from school to school to attempt to

avoid these labels actually reinforced them. Despite careful inpatient assessment, and specialist medical and educational advice, the schoolteacher in his local school still refused to countenance him in normal school as she felt 'unable to be responsible for what he might do!'

True organic impairments

In DSM III (APA, 1980) under Organic Personality Syndrome are listed four characteristics: (i) emotional lability, temper outbursts, and sudden crying; (ii) impairment of impulse control; (iii) marked apathy and indifference; (iv) suspiciousness and paranoid ideation. These characteristics, to a greater or lesser degree, and in various permutations, actually provide for nearly all the so-called specific associations between epilepsy and behaviour such as the hyperkinetic syndrome (Kramer and Pollnow, 1932) or schizophrenia-like psychoses (Slater, Beard, and Glithero, 1963).

However, much the more important work comes from neuropsychology (Hermann, 1981, 1982; Flor-Henry, 1983). There are emerging numbers of deficits in higher-order skills which, though they are not limited or specific to children with epilepsy, do form an understandable basis of some of their real-world problems.

Problems in appreciating 'personal space' are among those which create social difficulties for children with epilepsy whose cerebral dysfunction seems to render them 'blind' to their intrusiveness.

F.G., at the age of 18, displayed a remarkable talent for pattern drawing which far outshone her other skills. Socially she was gauche and inept, and her emergent sexual feelings had on occasion been translated into rather direct approaches which embarrassed the recipients of her attentions but not her. Despite her several talents she was socially isolated and friendless among a group of young people with various special needs. She had marked obsessional ruminations and was preoccupied by inner voices; she had some rituals too.

Her epilepsy started with severe convulsions when aged 3, which led to a major regression in her language. Psychomotor seizures soon supervened, and persisted throughout her life. Her warm and caring parents treated her with great kindness and consideration. Her character at 18 showed many features of Asperger's syndrome (Wing, 1981). Though this is uncommon in girls it is more likely to be seen in girls who have clear-cut brain damage.

THE SOCIOLOGY OF EPILEPSY

The aspects of sickness which are the traditional preserve of physicians cover the mode of development of the sickness within the individual and the individual's reaction and interpretation of that process. Social and epidemiological medicine are usually servants of that concern, and rarely real extensions of it. But another aspect of sickness concerns the interaction between the individual, the illness, and society. Sickness has a social presentation, it is often through failure to maintain their social role that children are recognized as sick, and indeed, severity is often described in terms of the extent to which a sickness precludes a greater part of the expected role.

Schneider (1953) usefully listed the categories under which the relationship of sociological factors to mental health could be summarized. This framework will be used here as headings to summarize the special significance of social factors to epilepsy.

Failure to meet role demands

Role means the parts people play in an interaction. People play different roles in various situations, and it is socially useful to have this flexibility. Apart from a complex professional role with its various expectations, the reader will also play roles such as spouse, mourner, friend, child, and parent. In each of these it is necessary also to sustain some elements of 'self' (like an actor's 'self' or his style which is incorporated in his many parts) and to respect the roles of others.

Some roles are optional, others obligatory; some have great scope, others are ritualized and narrow, and require precise performance. Childhood also requires roles to be played and sustained. Parents have expectations of children, fantasies that they hope to see fulfilled, which sickness can destroy. They will be concerned if their child fails to understand how to be a friend, or a guest as opposed to a host, how to receive a gift, decline an offer. These are complex skills.

Being sick is usually a transient role, and in childhood occasional illness allows worthwhile regressions in the more delicious aspects of sickness, renewals of closeness to mother, and rehearsals for future nurturant roles. Chronic sickness is usually an unlooked-for role, and in epilepsy the seizure may thrust a child unexpectedly into a very public performance. The constant replaying of the sick role may tend towards 'being a sick person' becoming a dominant theme, or the only role that works satisfactorily. Thus if school cannot be sustained without declaring the sick role, then schooling too can become deviated from normal and 'special education' required, which both confirms 'differentness' and provides an alternative culture. Epilepsy will also preclude certain roles; only recently have quite widespread restrictions upon marriage and parenting been rescinded, and still driving and using certain machines are proscribed. Children are often prevented from becoming 'swimmers' or 'cyclists', which may further limit other social roles.

Society has a set of projections, expectations about persons in a role, and that implies loss of credibility as to how someone would actually perform in a given role. Thus when it comes to obtaining a driving license a person will cease to be a graduate, employer, parent, and becomes instead a person with epilepsy, a transcendant, stigmatized, role which invalidates the would-be driver.

Failure to meet the demands of a given role requires the adoption of another. This will lead to social mobility, which presents its own problems.

> G.H., a 15-year-old boy, the first of a sibship of four in a well-placed middle-class family, suffered persistent seizures, memory difficulties and created problems within the family by his insistence upon having things his way or else having a temper outburst. He suffered post-traumatic epilepsy from early childhood and showed facial asymmetry as one neurological residuum of that trauma.
>
> He was a boy with performance abilities in the very superior range, and verbal skills in the average range. This was consistent with his more limited skills in verbal explanation and social exchanges. But the real expectation of this boy was that he would succeed, through verbal skills and scholastic excellence, in the social circle his family moved in. He used massive denial to protect against the derision, pranks, jokes, and bullying to which he was subject by his peers. One device was to 'forget' or 'misunderstand' things which were unpleasant. This exaggerated his organic memory impairments. His basic high intelligence was unlikely to suffice to allow him to achieve the sort of role which the family would have expected, and these behavioural skirmishes were probably the first part of a negotiation of more limited expectations. They were also a summary of the general sense of guilt and dissatisfaction already experienced but currently largely denied.

Membership in an underprivileged group

An alternative to continual social mobility, or an eventual outcome of social mobility, will be membership in an underprivileged group. A banal but important underprivilege comes with the difficulty of finding babysitters for a child with epilepsy. It has been more difficult for people with epilepsy to obtain life or health insurance, people with epilepsy are over-represented among the mentally handicapped and the chronic sick, who also tend to occupy underprivileged parts of health care organizations. Hence certain health care facilities and individuals with epilepsy mutually stigmatize each other.

Taylor and Harrison (1976) showed a social polarization among people with epilepsy in their long-term follow-up as, more recently, have Ounsted and colleagues (1987). In the Isle of Wight study (Rutter, Graham, and Yule, 1970) the children of parents in non-manual occupations were under-represented among children with epilepsy with psychiatric disorder. Patients selected for temporal lobectomy for the relief of epilepsy (Taylor and Falconer, 1968) were shown to be skewed towards low social class before surgery. But patients who relied upon public service agencies for their referral, i.e. those separated from their parents for various reasons, were far less likely to be referred for treatment than those with their parents if they were heavily socially handicapped. Underprivilege thus tended to be self-perpetuating, with each loss tending to limit future chances of finding a way out of their predicament.

Current social policy in England and Wales leading to the relocation of mentally handicapped persons in long-stay hospitals into hostels in the community has led to a relative retention of patients with epilepsy on long-stay hospital wards.

Forced abrupt transition from one social situation to another

For most people social transitions are pre-planned and organized, and even then they count as 'life events'. A common and real 'transition' is the seizure itself, since the sufferers come to themselves in a different situation from that obtaining before the seizure, including at times removal to a hospital and separation from personal belongings and from a work schedule. But children may be serially passaged through a wide variety of locations in the name of 'diagnosis', 'treatment', 'management', 'surgery', and 'schooling'.

Although the eventual outcome was satisfactory the following case reveals a number of transitions in care and also failure to meet demands, and underprivileged group membership.

H.I.'s unmarried mother suffered pre-eclampsic toxaemia before his birth in August 1978. Birth weight was 6 lb 1 oz, and in the special care baby unit two seizures were described. After leaving the hospital his mother found him hard to feed, hard to manage, and very wakeful. As mother's relationship with him broke down, care was shared with his maternal grandmother. From the time he started to walk he was regarded as overactive, distractable, oppositional, and bad-tempered. In early childhood 'attacks' which were attributed to breath-holding were described. By 1985 mother reported to a neurologist that 'petit-mal' attacks had been occurring for the past year in association with a worsening behavioural problem. No abnormality was seen in his EEG. Social workers concerned about child abuse had given charge of him to his grandmother. Behavioural management by psychologists was attempted but failed. Psychiatric advice was sought.

In the presence of his mother he was wildly distractable, endlessly and dangerously restless, frantic, noisy, and disinhibited. These traits were reduced in her absence and he could be quieted. He showed high levels of anxiety. His attacks were clearly psychomotor in type, and there was an aura and mumbling of gibberish.

His EEGs showed a left temporal focus. His WISC scores were Verbal IQ=92, Performance IQ=85. He was left-handed. Scans revealed a deep lesion in the mesial aspects of the left temporal lobe. After several weeks of psychological preparation of mother and child this was removed in May 1986 without sequelae. It was an oligodendrioglioma. Rehabilitation was in the psychiatric unit for 3 weeks, when he was returned to the care of his mother. By September he and his mother sat quietly for an hour during a revisit to the unit; they seemed to be enjoying their relationship. He had no further seizures.

But since our follow-up is brief it is possible that this child might yet exceed the capacity of his mother to cope, and he will then experience a transition to a special facility for children with epilepsy as a boarder. In role terms it is like learning to play a part in a drama where the lines, the scenery and the other actors are constantly being changed.

Disorganization of the social system

Psychiatric disorder increases during periods of social disorganization and in areas prone to social disorganization. Underprivileged persons tend to aggregate in disorganized parts of the social system. In the series of children with temporal lobe epilepsy described by Ounsted *et al.* (1966) 27 per cent of the homes were regarded as 'disordered', which was rated when one or more of five features were noted: gross poverty, death of mother, grossly aggressive father, psychosis or severe neurosis in either parent. In the very long term this constellation of events did not prove to be an independent factor leading to poor outcome. The pathway of association of these sorts of phenomena are clearly complex, leaving out of consideration the concept of 'invulnerability' and the overriding nature of certain other physical criteria. Yet descriptively they point to a number of patients in complex disorganized situations. A recent study of depression in epilepsy by Mendez, Cummings, and Benson (1986) revealed, incidentally, the high levels of disorganization of persons with epilepsy and others using vocational services for the disabled in their Los Angeles study, though individuals with epilepsy were more prone to depressive phases under such stress.

Social disorganization increases the difficulty of finding and maintaining adequate health care.

I.J., then aged 11 years, arrived at outpatients having leapt out of the bedroom window 12 feet from the ground into the street. On the previous day he had burned down the family house. He paced around the room sniffing it like a dog. He was vacant-eyed and speechless. Status of minor epilepsy was diagnosed and his condition responded at once to i.v. diazepam, when he was admitted as an inpatient. It relapsed next day but no status could be detected in the EEG, though the record was markedly abnormal, showing widespread slow waves and focal spike activity. The episode was the most florid declaration of his emergent organic psychosis which might have been present for many months.

His parents were emigrants from another country of very different culture. They were alienated and unemployed. Their few belongings had been destroyed in the fire. They were first cousins. Their first child was stillborn, there were several miscarriages, but they had two healthy daughters whose social worth was scarcely considered in comparison with this only son. He was born by Caesarean section weighing 5 lb 15 oz, and his infancy and childhood were puncuated with evidence of his overactivity and dangerousness. He was in a special school. At the age of 10 he was severely injured in a road traffic accident, and epilepsy was noted publicly in hospital 5 weeks later, though it was unclear whether this was the first attack.

Language and culture combined to make an accurate history almost impossible. Expectations of the child were very high. Neither parent was able to manipulate the social system to their, or their child's, advantage and each step the child's disorder took increased their alienation, with deleterious effects on the child.

Inability to attain social acceptance

Rejection is the active term in the process of prejudice and stigmatization. The repercussions of stigmatization are concrete difficulties for sufferers, inability to maintain group membership, loss of opportunities to compete and to succeed in certain sports and at certain levels of education. The commonest device to avoid rejection is to avoid declaration of disability.

It is at work that the failure of the person with epilepsy to gain acceptance has its most serious consequences. In failing to gain employment the individual with epilepsy is not merely deprived of livelihood; he or she is deprived of all the symbolic value of work. The symbolic value covers social needs, the habit of work, and the sense of community which it gives; it covers psychological needs, such as a sense of fulfilment and self-realization; also responses to moral pressure, from the feeling of duty or the desire to serve others. A place in normal school serves similarly.

The chronically sick are relieved, by virtue of their illness, of some of the symbolic and economic inducements to work. Unemployment in epilepsy is thus a problem of two main types. Either the individual is willing to work but is deprived of the opportunity in any area compatible with his sense of values, or the person with epilepsy is unwilling to work because none of the symbolic aspects of work have very much significance for him or her. Economic factors seem rarely to be significant inducement for success, seizure frequency a rare cause of work failure.

J.K., a boy of 9, was referred for severe conduct disorder at home and at school. He was defiant, rude, foul-mouthed and oppositional. 'Absences' were described but these seemed descriptively more like episodes of 'dumb insolence' than true seizures. In the course of the interview, however, his father's epilepsy was declared. This man had experienced the sudden onset of sporadic grand mals 5 years before, in his 30s. His first seizure was in the street, and led to immediate hospitalization. A family history of epilepsy and mental handicap led to him being placed immediately on treatment. As a person with epilepsy in treatment he was regarded as unable to work. His wife, rather triumphantly, claimed the role of breadwinner, and he was relegated to be a baby-sitter for the boy whose conduct had now come into question. Father's medical treatment seemed to have been associated with severe side-effects from the start, which were noticed at the interview. They added to the stigma of his epilepsy, his loss of role as worker, provider, and proper father. The net loss to the family was substantial, the boy was stigmatized at school as his sick father's son, and at home his devalued father failed to parent him. By mimicking his father's epilepsy the boy sought one alternative role that might work while his awful behaviour drew attention to his and his family's distress.

Subjective or objective mobility in the class structure

Many sicknesses are unequally distributed throughout the class structure. Two theories contend to explain this: a theory of social genesis in which factors which are associated with lower social status, poverty, malnutrition, reduced health care, smoking, contribute to the genesis of the disorder, and a theory of social drift whereby people of reduced or limited function are unable to maintain or achieve privileged places in the social hierarchy. These theories have been regarded as crucial in the genesis of schizophrenia but through the 'life events' research they can also be seen to be germane to the life of people with epilepsy. Young people entering upon their working careers find a point of entry into a working life, if they find one at all, very different from that which their family might have expected. Not only seizures but cognitive and personality problems militate against success, and in the diligent begin immediately to produce job changes interspersed with unemployment.

K.L. was referred at the age of 14 for treatment of his habit of grossly abnormal and wild motor threshings, punchings, and shoutings, which were almost always nocturnal or during dozing episodes by day. They had a 'grossly hysterical' flavour and always wrecked any EEG being made synchronously. Even so he had had some genuine epilepsy since early childhood. His middle-class parents were over-neat, meticulous, tense. Their sexual lives had ceased soon after the boy's birth. Family factors were regarded as contributing to the distress.

Initial examination of the boy revealed his learning problems but also exposed his clumsiness, his outspoken soft neurological signs. Over the years until school-leaving, supportive therapy as well as continuing drug treatment allowed many epochs of several months without nocturnal events. As soon as the question of work arose there was an upsurge of these, which proved to be frontal seizures with retained partial awareness, terror, and fighting movements. Despite excellent middle-class socialization his real skills were extremely poor, his evaluation of social nuance very low and his motor ineptitude a serious handicap. Several spells in various epilepsy treatment facilities were needed, and much support. Eventually he settled somewhat whilst training as a gardener.

L.M. suffered psychomotor epilepsy mainly of right temporal origin, but often bilateral abnormalities were seen in the EEG. She was not a favoured subject for surgical treatment. Though of excellent appearance and general intelligence, she disconcerted people socially by entering too closely into their personal space and claiming a whispered pseudo-intimacy in which she would share her vaguely formulated paranoid interpretation of the world. If asked her views she would make very accurate but socially inappropriate observations with considerable vehemence. She was an adopted child and throughout her rearing she had clearly mystified her adoptive parents for whom she had little respect.

She worked well and kept largely seizure-free in her jobs. But as soon as her sporadic epilepsy gave rise to a chance to discharge her she lost her job, not just because of her non-declaration of her illness, or the 'danger to other people' but because her interpersonal relationships had been marked more by her acerbic accuracy than the warmth that might have saved her job.

Several work failures led to rootlessness, a return to the unsatisfactory adoptive home and thence to epilepsy centres in search of surgery and a once for all cure.

Incompatible values

Marked differences between expectation and achievement exist in several areas of life for the parents of children with epilepsy, and for their chlidren. The parents have expectations about their child, even before it is born, that the child will be healthy and not sick, be at least as clever as they, and maintain their standards. Parents cleave to these beliefs even in the face of overwhelming information that they cannot be sustained. It is probably appropriate that they should. It is necessary to sustain hope, since abandoning a child who is sick will itself have deleterious consequences. However, it will produce belief systems, like the 'hyperpaedophilia' discussed above, which can militate against the child's best interests eventually. Sustaining these extreme beliefs in the face of contrary evidence is exhausting to parents who seem to have to commit themselves so heavily to those beliefs.

M.N. was just 12 years old when she became ill for the first time. She came of a happy normal healthy family. On a caravan holiday she became listless and suffered severe headaches. Influenza was diagnosed but she became progressively less able to move at all, and suffered her first major convulsion whilst being encouraged to eat. Series of convulsions followed and encephalitis was the diagnosis made but no vital evidence of that was adduced. In the course of a long illness punctuated by severe seizures she regressed to infantile levels. Over the next few years marked developmental recovery was made but epileptic fits persisted. These provide inadequate warning for protective action and injuries are common.

Now aged 15, M.N. can see that her former peers are in classes 3 years beyond the one she is in, and even then she performs comparatively poorly. Her young classmates shun her whenever pairing for activities is required. She can see herself 'adrift', distanced from her year group, unacceptable to her classmates. Similar circumstances obtain in her family. They might have expected her death or profound handicap, but they are curiously placed having to live with a girl whose identity is spoiled but who is well enough for them to be 'grateful'. The family place overwhelming faith in stopping her seizures (which has proved impossible), as this will constitute their idea of a good outcome.

In essence the spoiled child is incompatible with their image of the child she was to have been. The child is also incompatibly placed, by her years of illness, in her developmental schedule. She has several years of her adolescent psychosexual development to make up despite her chronological age, indicating that much work has to be done.

Social isolation

Harré (1979) provided a broad social psychological perspective on the construction of 'social being'. Social behaviour requires cognitive and interpersonal skills of a high order to negotiate social encounters. Without these skills the individual will be categorized and stigmatized and accorded some social recognition, but only as a devalued person; in one sense they are admitted to society, but the dues are heavy. Some people cannot sustain even these engagements, cannot psychologically afford the dues, or react intransigently to their situation; such persons are socially isolated, and without active and forceful habilitation they remain seriously handicapped.

N.O. was aged 16 when he was seen on a consulting visit to a facility for children with epilepsy. He had been there for about a year when one night he rose at 2 a.m. and started to demolish the furnishings in the villa in which he lived. He was found to be hallucinating and, though largely incoherent, he expressed paranoid ideation. The episode settled with antipsychotic drugs. The consultation was a follow-up.

It emerged that he was isolated from his family and had been separated from them in three different treatment centres for the past 8 years. His natural mother had died. He had really no attachments to the outside world and had no long-term affiliations in the institution. This was true anomie, and although his psychotic episode was unarguably a real change in the dynamics of his cerebration it was possible to see it, in social and psychological terms, as being not so different from his usual state in the world, bereft, lost, adrift, lonely and isolated.

It was important and interesting that the excellent and caring establishment he was in, and the helpful and caring public service who had arranged for him to be there, were unaware that this boy had lost his life history, that he existed in a state of anomic and that, in a sense, the sort of care he had been receiving had contributed to that. The very best sorts of care for the handicapped retain an awareness of the potential social isolation and work hard against it, but in actual practice abandonment is hard to counter.

CONCLUSION

The psychosocial issues surrounding childhood epilepsy are under-researched and deserving of much more attention. One of the finest textbooks on children's epilepsy scarcely refers to the huge consequences in psychosocial terms of these potentially tragic, chronic diseases (Aicardi, 1986). The lack of research has to do with the motivation for research and the styles of research which are likely to gain funding. The motivation for much of the research seems to relate either to achieving a categorization or else attempting to destigmatize children who have been so categorized. There is actually no need to argue about causation or to attribute variance. There is no need to assume that there are 'general rules' which operate under so vast a rubric as epilepsy. It is necessary to break down that category into small, accurate, worthwhile, biomedical fragments if any meaningful psychosocial predictions are to be made. And it is necessary to understand that psychosocial prediction and understanding is very highly contingent upon a very diverse set of data, so that the predicament of one person will be radically different from another, although they share many of the measured characteristics. The styles of research which gain funding are those which test robust hypotheses rather than those which, in a more preliminary way, simply begin to order our experience of the world. This phase is still necessary for childhood epilepsy.

An attempt has been made in this chapter to refer to some of the nuances and to relate them using biographical vignettes. These biographies contain data about childhood epilepsy which are extremely difficult to synthesize into a probabilistic or epidemiological science. It is seen as one of the weaknesses of social science that it fails to generate robust hypotheses. Yet it can be said, and it is argued in this chapter, that childhood epilepsy is a category, and entering into that category opens up a set of contingencies which would either not exist at all, or would otherwise exist at much lower levels of liability. It is possible to *understand* the psychosocial risks to the child with epilepsy in the Jasperian sense, from having had or having read appropriate experiences of it, without necessarily being able to be mathematically precise about the levels of risk involved.

In essence the message of this chapter is that, although the seizure mechanism might be triggered in brains which are otherwise unimpaired, it is more likely that persistent recurrent (i.e. chronic) epilepsy will be associated with impairment. This impairment may not produce significant psychosocial disadvantage but the category 'epileptic' is one which generally carries a good deal of opprobrium and generates much anxiety among other people. The negative outcomes of diseases associated with epilepsy occur sufficiently often to produce intermittent (i.e. powerful) reinforcement, of its negative image. Several of the origins, psychological as well as social, of these negative images are described in this chapter. People hoping to help children with epilepsy need to be aware of the wide variety of potential negative outcomes, which affect very many different aspects of life and which are highly contingent, if they are to be successful in their interventions. They need, in particular, to remember that they form part of the social structure which has these negative images; and that they are among the humans who have such a lot of trouble in tolerating seizures.

REFERENCES

Aicardi, J. (1986). *Epilepsy in Children*, Raven Press, New York.

American Psychiatric Association (1980). *Quick Reference to the Diagnostic Criteria from Diagnostic and Statistical Manual of Mental Disordrs*, 3rd edn, APA, Washington, DC.

Baumer, J.H., David, T.J., Valentine, S.J., Roberts, J.E., and Hughes, B.R. (1981). Many parents think their child is dying when having a first febrile convulsion. *Developmental Medicine and Child Neurology*, **23**, 462–464.

Daly, M., and Wilson, M. (1978). *Sex, Evolution and Behaviour*, Duxbury Press, Massachusetts.

Fenwick, P., and Fenwick, E. (1985). *Epilepsy and the Law*, Royal Society of Medicine, London.

Ferguson, S.M., and Rayport, M. (1965). The adjustment to living without epilepsy. *Journal of Nervous and Mental Disease*, **140**, 26–37.

Flor-Henry, P. (1983). *Cerebral Basis of Psychopathology*, John Wright, London.

Goffman, E. (1963). *Stigma: Notes on the Management of Spoiled Identity*, Prentice Hall, Englewood Cliffs, NJ.

Green, M., and Solnit, A.J. (1964). Reactions to the threatened loss of a child: a vulnerable child syndrome. *Pediatrics*, **34**, 58–66.

Gunn, J.C. (1969). The prevalence of epilepsy among prisoners. *Proceedings of the Royal Society of Medicine*, **62**, 60–63.

Hackney, A., and Taylor, D.C. (1976). A teacher's questionnaire description of epileptic children. *Epilepsia*, **17**, 275–281.
Harré, R. (1979). *Social Being*, Basil Blackwell, Oxford.
Hermann, B.P. (1981). Deficits in neuropsychological functioning and psychopathology in patients with epilepsy: a rejected hypothesis revisited. *Epilepsia*, **22**, 161–168.
Hermann, B.P. (1982). Neuropsychological functioning and psychopathology in children with epilepsy. *Epilepsia*, **23**, 545–554.
Jaspers, K. (1962). *General Psychopathology*, translated by J. Hoenig and M.W. Hamilton, Manchester University Press, Manchester.
Kramer, F., and Pollnow, H. (1932). Uber eine hyperkinetische Erkranktung im Kindesalter. *Monatsschrift fur Psychiatrie und Neurologie*, Berlin.
Lockyer, D. (1981). *Symptoms and Illness: The Cognitive Organization of Disorder*, Tavistock Publications, London.
MacArthur, R.H. (1962). Some generalised theorems of natural selection. *Proceedings of the National Academy of Sciences*, **48**, 1893–1897.
Mendez, M.F., Cummings, J.L., and Benson, D.F. (1986). Depression in epilepsy. *Archives of Neurology*, **43**, 766–770.
Ounsted, C. (1955). The hyperkinetic syndrome in epileptic children. *Lancet*, **ii**, 303–311.
Ounsted, C. (1971). Some aspects of seizure disorders. In D. Gairdner and D. Hull (eds), *Recent Advances in Paediatrics*, 4th edn, J. & A. Churchill, London.
Ounsted, C., Lindsay, J., and Norman, R. (1966). *Biological Factors in Temporal Lobe Epilepsy*, Spastics Society Medical Education and Information Unit/Heinemann Medical Books, London.
Ounsted, C., Lindsay, J., and Richards, P. (1987). *Temporal Lobe Epilepsy 1948–1986: A Biographical Study*, MacKeith Press, London.
Rutter, M., Graham, P., and Yule, W. (1970). *A Neuropsychiatric Study in Childhood*, SIMP/Heinemann, London.
Schneider, E.V. (1953). Sociological concepts and psychiatric research. In: *Interrelations between the Social Environment and Psychiatric Disorders*. Millbank Memorial Fund, New York.
Slater, E., Beard, A.W., and Glithero, E. (1963). The schizophrenia-like psychoses of epilepsy. *British Journal of Psychiatry*, **109**, 95–150.
Taylor, D.C. (1969a). Some psychiatric aspects of epilepsy. In R.N. Harrington (ed.), *Current Problems in Neuropsychiatry*, Headley Brothers, Ashford.
Taylor, D.C. (1969b). Aggression and epilepsy. *Journal of Psychomatic Research*, **13**, 229–236.
Taylor, D.C. (1971). Psychiatry and sociology in the understanding of epilepsy. In M.G. Gelder and B.M. Mandelbrote (eds), *Psychiatric Aspects of Medical Practice*, Staples, London.
Taylor, D.C. (1972). Mental state and temporal lobe epilepsy: A correlative account of 100 patients treated surgically. *Epilepsia*, **13**, 727–765.
Taylor, D.C. (1973). Aspects of seizure disorders: II. On prejudice. *Developmental Medicine and Child Neurology*, **15**, 91–94.
Taylor, D.C. (1979). The components of sickness: diseases, illnesses and predicaments. *Lancet*, **ii**, 1008–1010.
Taylor, D.C. (1982). Epilepsy: a model of sickness. In M. Sandler (ed.), *Psychopharmacology of anticonvulsants*, Oxford University Press, Oxford.
Taylor, D.C. (1982). The components of sickness: diseases, illnesses and predicaments. In J. Apley and C. Ounsted (eds), *One Child*, Spastics International Medical Publications, London.

Taylor, D.C. (1985). Psychological aspects of chronic sickness. In M. Rutter and L. Hersov (eds), *Child and Adolescent Psychiatry—Modern Approaches*, 2nd edn, Blackwell Scientific Publications, Oxford.

Taylor, D.C. (1987). Epilepsy and prejudice. *Archives of Disease in Childhood*, **62**, 209–211.

Taylor, D.C., and Falconer, M.A. (1968). Clinical, socio-economic, and psychological changes after temporal lobectomy for epilepsy. *British Journal of Psychiatry*, **114**, 1247–1261.

Taylor, D.C., and Harrison, R. (1976). Childhood seizures: a 25-year follow up. *Lancet*, **i**, 948–951.

Walker, A.E. (1961). Murder or epilepsy? *Journal of Nervous and Mental Disease*, **133**, 430–437.

Wing, L. (1981). Asperger's syndrome: a clinical account. *Psychological Medicine*, **11**, 115–129.

Chapter 9

Correlates of Behavior Problems and Social Competence in Children with Epilepsy, Aged 6–11

Bruce P. Hermann, Steven Whitman and Jade Dell

Much has been written concerning the incidence and nature of behavioral pathology and personality change in individuals with epilepsy. While the bulk of the literature and the ensuing controversy concerns adults with epilepsy, a growing amount of work has inquired into behavioral problems of children and adolescents with epilepsy. We will very briefly review some of the existing literature and highlight several methodological difficulties and conceptual issues inherent in this field of research. This discussion and review will set the stage for the remainder of the chapter, in which we will present a conceptual model for understanding the determinants of psychopathology in children with epilepsy, and subsequently test the model's utility in an empirical investigation of children (aged 6–11) with epilepsy.

REVIEW OF PREVIOUS RESEARCH

Considerable evidence indicates that behavioral problems are overrepresented in children with epilepsy relative both to healthy controls and children with other chronic disorders. For instance, in the Isle of Wight study, Rutter, Graham, and Yule (1970) reported that 29 percent of the 63 children with uncomplicated epilepsy manifested a psychiatric disorder relative to 12 percent of the 138 children with chronic but non-neurological disorders. Mellor, Lowit, and Hall (1974) reported that 27 percent of 308 children (aged 5–13) with epilepsy manifested a behavior disorder relative to 15 percent of healthy controls. Such general data are certainly helpful in pointing out the increased psychiatric risk associated with childhood epilepsy, but more clinically relevant information might involve the identification of specific social and biological variables which predispose the child with epilepsy to significant behavioral dysfunction.

Childhood Epilepsies: Neuropsychological, Psychosocial and Intervention Aspects
Edited by B. Hermann and M. Seidenberg

Several investigations have attempted to elucidate factors associated with an increased risk of behavioral pathology in children with epilepsy, and some representative studies will be reviewed here. Holdsworth and Whitmore (1974), in an investigation of 85 children with epilepsy attending ordinary schools, employed medical information derived from school personnel and school health service files. They reported that 18 children (21 percent) presented with noticeably deviant behavior. They found that disturbed behavior was significantly associated with frequent seizures during the previous 12 months, educational retardation and the absence of phenobarbital as the anticonvulsant medication. Stores (1978, 1980) investigated behavioral functioning in four groups of children with epilepsy, identified through the EEG Department of The Park Hospital for Children, Oxford, and classified according to EEG criteria: a 3/s spike and wave group (N=17); an irregular spike and wave group (N=17); a right temporal lobe spike group (N=16); and a left temporal lobe spike group (N=20). Boys with epilepsy, in particular those with an epileptogenic focus in the left temporal lobe, were reported to be at increased risk for behavioral pathology. Ounsted (1969) reported on a consecutive series of 100 children with temporal lobe epilepsy (TLE) obtained through family physicians, health visitors, and the paediatric departments of Oxford, Northampton, and Swindon. Seizure type was classified by employing both clinical and EEG criteria. It was noted that the age of onset of seizures, the presence of a 'disordered home', and aetiological factors such as neurological insult by trauma or direct infection, were associated with rage outbursts.

The potential adverse effects of some anticonvulsant medications, particularly the barbituates, on behavioral adjustment in general and depression in particular, are now being identified with greater precision (e.g. Brent, Crumrine, and Varma, 1987; Ferrari, Barabas, and Matthews, 1983). Additionally, the more general behavioral and cognitive side-effects of polytherapy are the subject of increasing scrutiny (Cull and Trimble, Chapter 6 in this volume).

It is relevant to note that, in the adult literature, a significant controversy surrounds the issue of whether or not the presence of TLE predisposes to significant psychopathology. Some argue that TLE predisposes to psychosis, pathological aggression, sexual dysfunction, and/or a variety of personality characteristics (Blumer, 1975; Bear and Fedio, 1977; Waxman and Geschwind, 1975). Other studies have failed to demonstrate increased psychopathology in adults with TLE (Standage and Fenton, 1975; Matthews and Klove, 1968; Hermann and Whitman, 1984; Rodin and Schmaltz, 1984; Mungus, 1982).

In the paediatric literature, few comparisons between children with TLE or psychomotor seizures relative to those with other seizure types—for example, primary generalized epilepsy (GE), have been reported. In a retrospective review of available case material from the Maudsley Hospital, Nuffield (1961) reported that children with 3/s spike and wave activity were characteristically shy, retiring or neurotic, in contrast to those with temporal lobe spike discharges, who were aggressive or antisocial in other ways. No distinctions were made in his study for laterality of lesion or gender. Rutter *et al.* (1970), in the epidemiological Isle of Wight study, reported that children with clinically diagnosed psychomotor seizures were more likely to manifest behavioral pathology. Their sample of such children was, however, extremely small ($N=8$). Similarly, Hoare (1984) found increased psychopathology among children with complex partial seizures. Finally, other investigations (e.g. Whitman, Hermann, Black, and Chhabria, 1982) have failed to find seizure-type effects on standardized measures of psychopathology in children with epilepsy.

Studies investigating the relationship between epilepsy and psychopathology are very difficult to conduct in a methodologically and conceptually sound manner because of the large number of potentially confounding variables. For example, possible relevant considerations in epilepsy/psychopathology investigations include subject variables (e.g. age, gender, education, IQ); seizure-related variables (e.g. age at onset, duration of disorder, seizure control); EEG variables (e.g. frequency and topographical distribution of epileptiform activity, presence/absence of other wave forms such as diffuse or focal slow waves, adequacy of the EEG investigations); societal considerations (e.g. reactions of others to the individual's seizure disorder, job discrimination); and treatment variables (e.g. number of medications, type and dosage of various anticonvulsants), as well as a host of other possible sources of variance. The control of all these variables would be a large-scale and difficult undertaking, but failure to control for any, or for only a small number of, variables, leaving the others uncontrolled/unaccounted for, invites spurious findings and doubtless contributes to the many conflicting and contradictory reports in the literature.

The purpose of the investigation to follow is an attempt to identify the multietiological correlates/determinants of psychopathology and social competence in a sample of children aged 6–11 with epilepsy. This task is undertaken in the context of a broad model of psychopathology in epilepsy, using statistical procedures designed to identify the most robust predictors of problem behavior and social difficulties in order to begin to set the stage for prevention efforts.

This chapter will proceed as follows. First, we will briefly present a model which we have been utilizing to study psychopathology in adults with epilepsy. We believe that this model also has applicability to children with epilepsy. Second, we will present the results of an investigation which utilized this model in the search for the high-risk variables associated with the presence of behavioral and social problems in children (aged 6–11) with epilepsy. Finally, we will review the implications of our findings for clinical practice, theoretical research, and efforts aimed at the prevention of behavioral problems and social difficulties in children with epilepsy.

A MULTIETIOLOGICAL MODEL OF PSYCHOPATHOLOGY IN EPILEPSY

We have recently suggested that it might be helpful to develop a model of psychopathology in epilepsy which would simultaneously consider many potential etiological factors (Hermann and Whitman, 1986). Such a model might facilitate empirical investigations which would help to resolve many of the existing controversies and, additionally, facilitate the development of treatment interventions.

Building upon the work and writings of previous investigators, it has been suggested that there are four general forces, or hypotheses, which represent potential etiologies of psychopathology in epilepsy. These broad factors include biological, psychosocial, medication, and demographic factors. Many, if not all, of the specific variables which are known or suspected to be of etiological importance can be subsumed under one of these four guiding hypotheses (see Table 9.1).

The biological hypothesis encompasses those variables thought to be related to the cause, or outcome of the individual's epilepsy, and includes factors such as seizure type, etiology, and duration of epilepsy. The psychosocial hypothesis generally concerns those factors thought to be related to the stress and tension associated with living with the disorder, the widely discussed stigma and discrimination, as well as other factors such as social support and adjustment to epilepsy. The medication hypothesis reflects the perspective that while anti-epilepsy drugs have a positive effect on seizure frequency, *some* medications may predispose *some* individuals to specific behavioral problems. Finally, the demographic hypothesis reflects the fact that there is a well-known contribution of several demographic factors (e.g. age, education, sex) to a variety of psychopathologies.

It is interesting to note that although several of the specific variables included in these four hypotheses have been examined as risk factors for psychopathology in epilepsy, there are very few investigations in which variables from more than one hypothesis have been allowed to 'compete' with each other in data-based investigations in order to determine their relative explanatory power.

Table 9.1 is not meant to be exhaustive; rather, it is meant to be illustrative. The use of such a conceptual grouping of specific risk factors and hypotheses may have several benefits. First, it may facilitate empirical investigations inquiring into the overall relative explanatory power of the biological versus psychosocial hypotheses. Second, within each hypothesis it may be possible to generate an ordering of the variables in terms of their statistical explanatory value in relation to specific behavioral problems. Third, there is known intercorrelation among several of the variables within each of the four hypotheses, and the use of multivariate statistical techniques should allow the identification of *independent* risk factors in relation to specific psychopathologies.

Table 9.1
Potential etiological factors grouped according to specific hypotheses

Biological	Psychosocial	Medication	Demographic
Seizure type	Locus of control	Polytherapy	Age
Etiology	Stigma	Medication type	Sex
Duration of epilepsy	Discrimination	AED levels	Education
Number of seizure types	Social exclusion		
EEG characteristics	Family environment		
Related neuropsychological deficits	Negative life events		
Number of episodes of status epilepticus	Social support		
Age at onset of epilepsy	Fear of seizures		

The investigation to follow has selected factors from each of the four hypotheses shown in Table 9.1, and will examine their comparative explanatory value when attempting to identify independent risk factors for psychopathology and social difficulties among children with epilepsy.

METHOD

Subjects

Children between the ages of 6 and 11 years referred to the Pediatric Neurology Section of the Department of Neurology at the University of Illinois Medical Center composed the subject pool. This tertiary-level clinic provides diagnostic and treatment services to children and adolescents with poorly controlled seizures, and children with known or suspected epilepsy with significant emotional, educational, or social problems. Children excluded from the regular school system because of mental handicap (i.e. placed in educationally mentally handicapped or trainable mentally handicapped settings) were excluded from consideration for this investigation. However, children attending alternative schools because of behavioral dysfunction were included in the subject pool, as were children who attended special learning-disorder classes as part of their regular educational programming. The final sample consisted of 44 boys and 57 girls aged 6–11 (Table 9.2). Details concerning the children are provided below.

Table 9.2
Sample characteristics (boys and girls, age 6–11)

Characteristics	Boys (n = 44)		Girls (n = 57)	
	No.	%	No.	%
Parental marital status				
Married	24	55	26	46
Other	20	45	31	54
Seizure type				
Partial	22	50	20	35
Generalized	19	43	33	58
Mixed	3	7	4	7
Number of different seizure types				
1	31	71	34	59
2	7	16	16	28
3	5	11	6	11
4	1	2	1	2
Etiology				
Idiopathic	32	73	34	60
Symptomatic	9	20	8	14
Unknown	3	7	15	26
Seizure control				
Good	17	39	22	39
Fair	15	34	11	19
Poor	12	27	24	42
Medications				
None	7	16	10	18
Monotherapy	25	57	30	52
Polytherapy	12	27	17	30
Average age (years)	9.4		9.0	
Average age at onset (years)	5.4		5.0	
Average duration (years)	4.0		4.0	
Average median family income	$17,424		$17,361	

Procedure

The behavioral and emotional status of each child was assessed through an interview with the child's parents using a standardized behavioral assessment inventory, the Child Behavior Checklist, a widely used inventory of high reliability and validity (Achenbach and Edelbrock, 1983). The interviewer was blind to the child's neurologic status in general, his/her seizure type in particular, and the EEG results.

Each child received an evaluation by a pediatric neurologist who was blind to the results of the psychological data. As part of the neurological evaluation each child underwent an EEG. Electrodes were applied according to the 10–20 international system of electrode placement, and records were run on a

Table 9.3
Method for determining seizure control

Seizure severity defined	
Severe:	Generalized tonic–clonic (including partial evolving into generalized tonic–clonic)
Moderate:	Complex partial seizures; generalized tonic only; generalized clonic only
Mild:	Simple partial seizures; generalized absence; myoclonic; atonic
Seizure control defined	
Good:	0–1 severe seizures/year 0–5 moderate seizures/year 0–2 mild seizures/year
Fair:	2–12 severe seizures/year 0.5–4 moderate seizures/month 2–60 mild seizures/month
Poor:	more than 1 severe seizure/month more than 4 moderate seizures/month more than 2 mild seizures/day

10-channel EEG machine. The standard 22 electrodes were used with many different referential and bipolar montages during wakefulness, hyperventilation, photic stimulation, and sleep. All EEGs were read and interpreted by the Director of the EEG Laboratories, who was blind to results of the psychological data.

For the purposes of this investigation six biological variables (age of onset, duration of disorder, seizure type, number of seizure types, seizure control, etiology), two psychosocial variables (parental marital state, family income), one medication variable (monotherapy/polytherapy) and one demographic variable (age) were evaluated as potential risk factors for psychopathology in epilepsy. The special coding system for the seizure control variable is presented in Table 9.3. The other variables were coded in the manner described in detail by Hermann *et al.* (1988). Table 9.2 provides information concerning the distribution of the biological, psychosocial, and medication variables for the sample of boys and girls. These variables were selected for investigation because they are among the pool of factors identified or suspected to be precursors of psychopathology in epilepsy.

Behavioral measures

The social competence and behavioral functioning of each child was assessed by means of an interview with the child's mother or guardian, using the Child Behavior Checklist (CBCL) (Achenbach and Edelbrock, 1983). This behavioral assessment inventory was designed to record, in a standardized format, the behavioral problems and social competence of children aged 6–16

Table 9.4
CBCL Behavior problem scales (narrow-band factor scores) for children age 6–11

Boys	Girls
Depressed	Depressed
Social withdrawal	Social withdrawal
Somatic complaints	Somatic complaints
Hyperactive	Hyperactive
Delinquent	Delinquent
Aggressive	Aggressive
Schizoid	Schizoid–obsessive
Uncommunicative	Sex problems
Obsessive compulsive	Cruel

years. The CBCL consists of 20 social competence and 118 behavior problem items.

Factor analysis of the CBCL items has resulted in the derivation of both broad-band (externalizing versus internalizing psychopathologies) and narrow-band (e.g. aggression, hyperactivity, depression) behavior problem scales, as well as three social competence scales, all of which have been demonstrated to be of significant discriminatory value. Scores for these behavioral problem and social competence scales are converted to standardized age- and sex-corrected T scores. Extensive information concerning the reliability and validity of the CBCL is documented in the test manual and summarized in previous reports from our group (Achenbach and Edelbrock, 1981, 1983; Whitman *et al.*, 1982; Hermann *et al.*, 1988).

For the purposes of this investigation the narrow-band factor scores for boys and girls aged 6–11 were utilized as the dependent measures. Table 9.4 shows the behavioral problem scales which were utilized for each gender. Because the narrow-band factor structure differs for boys and girls, the gender groups were evaluated separately. Additionally, the three social competence scales (Activities, Social, School) were utilized to assess specific areas of social competence for both boys and girls.

In previous investigations of our sample we have inquired into broad-band factors (Internalizing, Externalizing), or overall summary measures (Total Behavior Problems, Total Social Competence). Because of variations in narrow-band factor scores as a function of chronological age and gender, a large overall sample is needed. This report therefore reflects our first investigation of narrow-band factor scores in our sample of children with epilepsy.

Data analyses

Stepwise multiple regression analyses were computed for each dependent measure (i.e. each narrow-band factor score) using the 10 independent variables that are presented in Table 9.2. This was done independently for boys and girls. The assumptions underlying regression analysis (homogeneity of variance, independence, and normalcy of error variance) were verified both graphically and statistically. In no case was a transformation of the data necessary. For these analyses only variables which reached conventional levels of statistical significance ($p < 0.05$) were taken to indicate a significant result.

RESULTS

Boys

Table 9.5 provides a listing of the specific behavior problem and social competence scales, the variables which were found to be significant independent predictors for each scale, p-values for the significant predictor variables, and the overall multiple R (and R^2) values for the regression analyses.

As can be seen in Table 9.5, the results indicate that seizure control and parental marital status were the most frequent significant predictor variables. Most of the behavioral problems were associated with inadequate seizure control (i.e. fair to poor seizure control), and divorced/separated parents. The use of polytherapy was associated with poorer scores on the Social Withdrawal, Hyperactivity, and School Achievement scales. In only one instance was seizure type a significant predictor, with fewer somatic complaints associated with partial seizures. Multiple R values ranged from 0.31 to 0.64, accounting for 10–41 percent of the variance in the behavior problem/social competence scales.

Girls

Table 9.6 provides the results for the girls. Again, inadequate seizure control (fair/poor) and disrupted marital status (divorced/separated parents) were the most frequent predictors of problem behaviors. Lower median family income was associated with two behavior problems (Sex Problems, Schizoid-Obsessive), and lower median family income was associated with worse scores on one social competence scale (Social).

The use of polytherapy was associated with worse scores on the Hyperactivity and Activities scales. Earlier age at onset of epilepsy was associated with worse scores on the Cruel and Activities scales. A longer duration of epilepsy was associated with worse scores on the School Achievement scale. Finally, poor scores on the Activities scale were significantly correlated with epilepsy of symptomatic etiology, and partial/mixed seizure types.

Table 9.5
Results of regression analyses for boys, age 6–11

Dependent variable	Significant predictors[1]	*p*-value	*R*	R^2
Depressed	Inadequate seizure control	0.005	0.51	0.26
	Divorced/separated parents	0.01		
Social withdrawal	Polytherapy	0.005	0.51	0.26
	Divorced/separated parents	0.04		
Somatic complaints	Generalized/mixed seizure types	<0.001	0.64	0.41
	Divorced/separated parents	0.003		
	Inadequate seizure control	0.009		
Hyperactive	Polytherapy	0.001	0.47	0.22
Delinquent	Inadequate seizure control	0.02	0.35	0.12
Aggressive	Inadequate seizure control	0.01	0.39	0.14
Schizoid	Divorced/separated parents	<0.001	0.58	0.34
	Inadequate seizure control	0.02		
Uncom-municative	Inadequate seizure control	<0.001	0.58	0.34
	Divorced/separated parents	0.01		
Obsessive–compulsive	Inadequate seizure control	<0.001	0.61	0.38
	Divorced/separated parents	0.006		
School	Polytherapy	0.04	0.31	0.10
Activities	No significant predictors			
Social	No significant predictors			

[1] Variables listed are predictive of higher (worse) behavior problem scores and lower (worse) social competence scores. Social competence scales are: School, Activities, and Social.

Boys and girls combined

Table 9.7 provides a summary of the 37 instances where significant predictors of behavior problem/social competence scale scores were obtained. This table collapses the findings across all scales, and is arranged in order of most predictive to least predictive. As can be seen, seizure control, parental marital status, and polytherapy/monotherapy were the most common significant predictor variables.

Table 9.8 provides a summary of the frequency of significant variables across gender, and all behavior problem/social competence scales arranged according to the model described earlier. As shown in that table, the biological hypothesis was most predictive, the psychosocial hypothesis second, and medication third. No demographic variable was a significant predictor of any behavioral problem or social competence scale.

Table 9.6
Results of regression analyses for girls, age 6–11

Dependent variable	Significant predictors[1]	*p*-value	*R*	R^2
Depressed	Inadequate seizure control	0.005	0.43	0.18
	Divorced/separated parents	0.005		
Social withdrawal	Inadequate seizure control	0.008	0.35	0.12
Somatic complaints	No significant predictors			
Hyperactive	Inadequate seizure control	<0.001	0.47	0.22
	Polytherapy	0.04		
Delinquent	Monotherapy	0.04	0.27	0.07
Aggressive	Inadequate seizure control	<0.001	0.48	0.23
	Divorced/separated parents	0.03		
Schizoid–obsessive	Inadequate seizure control	0.01	0.46	0.21
	Lower family income	0.02		
Sex problems	Lower family income	0.001	0.42	0.18
Cruel	Earlier age at onset	0.004	0.46	0.21
	Divorced/separated parents	0.02		
School	Longer duration of epilepsy	0.005	0.37	0.14
Activities	Inadequate seizure control	<0.001	0.75	0.56
	Symptomatic etiology	<0.001		
	Partial/mixed epilepsy	0.002		
	Polytherapy	0.006		
	Earlier age at onset	0.04		
Social	Lower family income	0.04	0.37	0.14

[1] Variables listed are predictive of higher (worse) behavior problem scores and lower (worse) social competence scores.

Table 9.7
Summary of significant predictors of behavior problems and social competence in children with epilepsy, aged 6–11

Significant predictors	Boys	Girls	Total
Seizure control	7	6	13
Parents' marital status	6	3	9
Polytherapy/monotherapy	3	3	6
Family income	0	3	3
Seizure type	1	1	2
Age at onset	0	2	2
Etiology	0	1	1
Duration of epilepsy	0	1	1
			37

Table 9.8
Frequency of significant predictor variables grouped according to etiological category

Etiological category	Number of significant predictors	Specific predictors
Biological	19	Seizure control (13) Seizure type (2) Age at onset (2) Etiology (1) Duration (1)
Psychosocial	12	Parents' marital status (9) Family income (3)
Medication	6	Polytherapy/monotherapy (6)

DISCUSSION

In this section we will make some general observations on the results derived from our analyses, relate the overall pattern of findings to our multietiological model of psychopathology in epilepsy and, finally, review some particularly important specific findings.

When one collapses the results of the analyses across gender as well as across all behavior problem and social competence scales, the multietiological nature of our findings is apparent. As summarized in Table 9.8, biological factors, psychosocial factors, and medication factors, *in that order*, were significant predictors of psychopathology and social competence in children with epilepsy. We caution, however, against making too much of the relative power of biological, psychosocial, and medication factors, since our study was retrospective in nature, and we clearly had a less than comprehensive grouping of psychosocial and medication factors. For example, six biological variables were employed compared to only two psychosocial and three medication variables. Prospective investigations utilizing a more diverse and representative selection of psychosocial and medication factors would be of interest in order to examine the relative predictive power of these factors.

Within the major etiological categories some interesting trends were evident. Seizure control emerged as the most significant predictor variable in 14 regression analyses. It is relevant to raise the issue as to how seizure control exerts its effect. Is it truly a biological effect somehow related to poorly controlled seizures, or the extent of the underlying neuropathology, or do poorly controlled seizures subject the child to the many potential psychosocial consequences of epilepsy (stigma, social exclusion), or some combination of the above? Clearly, more investigation is needed to determine the manner whereby seizure control exerts such a strong effect on behavioral and social adjustment, especially as it has also been found by others to be related to behavioral adjustment in children with epilepsy (e.g. Hoare, 1984; Holdsworth and Whitmore, 1974).

Among the psychosocial variables the parents' marital status was the most frequent significant predictor overall, but seemed to be especially important for boys. For girls the median family income and parental marital status were equally important (Table 9.6). Clearly, a dissolved parental marriage is an important predictor, but cause/effect statements must again await further investigation. Does a child with epilepsy and associated behavioral problems contribute to the break-up of a marriage, and/or does divorce/separation have negative effects on the child? Clearly, both views have merit and deserve significant follow-up study in order to untangle the causal sequence, but the results at hand clearly suggest that this variable merits attention. Interestingly, over 30 years ago Grunberg and Pond (1957) found that environmental factors in general, and parental marital status in particular, were significantly associated with the behavioral adjustment of children with epilepsy.

Within the medication hypothesis the use of polytherapy was associated with behavioral and social difficulties. Specifically, polytherapy was associated with hyperactivity for both boys and girls. For boys, polytherapy was further associated with social withdrawal and poor school performance, while for girls it was associated with delinquency scores and decreased social activities.

At the present time our findings can be viewed as having some fairly specific clinical implications. First, it appears to be particularly important to attempt to obtain excellent seizure control, but through the use of monotherapy. Hence, effective up-to-date medical care is crucial. Second, it would appear that this is not enough in order to prevent behavior and social problems. The integrity of the child's immediate familial environment, that is, the status of the parents' marriage, is especially important. In summary, the centrality of comprehensive, multidisciplinary intervention in the context of modern medical management appears crucial if one is to attempt to prevent behavioral problems and enhance social competence.

The multifactorial nature of the determinants/correlates of problem behavior is further suggested by the results seen in Tables 9.5 and 9.6. For boys the *combination* of seizure control and parental marital status were significant predictors of five behavior problem scales, and operated alone or in combination with other variables on three other scales. Hence, the importance of multidisciplinary involvement is reinforced.

Two further important methodological observations must be considered. First, if the correlations between dependent variables are high, then we would expect similar risk factors to emerge as significant predictors for these dependent variables. We have examined the correlation matrix among the dependent variables utilized in this study and such high intercorrelations did indeed exist. For example, among the 66 intercorrelations (for the 12 dependent variables) for girls, 49 (74 percent) were statistically significant ($p < 0.05$), and 37

(56 percent) were significant beyond $p = 0.01$. Significant correlations ranged from 0.26 to 0.76. A similar situation existed for the boys. These intercorrelations suggest that the repeated findings of similar high-risk factors are not totally independent. This serves to weaken the importance of this consistency, but does not mitigate any of the main conclusions drawn from these analyses.

Second, it must be remembered that these children were studied at a tertiary-level medical setting, specializing in the more complicated and difficult cases of childhood epilepsy. Whether the results obtained here can be generalized to the broader population of children with epilepsy is a matter for future research.

CONCLUSION

As reviewed at the beginning of this chapter, children with epilepsy, on the average, appear to be at increased risk for psychopathology relative to various control populations. As is often the experience, these general statements do not always prove helpful when dealing with individuals—in this case, children with epilepsy. It has been our experience that while many children with epilepsy may manifest significant emotional and behavioral problems, others seem remarkably well adjusted. As reflected both in our selected review of the literature and the results of our investigation, a constellation of risk factors, multietiological in nature, appear to be emerging as potential determinants of psychopathology in children with epilepsy. Considerable research efforts are needed in order to gain a more complete and thorough quantitative understanding of the psychosocial situation of childhood epilepsy as so eloquently described by Taylor in this volume (Chapter 8). Such an understanding should be well worth the effort, as significant strides toward prevention of psychopathology in children with epilepsy could then begin in earnest.

REFERENCES

Achenbach, T.M., and Edelbrock, C.S. (1981). Behavioral problems and competencies reported by parents of normal and disturbed children aged four through sixteen. *Monograph of the Society for Research in Child Development*, **46**, Serial No. 188.

Achenbach, T.M., and Edelbrock, C. (1983). *Manual for the Child Behavior Checklist and Revised Child Behavior Profile*, University of Vermont, Burlington.

Bear, D.M., and Fedio, P. (1977). Quantitative analysis of interictal behavior in temporal lobe epilepsy. *Archives of Neurology*, **34**, 54–67.

Blumer, D. (1975). Temporal lobe epilepsy and its psychiatric significance. In D.F. Benson and D. Blumer (eds), *Psychiatric Aspects of Neurological Disease*, Grune and Stratton, New York, pp. 171–198.

Brent, D.A., Crumrine, P.K., and Varma, R.R. (1987). Phenobarbital treatment and major depressive disorder in children with epilepsy, *Pediatrics*, **80**, 909–917.

Ferrari, M., Barabas, G., and Matthews, W.S. (1983). Psychologic and behavioral disturbance among epileptic children treated with barbituate anticonvulsants. *American Journal of Psychiatry*, **140**, 112–113.

Grunberg, F., and Pond, D.A. (1957). Conduct disorders in epileptic children. *Journal of Neurology, Neurosurgery and Psychiatry*, **20**, 65–68.

Hermann, B.P., and Whitman, S. (1984). Behavioral and personality correlates of epilepsy. A review, methodological critique and conceptual model. *Psychological Bulletin*, **95**, 451–497.

Hermann, B.P., and Whitman, S. (1986). Psychopathology in epilepsy: A multietiologic model. In S. Whitman and B.P. Hermann (eds.), *Psychopathology in Epilepsy: Social Dimensions*, Oxford University Press, New York, pp. 5–37.

Hermann, B.P., Whitman, S., Hughes, J.R., Melyn, M.M., and Dell, J. (1988). Multietiological determinants of psychopathology and social competence in children with epilepsy. *Epilepsy Research*, **2**, 51–60.

Hoare, P. (1984). The development of psychiatric disorder among school children with epilepsy. *Developmental Medicine and Child Neurology*, **26**, 3–13.

Holdsworth, L., and Whitmore, K. (1974). A study of children with epilepsy attending ordinary schools. I. Their seizure patterns, progress, and behavior in school. *Developmental Medicine and Child Neurology*, **16**, 746–755.

Matthews, C.G., and Klove, H. (1968). MMPI performances in major motor, psychomotor, and mixed seizure classifications of known and unknown etiology. *Epilepsia*, **9**, 43–53.

Mellor, D.H., Lowit, I., and Hall, D.J. (1974). Are epileptic children behaviorally different from other children? In P. Harris and C. Maudsley (eds), *Epilepsy: Proceedings of The Hans Berger Centenary Symposium*, Churchill-Livingstone, Edinburgh, pp. 313–316.

Mungus, D. (1982). Interictal behavioral abnormality in temporal lobe epilepsy: A specific syndrome or non-specific psychopathology. *Archives of General Psychiatry*, **39**, 108–111.

Nuffield, E.J.A. (1961). Neuro-physiological and behavioral disorders in epileptic children. *Journal of Mental Science*, **107**, 438–458.

Ounsted, C. (1969). Aggression and epilepsy: rage in children with temporal lobe epilepsy. *Journal of Psychosomatic Research*, **13**, 237–242.

Rodin, E., and Schmaltz, S. (1984). The Bear–Fedio personality inventory and temporal lobe epilepsy. *Neurology*, **34**, 591–96.

Rutter, M., Graham, P., and Yule, W.A. (1970). *A Neuropsychiatric Study in Childhood*. J.B. Lippincott, Philadelphia.

Standage, K.F., and Fenton, G.W. (1975). Psychiatric symptom profile of patients with epilepsy: a controlled investigation. *Psychological Medicine*, **5**, 152–160.

Stores, G. (1978). School children with epilepsy at risk for learning and behavioral problems. *Developmental Medicine and Child Neurology*, **20**, 502–508.

Stores, G. (1980). Children with epilepsy: psychosocial aspects. In B.P. Hermann (ed.), *A Multidisciplinary Handbook of Epilepsy*, Charles Thomas, Springfield, pp. 224–242.

Waxman, S.G., and Geschwind, N. (1975). The interictal behavioral syndrome of temporal lobe epilepsy. *Archives of General Psychiatry*, **32**, 1580–88.

Whitman, S., Hermann, B.P., Black, R.B., and Chhabria, S. (1982). Psychopathology and seizure type in children with epilepsy. *Psychological Medicine*, **12**, 843–853.

Chapter 10

Epilepsy and Its Effects on the Family

Michael Ferrari

INTRODUCTION

Some case notes

Ken. At age 34, Ken had just returned home to live with his parents, both of whom were nearing retirement. Having just moved into a smaller house since all of their children had married and were living on their own, Ken's parents were somewhat ambivalent at the prospects of Ken's return to their domicile. After all, Ken's father reasoned, this was to be the time that he and his wife were to work on their own relationship, renewing their love and affection, reflecting on their lives together, and enjoying their grandchildren. Yet Ken needed a place to stay and, most importantly, people who cared about him.

Ken's mother also had some second thoughts about her quick invitation to her son to return to live with them if things did not work out otherwise. Ken had been so seemingly well adjusted to his life before his seizures had reappeared. After temporal lobe surgery he went for nearly three years without the reoccurrence of even a single seizure. He had gotten married, had two lovely children, and was for the first time in his life happy with himself. Yet when the seizures came back, Ken had gotten really depressed and began to drink. Soon after, he lost his job, his driver's licence, and now he was even isolated from his wife and children. Ken's mother felt obligated to open the doors of her house to her son, but silently, she wondered whether this is the right move for *anyone* in the family.

Monica. At 7 years, 8 months of age Monica is to all that see her the picture of health. She is good-looking, physically fit, and a delightful child in social interaction. Her strong peer interactive skills have repeatedly been rewarded by continued popularity at school. Her teachers speak of her as the

Childhood Epilepsies: Neuropsychological, Psychosocial and Intervention Aspects
Edited by B. Hermann and M. Seidenberg

'model student' and often relate praises to her parents for Monica's growing list of academic achievements. Few people, other than teachers or significant adult figures, know that Monica has a history of grand-mal seizures which were diagnosed by the age of 3 years, 7 months.

On this particular day, Monica's parents are expressing their pride in their daughter and resonating to other parents of children with epilepsy that they must be careful not to lower their expectations for their children. They tell of their grief and fears, but balance these expressed concerns with hope that through the challenges of coping with epilepsy their family can be strengthened and enriched. They report that in some ways epilepsy in their child has led them closer to each other and to God. They tell how appreciative they are of the support from friends and family that they receive.

Gary. At 12 years of age, Gary lives with his mother and his two brothers. Although often perceived by others as someone who is 'not all there', Gary has tested in the average range of intellectual ability. Gary does, however, have difficulties with tasks that require attentional vigilance and has repeatedly had school problems ranging from school failure to phobic avoidance of classes.

Gary's appearance suggests a young man with generally poor hygiene. He reportedly has no friends and tends to spend his time watching television at home and trying to interact with the friends of his older brothers. Seizure records indicate that Gary has had multiple types of seizure episodes. Each day he usually has four or five complex partial and numerous petit-mal seizures. Occasionally he has been known to have generalized episodes, but these have been less frequent in recent years. Family members contend that Gary cannot be trusted to tell you honestly about his seizures. When interviewed separately, each member of the family related that Gary sometimes fakes seizures to get what he wants and often lied about taking his medicine.

Gary's family believes that his seizures are indications of 'something wrong with his brain'. They claim that they do not think he is retarded but sometimes feel as if he is 'crazy'. Gary's one surviving grandparent, his maternal grandmother, has told the family she will not be left alone with Gary at any time. No-one quite knows why this is so, but Gary's mother believes that it is because she thinks Gary is unpredictable and could not be responsible for what he might do. Gary believes that he has a brain tumor that has simply eluded diagnostic testing. He claims that sometimes when he has seizures his family doesn't believe him, and this makes him very angry and he doesn't want to tell them about his seizures at all.

Comments

These three persons drawn from case files all have at least two things in common. First, they all have seizure disorders and second, each lives in a family environment. Yet the differences are far more strikingly present than any of the similarities. Ken has had an extremely difficult time living out on his own. His relationship with his wife has deteriorated, and he feels that his children cannot understand him and are at risk with his presence because of frequent anger outbursts accompanying his seizures. His move in with his parents now complicates their developmental transition into retirement.

Young Monica appears by all indications as well adjusted and well accepted. Her family is allied to a position of advocacy and acknowledge a strengthening of their family bonds because of her seizures. On the other hand, Gary's life appears greatly problematic. His mother has a small support network, limited education, and few effective coping skills. Because of his seizures, Gary is often seen as 'crazy' and has experienced considerable intrafamilial rejection and social ostracism. He has developed school avoidance and refusal and may have learned to use his seizure disorder as a means of manipulating others in the environment.

HOW DOES EPILEPSY AFFECT THE FAMILY?

Our review of cases seems to clearly illustate that there is no single answer to this question, and it is probably unproductive to search for one. Variations in family structure, differing manifestations of seizures and co-occurring conditions, social network support systems, and developmental variables are but a few of the multitude of mediating influences of the effects of epilepsy on the family. Collectively, these variables and others interact in ways that likely preclude the formulation of any sweeping generalizations concerning uniform effects of epilepsy on the family. Yet we know from the clinical and research literatures that there are some common denominators across families in which there is a person with epilepsy. We need to recognize, however, that these common factors are probably best conceptualized as areas of risk for families rather than inevitable outcomes.

Adults

The literature suggests that, in adults, one of the first classes of family-based effects relates to the likelihood of marriage and the quality of marital adjustment. Studies have shown that adults with epilepsy have a decreased likelihood of getting married when compared to rates for the general population (Dansky, Andermann, and Andermann, 1980). This decreased likelihood is primarily attributable to lowered rates of marriage in males since the rate for women with epilepsy is only slightly below that for population norms (Lechtenberg, 1984). This difference in rates for males and females is important, since research has shown that marriage itself seems to be correlated with better adjustment in men than remaining single (Bernard, 1972). While, admittedly, there are limitations present in establishing causal links, men who marry tend to live longer (Fehr and Perlman, 1985), enjoy better physical and mental health (Bloom, White, and Asher, 1979; Verbrugge, 1979), and have higher life satisfaction (Glenn, 1975; Veroff, Douvan and Kulka, 1981) than men who do not marry.

At this time there is not much data available concerning the ongoing adjustment of persons with epilepsy after they marry. There is some suggestion from follow-up studies (Lindsay, Ounsted, and Richards, 1979) that epileptic member marriages are more likely to end in separation and divorce than general norms; however, only adults with temporal lobe seizures have been successfully followed. Blumer (1975) has made the point that it would be inappropriate to generalize findings from these studies of persons with temporal lobe epilepsy to all adults with epilepsy, since temporal lobe patients often have difficult seizures to control and are represented by only a small number who do not have other seizure types as well. It is noteworthy that in one recent report, by Britten, Wadsworth, and Fenwick (1986), in which 46 subjects were followed until the age of 36, no differences were found in the marital status of persons with symptomatic versus idiopathic epilepsy. Unfortunately, there is no way to determine from the report what base rate of separation and divorce occurred among their sample or a determination of separated or divorced subjects by specific seizure type or focus.

There are several reports suggesting that the marital adjustments of adults with epilepsy are more likely to be complicated by sexual problems and fears relating to sexual performance (Remillard, 1983). Blumer (1975) has shown rates of hyposexuality in persons with complex partial seizures in up to 50 percent of the sample studies. There are many complicating factors, however, as such things as the effects of surgery on sexuality are as yet uncertain. Kolarsky (1976) and others (e.g. Lindsay *et al.*, 1979; Waxman and Geschwind, 1975) have also reported on the increased likelihood of sexual deviations in adults with epilepsy, particularly males.

Another area affecting sexuality in the marital relationship involves fears of seizures. Mittan (1986) has presented data indicating that a common 'family-related' fear reported by persons with epilepsy is whether sexual activity will precipitate seizures. Strauss, Risser, and Jones (1982) also reported significantly higher frequencies of sexual fears in men and women with left temporal lobe seizures relative to healthy controls, in their study of interictal fearfulness. This frequency of sexually related fears may perhaps be a significant reason for some of the sexual problems reported by adults with epilepsy; however, there is little data now available to support or refute this hypothesis.

It is also should be noted that until relatively recently there was little attention given to the concerns adults might have regarding the likelihood that having seizures might affect their children. Studies by Janz (1982) and Mittan (1986) report that a substantial number of adults with epilepsy are very frightened about the potential heritability of seizures and the possibilities that anticonvulsant medicine might cause their offspring to have birth defects.

The child and the family

How the child with epilepsy deals with his or her seizures is a variable of obvious import to the functioning of the family (Ferrari, Matthews, and Barabas, 1983; Livingston, 1970, 1972; Matthews, Barabas, and Ferrari, 1982). Other chapters in this volume have illustrated well that epilepsy in childhood is so much more than just a neurological condition. This literature will not be reviewed here. However, the importance of a comprehensive examination of epilepsy and its associated conditions cannot be understated. We know quite conclusively that seizures in children are, at times, correlated with learning and achievement difficulties, behavioral problems, and a broad range of psychosocial outcomes. As such, each of these dimensions of epilepsy must be considered as both a potentiator and buffer of family coping challenges.

We know from research that poorly controlled seizures in children can be a major disrupting psychosocial event for the family (Berg, 1982; Ferrari *et al.*, 1983). Yet the severity of the epilepsy alone is not a good predictor of family disruption (Breger, 1975; Hodgman, *et al.*, 1979; Golding and Margolin, 1975). Apparently factors such as each family member's perceptions of the degree of disruption may be more important than the actual level of disruption itself (Appolone-Ford, Gibson, and Driefuss, 1983; Appolone, 1978).

Children with epilepsy have been found to show increased levels of dependency (Stores and Piran, 1978; Hartlage, Green, and Offutt, 1972), perceived impairments of emotional and cognitive control (Matthews *et al.*, 1983; Ziegler, 1983) and to be generally attached to their parents (Mulder and Suurmeijer, 1977). An interactional study by Ritchie (1981) of 15 families with a child with epilepsy and 15 matched families with no chronically ill member showed that children with epilepsy took a more passive role in family interaction and demonstrated a reduced level of family involvement in decision-making. Mothers of children with seizures were more likely than control mothers to take a very prominent role in family discussions, and to be very strongly linked to the child.

Overprotectiveness on the part of the parents, a risk to parent–child relationships in many chronic illnesses and disabling conditions (Versluys, 1984; Burden, 1980; Fife, 1978; Meyerson, 1983; Seligman, 1983; Yurn and Zuckerman, 1979), has been found in the parent–child relationships in families with a person with epilepsy as well (Ferrari *et al.*, 1983; Pond, 1981; Wolf, Thorbecke, and Even, 1986; Ziegler, 1981). Safilios-Rothchild (1970) has shown that parents who expect to care for their children later in life are less likely to facilitate the development of independent behaviors. In epilepsy the presence of data that has suggested child dependency and parental overprotection may be indicating that parents of children with epilepsy have expectations that their children will need to remain dependent upon them for extended periods of time. There is now some data to suggest that parents of children with epilepsy are more likely to feel embarrassed by their child than are normal controls (Ritchie, 1981; Schneider and Conrad, 1983) as well as more likely to have lowered expectations for their child's level of achievement (Bagley, 1972; Long and Moore, 1979; Yule, 1973). Thus, it would not be surprising that part of the lowered levels of academic achievement witnessed in children with seizures (Ferrari *et al.*, 1983; Yule, 1973) is due to lowered expectations on the part of the families. To date, there have been only a few limited studies of parental expectations of their children with seizures.

A CONTROLLED STUDY

In order to investigate the expectations and attitudes of parents of children with epilepsy further, a study of 21 families in which a child with epilepsy lived was undertaken.

Method

Subjects

Thirty-six families were originally requested to take part in the study. Families contacted were identified through their physicians, schools, and referrals from the Delaware Epilepsy Association. Of the 36 families contacted, 26 replied affirmatively to the invitation to participate. Study famililes included only two parent families in which one child had epilepsy, and there was at least one sibling no more than 4 years older or younger than the child with epilepsy who was generally healthy and did not have seizures.

Twenty-one of the 26 families actually partook in the study. The five families who did not participate were excluded because, in four, the siblings' age spacing was too large, and in one, the biological sibling did not live at home.

Table 10.1 depicts the demographic data on the sample under study. In nine of the 21 sibling pairs the child with epilepsy was the older child. The mean age for older siblings was 11.6 years, for younger siblings 9.2 years.

The children with epilepsy in the study had varied seizure manifestations. Eight had generalized tonic–clonic seizures but six of the eight also had other seizure types. One child had Jacksonian seizures, five had complex partial seizures, three had petit-mal and the remaining four had mixed seizures. No

Table 10.1
Subjects of the study

	Children with epilepsy	Comparison sibling
Sample size	$N = 21$	$N = 21$
Mean age	10.47 years	10.34 years
(SD)	(2.19)	(1.98)
Sex		
Female	14	11
Male	7	10

subjects were included in the study that had a diagnosed DSM-III psychiatric disorder. Three of the children with epilepsy were receiving some type of special educational assistance. One of the comparison siblings was also a special education student in his school.

Procedure

All data was collected in a single visit with the family. Following the collection of background demographic information on the children, parents were requested to complete a 10-item questionnaire which required them to make predictive ratings of each of their children's performance in varied personal–social and academic domains 3 years in the future. This questionnaire was adapted from the work of Long and Moore (1979) and is presented in Table 10.2.

Parents were instructed to complete the questionnaire on their child with epilepsy and on the comparison sibling chosen for the study. The order in which parents were asked for their ratings was counterbalanced within the group, so that approximately half of the subjects' parents were asked to complete the questionnaire on the child with epilepsy first, while the other half completed the questionnaire first on the comparison sibling.

Results

Fathers of the children in the study were present for only seven of the 21 visits with the study families. All of the mothers were present during data collection, and as such only the raw data from the mothers' predictions will be presented here.

A preliminary analysis of the data included a group (child with epilepsy vs. comparison sibling) × birth order (older vs. younger siblings) × sex (male vs. female) analysis of variance. Sex of child did not emerge as significant on any of the items on the questionnaire, nor a total questionnaire score, and thus was eliminated from further analyses. Group × birth order (2 × 2) analyses of

Table 10.2
Predictions questionnaire

Key: Excellent — Above average — Average — Below average — Poor
1 . . . 2 . . . 3 . . . 4 . . . 5 . . . 6 . . . 7

In three years, I predict my child will:

1 . . . 2 . . . 3 . . . 4 . . . 5 . . . 6 . . . 7
'do well at school'

1 . . . 2 . . . 3 . . . 4 . . . 5 . . . 6 . . . 7
'do well at sports'

1 . . . 2 . . . 3 . . . 4 . . . 5 . . . 6 . . . 7
'be a moody person'

1 . . . 2 . . . 3 . . . 4 . . . 5 . . . 6 . . . 7
'have a wide choice of jobs'

1 . . . 2 . . . 3 . . . 4 . . . 5 . . . 6 . . . 7
'make friends easily'

1 . . . 2 . . . 3 . . . 4 . . . 5 . . . 6 . . . 7
'have emotional problems'

1 . . . 2 . . . 3 . . . 4 . . . 5 . . . 6 . . . 7
'enjoy his/her own company'

1 . . . 2 . . . 3 . . . 4 . . . 5 . . . 6 . . . 7
'be trusting of other people'

1 . . . 2 . . . 3 . . . 4 . . . 5 . . . 6 . . . 7
'be aggressive'

1 . . . 2 . . . 3 . . . 4 . . . 5 . . . 6 . . . 7
'be a reliable person'

variance were then undertaken on all variables. Post-hoc Scheffe's multiple comparisons were used in the evaluation of significant mean differences.

Table 10.3 illustrates the results of the analyses which showed main effects of group (child with epilepsy vs. comparison sibling) in the mother's ratings. As can be seen, on eight of the 10 factors the children with epilepsy were given significantly lower ratings by their mothers. The pattern of the ratings were uniformly *lower* competence and health among the epileptic children. Mothers predicted their children with epilepsy to be less reliable, less trusting of others, to have a greater likelihood of emotional problems, show lower school performance and performance in sports, be more moody, derive less enjoyment from their own company, and be less adept as making friends than their siblings. Only on two of the variables was there no significant difference found in the mother's prediction. These were the likelihood of being aggressive and the likelihood of having a wide choice of jobs.

It is noteworthy that birth order (younger or older sibling) emerged as a significant factor only on one of the dependent measures, namely, 'Ease at making friends.' On this measure younger children were predictively rated by their mothers as more likely to have ease at making friends than older children

Table 10.3
Mean maternal ratings by group

Variable	Group		F value
	Child with epilepsy	Sibling	
School performance	4.29	2.86	$F(1,38) = 15.29, p<0.0004$
Sports	4.23	3.33	$F(1,38) = 5.78, p<0.02$
Be a moody person	4.29	3.24	$F(1,38) = 6.81, p<0.01$
Choice of jobs	3.95	3.29	n.s.
Ease making friends	4.09	3.00	$F(1,38) = 10.78, p<0.022$
Have emotional problems	4.14	2.86	$F(1,38) = 9.91, p<0.003$
Enjoy own company	3.90	2.95	$F(1,38) = 7.15, p<0.01$
Trusting of others	3.62	2.90	$F(1,38) = 4.38, p<0.04$
Be aggressive	4.00	3.29	n.s.
Be reliable	3.48	2.38	$F(1,38) = 9.39, p<0.004$

($F(1,38) = 4.11$, $p < 0.05$). It is also of note that there were no significant interactions on any of the dependent measures evaluated.

Discussion

Findings from the present study indicate that within-family comparisons of personal–social and academic predictors for children with epilepsy and their healthy siblings reveal diminished expectations of performance for the child having seizures. This finding is consistent with some previous research and observation (cf. Long and Moore, 1979; Mulder and Suurmeijer, 1977) that has shown the parents of children with epilepsy to have generally lowered expectations for their child's future and personal adjustment.

Perhaps more striking in the results of the present study is the degree to which children with epilepsy are perceived by their mothers as less likely to do well in the future. The question arises as to why this is so. Potentially, the answer to this query may involve a number of factors that interact with the presence of epilepsy as it presents in the child. Are mothers responding merely to the epilepsy in making their lowered predictions? Or are they responding to conditions they perceive as associated with the epilepsy, such as learning problems and personal–social difficulties? Although only three of the subjects with seizures were receiving special educational assistance, only a systematic evaluation of learning potential could adequately answer this question. Clearly, with 80 percent of the items on the questionnaire rated as significantly lower for the child with seizures, irrespective of age relationships to sibling and sex of child, factors that relate to the child are the basis for lowered expectations.

EPILEPSY AS A FAMILY VARIABLE

Thus far, our focus has been on the family and epilepsy literature that has pertained to seizures in the family lives of adults and children, and in parent–child relationships. There has also been an examination of some of the illness-related variables that may influence the family as a growth-producing psychosocial environment for children and adults. The study reported herein has also demonstrated how parents' responses to the presence of epilepsy in their children can greatly influence their expectations for their child, and as such may play a significant role in the underachievement and adjustment problems of children with seizures. I have not yet, however, addressed epilepsy as a family variable which occurs in the normative developmental cycles of individuals and families. Yet this is an important point of focus, despite the fact that, to date, family developmental factors have been greatly understudied (Ferrari, 1986). Clearly, the responses of the family to the presence of a member with a seizure disorder must be considered within a framework that includes the strong developmental needs and processes existent in the family.

Developmental issues in families

Why are the challenges posed for 34-year-old Ken's family so much different than for 12-year-old Gary's family? The research reviewed in this chapter, and throughout this book, tells us there is no easy answer. One of the reasons may relate to the differing seizure manifestations of the two persons, or the somewhat different responses each has received from the families. The clinical courses of their seizures have also been different, as well as the medical interventions. Clearly, however, Ken is faced with developmental challenges far removed from those faced by Gary and his family. Ken's family of origin has launched all of its children; fostering and supporting their independence. His parents are preparing for retirement from work and have already begun a process of renegotiating aspects of their spousal relationship now in the absence of their children.

Gary's single-parent family has very different developmental challenges. In addition to her role as provider, Gary's mother must be nurturant and willing to provide a great deal of guidance to her growing children. Gary should be busily achieving in school, learning of his culture, and developing a unique sense of self. His behavior problems, his belief systems, and his failures in forming significant emotional relationships are all intimately tied to his illness and the point in development in which it is presenting.

Family developmental considerations are very complex variables (Duvall and Miller, 1985). By their very nature they belong to individuals and families simultaneously. They consist of the potentiation of individual members' emotional needs, intellectual statuses, strengths and process, biomaturational markers, and intra- and extrafamilial relationships.

When epilepsy presents in childhood, it comes at a time when, developmentally, the typical nuclear family is challenged to adjust the marital unit to allow space for children and renegotiable existing extended family relationships. As the children grow, the marital system becomes increasingly recognized for its parenting role, and with it the needs to nurture and guide the children. I have previously covered some of the literature that has maintained that one common response of parents to epilepsy in their children is overprotection. In the light of a developmental framework it is not surprising that this is so, given the significant role of the parents in protecting their offspring. However, it is likely that this typical response becomes dysfunctional when it is carried to an extreme degree (e.g. not allowing the child to be alone at any time) or continued into later developmental stages. For example, the developmental challenges of families with older children and adolescents revolve around striking a balance between connection to the family of origin and freedom to explore other relationships outside the family. When parental protectiveness continues in a heightened form well into adolescence and early adulthood, the developmental needs of the young adult to become significantly differentiated from the family are likely to become unfulfilled. This often leads to difficulties in later developmental periods, as the adult tries to form his/her own marital system, and develop other avenues of his/her life, such as a career focus.

How significant family developmental variables are for the ongoing development of the individual is not yet fully clear. Some have argued (e.g. Carter and McGolderick, 1980) that certain developmental periods, such as the adolescent period, are so powerful that the entire family truly experiences them. If this is the case, it is likely that the effects of epilepsy in these developmental periods might be most pervasive.

The family adjustment process

Also of importance to our overall consideration of the effects of epilepsy on the family is the idea that epilepsy, like other chronic illnesses, is a form of personal and family stressor that requires an adjustment response. There is considerable discussion and theory that relates the onset of illness symptoms to adaptational processes like those experienced in loss and grief (Austin, 1986; Gargiulo, 1985; Olshanky, 1962) although there may be more differences in the process then similarities.

While there are now some data on the family's typical responses to the presence of a member with seizures in the household, there is really very little data that concerns the ongoing coping responses of families (Lechtenberg, 1984; Ziegler, 1981). Ward and Bower (1978) interviewed 81 families of children with epilepsy, seeking to assess the effects of the diagnosis of epilepsy on the family. They reported parental heightened anxieties in most cases, and many reports by parents that they felt their child had died during a seizure and were considerably fearful. Roughly half of the parents also felt that epilepsy was a correlate of serious personality or behavior problems, and they also felt that normal aspects of the parent–child relationship (e.g. the need for discipline) might evoke a seizure. Like other findings that have already been reviewed here (i.e. overprotectiveness, lowered expectations, parental embarrassment) the findings of the Ward and Bower (1978) study of family adaptation are limited to a certain short period of time following the diagnosis of the epilepsy. How might we conceptualize the differences in the families of Monica, a child who was doing well along with her family, the pillar of support to many other families with epilepsy, against the striking contrast of Gary and his family? What variables might have facilitated the family adaptational processes in Gary's family? Unfortunately, at this time we have more questions than answers, although the formulation of the questions is a necessary first step in the process of answering them. What is clearly needed at this point are long-term longitudinal studies that can afford the richness of exploring the adaptation process in the full family system, and how we might best facilitate that process.

REFERENCES

Appolone, C. (1978). Preventative social work intervention with families of children with epilepsy. *Social Work and Health Care*, **4**, 139–148.

Appolone–Ford, C., Gibson, P., and Driefuss, F.E. (1983). Psychosocial considerations in childhood epilepsy. In *Pediatrics: Epileptology, Classification and Management of Seizures in the Child*, PSG Publishing Co, Littleton, MA.

Austin, J.K. (1986). Adult onset: the grieving process. Paper presented at the National Conference of the Epilepsy Foundation of America, Alexandria, VA.

Bagley, C. (1972). Social prejudice and the adjustment of people with epilepsy. *Epilepsia*, **13**, 33–45.

Berg, B.O. (1982). Prognosis of childhood epilepsy—another look. *New England Journal of Medicine*, **306**, 861–862.

Bernard, J. (1972). *The Future of Marriage*, Bantam Books, New York.

Bloom, B.L., White, S.W., and Asher, S.J. (1979). Marital disruption as a stressful life event. In G. Levinger and O.C. Moles (eds), *Divorce and Separation: Context, Causes, and Consequences*, Basic Books, New York.

Blumer, D. (1975). Temporal lobe epilepsy and its psychiatric significance. In D.F. Benson and D. Blumer (eds), *Psychiatric Aspects of Neurologic Disease*, Grune & Stratton, New York.

Breger, E. (1975). Psychiatric consultation to the epileptic child and his family: A study of 60 caess—Part 3: Follow-up study. *Maryland State Medical Journal, February*, pp. 47–50.

Britten, N., Wadsworth, M.E., and Fenwick, P.B. (1986). Sources of stigma following early-life epilepsy: evidence from a National Birth Cohort study. In S. Whitman and B.P. Hermann (eds), *Psychopathology in Epilepsy: Social Dimensions*, Oxford University Press, New York.

Burden, R.L. (1980). Measuring the effects of stress on the mothers of handicapped infants: must depression always follow? *Child Care, Health and Development*, **6**, 111–123.

Carter, E.A., and McGolderick, M. (1980). *The Family Life Cycle: A Framework for Family Therapy*, Gardner Press, New York.

Dansky, L.V., Andermann, E., and Andermann, F. (1980). Marriage and fertility in epileptic patients. *Epilepsia*, **21**, 261–271.

Duvall, E., and Miller, S. (1985). *Marriage and Family Development*, Harper & Row, New York.

Fehr, B., and Perlman, D. (1985). The family as a social network and support system. In L. L'Abate (ed.), *The Handbook of Family Psychology and Therapy*, Dorsey Press, Homewood, IL.

Ferrari, M. (1986). Relationships in epilepsy: getting stuck and why. Paper presented at the National Conference of the Epilepsy Foundation of America, Alexandria, VA.

Ferrari, M., Matthews, W.S., and Barabas, G. (1983). The family and the child with epilepsy. *Family Process*, **22**, 53–59.

Fife, B.L. (1978). Reducing parental overprotection of the leukemic child. *Social Science and Medicine*, **12**, 117–122.

Gargiulo, R.M. (1985). *Working with Parents of Exceptional Children*, Houghton Mifflin, Boston, MA.

Glenn, N.D. (1975). The contribution of marriage to the psychological well-being of males and females. *Journal of Marriage and the Family*, **37**, 594–600.

Goldin, G.J., and Margolin, R.J. (1975). The psychosocial aspects of epilepsy. In G.N. Wright (ed), *Epileptic Rehabilitation*, Little-Brown, Boston, MA, pp. .

Hartlage, L.C., Green, J.B., and Offutt, L. (1972). Dependency in epileptic children. *Epilepsia*, **13**, 27–30.

Hodgman, C.H., McAnarney, E.R., Myers, G.J., Iker, H., McKinney, R., Parmelee, D., Schuster, B., and Tutihasi, M. (1979). Emotional complications of adolescent grand mal epilepsy. *Journal of Pediatrics*, **95**, 309–312.

Janz, D. (1982). *Epilepsy, Pregnancy and the Child*, Raven Press, New York.

Kolarsky, A. (1976). Male sexual deviation: association with early temporal lobe damage. *Archives of General Psychiatry*, **17**, 735–743.

Lechtenberg, R. (1984). *Epilepsy and the Family*, Harvard University Press, Cambridge, MA.

Lindsay, J., Ounsted, C., and Richards, P. (1979). Long-term outcome in children with temporal lobe seizures. II. Marriage, parenthood and sexual indifference. *Developmental Medicine and Child Neurology*, **21**, 433–440.

Livingston, S. (1970). The physician's role in guiding the epileptic child and his parents. *American Journal of Diseases in Children*, **119**, 99–102.

Livingston, S. (1972). *Comprehensive Management of Epilepsy in Infancy, Childhood, and Adolescence*, Charles C. Thomas, Springfield, IL.

Long, C.G., and Moore, J.R. (1979). Parental expectations for their epileptic children. *Journal of Child Psychology and Psychiatry*, **20**, 299–312.

Matthews, W.S., Barabas, G., and Ferrari, M. (1982). Emotional concomitants of childhood epilepsy. *Epilepsia*, **23**, 671–681.

Meyerson, R.C. (1983). Family and parent group therapy. In M. Seligman (ed.), *The Family with a Handicapped Child: Understanding and Treatment*, Grune & Stratton, New York.

Mittan, R.J. (1986). Fear of seizures. In S. Whitman and B.P. Hermann (eds), *Psychopathology in Epilepsy: Social Dimension*, Oxford University Press, New York.

Mulder, H.C., and Suurmeijer, T.P. (1977). Families with a child with epilepsy: a sociological contribution. *Journal of Biosocial Science*, **9**, 13–24.

Olshansky, S. (1962). Chronic sorrow: a response to having a mentally retarded child. *Social Casework*, **43**, 190–193.

Pond, D. (1981). Psychosocial aspects of epilepsy—the family. In E.H. Reynolds and M.R. Trimble (eds), *Epilepsy and Psychiatry*, Churchill Livingstone, New York.

Remillard, G.M. (1983). Sexual ictal manifestations predominate in women with temporal lobe epilepsy: a finding suggesting sexual dimorphism in the human brain. *Neurology*, **33**, 323–330.

Ritchie, K. (1981). Interaction in families of epileptic children. *Journal of Children Psychology and Psychiatry*, **22**, 65–71.

Safilios-Rothchild, C. (1970). *The Sociology and Social Psychology of Disability and Rehabilitation*, Random House, New York.

Schneider, J., and Conrad, P. (1983). *Having Epilepsy*, Temple University Press, Philadelphia, PA.

Seligman, M. (1983). *The Family with a Handicapped Child: Understanding and Treatment*, Grune & Stratton, New York.

Stores, G., and Piran, N. (1978). Dependency of different types of school children with epilepsy. *Psychological Medicine*, **8**, 441–445.

Strauss, E., Risser, A., and Jones, M.W. (1982). Fear responses in patients with epilepsy. *Archives of Neurology*, **39**, 626–630.

Verbrugge, L.M. (1979). Marital status and health. *Journal of Marriage and the Family*, **41**, 267–285.

Veroff, J., Douvan, E., and Kulka, R.A. (1981). *The Inner American: A Self-portrait from 1957 to 1976*, Basic Books, New York.

Versluys, H.P. (1984). Psychological adjustment to physical disability. In C.A. Tromblay and A.E. Dell-Orto (eds), *The Psychological and Social Impact of Physical Disability*, Springer, New York.

Ward, F.W., and Bower, B.D. (1978). A study of certain social aspects of epilepsy in childhood. *Developmental Medicine and Child Neurology*, **20**, 1–63.

Waxman, S.G., and Geschwind, N. (1975). The interictal behavior syndrome of temporal lobe epilepsy. *Archives of General Psychiatry*, **32**, 1580–1586.

Wolf, P., Thorbecke, R., and Even, W. (1986). Social aspects of psychosis in patients with epilepsy. In S. Whitman and B.P. Hermann (eds), *Psychopathology in Epilepsy: Social Dimensions*, Oxford University Press, New York.

Yule, W. (1973). Epilepsy: education and enigma. *Special Education*, **62**, 205–218.

Yura, M.T., and Zuckerman, L. (1979). *Raising the Exceptional Child*, Hawthorne Books, New York.

Ziegler, R.G. (1981). Impairments of control and competence in epileptic children and their families. *Epilepsia*, **22**, 339–346.

Chapter 11

The Surgical Treatment of Epilepsy

Allen R. Wyler

INTRODUCTION

The surgery of epilepsy is an effective treatment for many seizure disorders which have not been adequately controlled with appropriate anticonvulsant medications. In this chapter the background and rationale of different surgical approaches will be discussed. In particular the following surgical procedures will be reviewed: (1) focal resections, (2) hemispherectomy, and (3) corpus callosum sectioning. Presently, referral of patients to centers that specialize in epilepsy surgery is grossly underutilized by physicians. This is primarily because of an inadequate knowledge of the potential benefits of surgery compared to the perceived risks. Present surgical techniques result in very good outcomes for carefully evaluated patients, with a very acceptable morbidity and mortality. Thus, epilepsy surgery should no longer be considered the 'Court of Last Resort', and surgery should be considered at the earliest possible age when it has become evident that medical management will not be sufficient to control a patient's seizure disorder.

BACKGROUND

The modern era of surgery for epilepsy was introduced in the later part of the nineteenth century by the British neurosurgeon Dr Victor Horsely. His first reported case was operated upon in 1886 while he was at a National Hospital at Queen Square, London. Horsely demonstrated that, for many cases of epilepsy, a focal point could be found on the surface of the brain that gave rise to the seizures, and if this focal region of brain was removed surgically the seizures would cease. These earlier cases were limited primarily to patients with diagnosable structural lesions, such as depressed skull fractures. Horsely's observations were not fully exploited until the 1950s, at which time Dr Wilder Penfield began to publish his series of patients who had been operated upon at

Childhood Epilepsies: Neuropsychological, Psychosocial and Intervention Aspects
Edited by B. Hermann and M. Seidenberg

the Montreal Neurological Institute. Penfield and his colleague, Herbert Jasper, made a major advance in surgery for epilepsy by introducing the use of the EEG within the operating room. By recording directly from the surface of the patient's cortex they could localize focal epileptogenic abnormalities that did not have associated structural abnormalities, thereby increasing the effectiveness and utility of the surgery. Shortly thereafter, the surgery of epilepsy became accepted as a therapy for patients not well controlled with medications. But even today, the surgery is grossly underutilized.

There are several reasons why many patients and physicians do not consider surgery as a therapeutic option. First, there are currently approximately seven drugs that are effective anticonvulsants. (Prior to 1938 when Dilantin was introduced, there had been only bromides and phenobarbital). Since many of these drugs are effective, the need for surgery is not perceived as great by many physicians. Second, many physicians remain unaware that this option is available, since there are few regional epilepsy centres where this type of specialized surgery is available. Third, the risks of surgery are often overestimated by patient and physician. Finally, many physicians do not understand the problems faced by the patient with epilepsy, and underestimate the problems that epilepsy can cause the patient who suffers from it. The physician may consider two seizures a month quite acceptable for the patient, whereas the patient may find this degree of seizure control unacceptable.

WHY CONSIDER SURGERY AT ALL?

There are several reasons to consider surgery when an aggressive attempt at controlling seizures medically has failed.

1. Continued convulsive seizures have a definite long-term effect on the patient's mental capabilities. More than 100 tonic–clonic seizures is associated with a decline in the IQ of patients with epilepsy (Dodrill, 1986).
2. Active epileptic attacks will usually cause social embarrassment to the patient which will ultimately result in poorer psychosocial development. This will have a compounding effect on through young adulthood, and will be reflected in the patient's long-term vocational and social outcome.
3. People with convulsive seizures have a significantly higher incidence of sudden death in comparison to people without seizures (Hauser, Annegers, and Elveback, 1980).

CRITERIA FOR SURGERY

The first and primary indication for epilepsy surgery is the failure to control the patient's seizures adequately with anticonvulsant medications. This indication is not often debated; however, what is debated is the definition of inadequate seizure control. Unfortunately one cannot define a numerical threshold between adequate and inadequate seizure control. This must be decided by considering the effect of the seizures upon the patient, his expectations, and his realistic psychosocial and vocational potentials. For example, one seizure a year could not be tolerated by a person who was making a career as an airline pilot, since that would result in the loss of his profession. On the other hand, three seizures a week might not adversely affect the psychosocial expectations of a mentally retarded and institutionalized patient. The most common mistake made by most physicians is to unilaterally decide for the patient what is 'acceptable seizure control'. This is truly the patient's decision, and not the physician's. In addition, the seizure's effect upon the patient's health is a consideration. For example, atonic seizures that result in abrupt falls can be much more serious in their consequences than brief absence seizures.

The second criterion for epilepsy surgery is that reasonable trials with the primary anticonvulsants have failed to control the patient's seizures. A 'reasonable trial' implies that the medication has been documented to be within the accepted therapeutic serum ranges during periods in which the patient was still having seizures. This criterion also assumes that the anticonvulsants appropriate for the patient's type of epilepsy have been tried. For the partial epilepsies this means phenytoin, carbamazepine (both alone and then in combination), and phenobarbital (which may be given as primidone). Drugs such as sodium valproate or ethosuxamide are inappropriate in attempts at controlling the partial epilepsies and should not be tried.

Before phenytoin or carbamazepine are considered failures, they should have been administered almost to the point of causing toxic side-effects. However, seizure control should not be obtained at the cost of chronic toxicity. In addition, secondary drugs such as diazepam should not be included in the drug trial. The length of time needed to verify a 'reasonable trial' depends on the patients' seizure frequency. For example, if a patient is having four seizures a week, then 2–3 weeks of treatment with phenytoin in the high therapeutic range is sufficient to document a failure if the seizures persist. However, if seizures occur at a rate of one per month, then a longer period of time is obviously needed to make the appropriate judgement. If a seizure disorder cannot be medically controlled within 2 years of aggressive therapy, then the chance of medical control is very low, and it is of little use trying various other combinations of drugs.

The third consideration for surgery is that the patient must have a reasonable chance of benefiting from the surgery, and that this chance is greater than the risks of a surgical complication. This last criterion will in large part depend on the data accumulated during the patient's workup.

THE PRESURGICAL EVALUATION

The foundation of the surgical workup is primarily dependent upon an adequate EEG evaluation. The other major components are: (1) neuropsychological assessment, (2) neuroradiological investigation, and (3) an intracarotid amytal test. All of these components are taken together to form a decision as to the appropriateness of elective surgery and the type of surgery best indicated. Each component will be discussed separately.

EEG Evaluation

The first stage of the workup is an evaluation of the patient's routine EEGs and clinical seizure history in order to classify his epilepsy into either primarily generalized (i.e. true absence seizures) or partial seizures. If the patient has partial seizures, then the next step is to determine if one or multiple foci are present. True petit-mal epilepsy is not well treated with any type of surgery, whereas focal or multifocal seizures can be successfully treated surgically. As a general rule, discrete foci are best treated with a focal resection whenever possible, and multifocal seizure foci respond to corpus callosum sectioning in selected cases.

All available previous routine EEGs for a patient should be evaluated. These past EEGs can help determine just what type of long-term EEG/video monitoring is necessary. In our center, if a straightforward case of unilateral temporal lobe epilepsy is suspected we routinely include the sphenoidal electrodes when monitoring patients. This is because these recording have been shown to be superior to standard recordings for disclosing discharges from mesial temporal structures (Sperling, Mendius, and Engle, 1986). The monitoring should include at least two clearly recorded spontaneous seizures that the patient's family deems representative of the patient's usual attacks.

If the onset of the EEG seizure does not precede or coincide with the onset of the clinical seizure, or if the epileptiform discharges are not clearly focal to one CNS region, one must consider the implantation of intracranial electrodes. It is not within the scope of this chapter to discusss the relative merits of intracortical depth electrodes (Bancaud *et al.*, 1965) or subdural strip electrodes (Wyler, Ojemann, Lettich, and Ward, 1984; Rosenbaum, Laxer, Vessely, and Smith, 1986), but both options have yielded excellent results. Spencer (1981) has reviewed the use of depth electrodes, and has emphasized that such recordings are needed for the more complex diagnostic cases, and that their use has enabled 36 percent more patients to be selected for surgery by defining an otherwise unidentifiable single epileptogenic focus. In addition, depth recordings could have prevented surgery for another 18 percent by demonstrating multifocal epilepsy that is known to have a poor surgical prognosis.

If the EEG has provided enough information to decide that surgery is an option for the patient, then additional data may be obtained. A standard set of non-contrast and intravenous contrast enhanced CT scans have usually been obtained in the course of the patient's initial workup. If several years have elapsed since the original scans, they should be repeated to insure that the patient does not have a slow-growing tumor such as a meningioma.

More recently, magnetic resonance scans (MRI) have proven useful in the evaluation of surgical candidates. These scans are complementary to X-ray CT images since they can often visualize small hamartomas that CT scans will miss (Sperling *et al.*, 1986). On the other hand, the CT scan should not be replaced by the MRI since the former will visualize many things the MRI will miss, such as bone erosion. Initially, it was hoped that MRI scanning would help diagnose subtle changes associated with mesial temporal lobe sclerosis. Unfortunately, that has not been the case. The major disadvantage of MRI is that each scan takes longers than a CT scan, and this makes scanning small children, who will not lay still, very difficult.

Neuropsychological evaluation

It has been the practice of many epilepsy centers to use extensive neuropsychological tests to help localize the focus. The rationale is that the neuropathology producing the epileptogenic focus may cause neuropsychological deficits. Thus, by careful neuropsychological assessment, these cognitive deficits might provide additional information with which to localize the focus. There is at present no consensus among neuropsycholgists as to which tests or test batteries should be used in order to maximise this potential. The more important issue is to use a battery of tests that provides a comprehensive evaluation of cognitive function so that deficits can be clearly identified if they exist.

In addition to helping to localize a focus, the neuropsychological evaluation can also be very useful for planning the patient's postoperative vocational rehabilitation when necessary. For example, a patient with a significant verbal memory deficit has a markedly different rehabilitation potential than one with visual spatial problems.

Intracarotid amytal (Wada) test

It is often desirable to know which side of the brain is dominant for speech. For this purpose the Wada test was devised (Wada and Rasmussen, 1952). There are many different methods for completing this test. In essence, sodium amytal is injected into each carotid artery for the purpose of suppressing each function. During unilateral hemispheric dysfunction (produced by the amytal), the patient can be tested in a variety of ways to ascertain speech and memory capability.

SURGICAL APPROACHES

Focal resections

Once the region of brain that contains the epileptogenic focus has been identified essentially two approaches can be used to remove the focus. The first approach is termed the 'tailored' resection, the second is termed the 'en bloc' resection. The first, or tailored approach, is very much similar to the strategy pioneered by Penfield and Jasper (1954). The preoperative workup determines the location of the focus; for example, temporal lobe. The surgery is done under local anesthesia (in adults) to insure that the patient is awake and cooperative so that the cortex can be functionally mapped to demonstrate regions such as motor strip and language-related areas. Prior to the functional mapping, electrocorticography is done to define the cortical regions that exhibit epileptogenic spiking. To provide the most accurate localization, strip electrodes (Wyler *et al.*, 1984) are used to explore non-exposed regions, such as uncus and hippocampus in the case of temporal lobectomy. After these data are obtained the cortical resection is then 'tailored' to provide the largest possible removal of epileptogenic cortex that can be safely carried out without jeopardizing critical neurologic function.

There are obvious problems to this surgical approach. First, the patient is awake, thus making the surgery impossible for most children under the age of 16 years. Moreover, craniotomy under local anesthesia can be very stressful to the surgeon. Second, the time allowed for corticography and functional mapping is limited to 1–2 hours. (This time is usually quite sufficient, though.) One solution to this problem has been developed by Goldring and Gregorie (1984). Two or three days prior to ablative surgery a craniotomy is done over the proposed resection site. A large grid of electrodes is placed over the exposed dura and the wound closed. This grid can be used both for stimulation of the underlying brain and EEG recordings. This allows the cortical region of interest to be mapped for important functions (i.e. language) and the regions of active spiking to be identified. During this testing the patient is within the familiar environment of the laboratory rather than the operating room. After the patient has been studied extensively he is returned to the operating room where the cortical resection can be done under general anesthesia. Thus, this technique is especially attractive for use with patients who, like children under age 16, would not tolerate operation under local anesthesia. The obvious disadvantage to this approach is the need for two separate operations, and the potential increased risk of infection. More recently, in our center, we have done all resections under general anesthesia without 'mapping' speech cortex unless the epileptogenic focus is suspected as being in lateral temporal lobe.

In contrast to the 'tailored resection' is the 'en bloc' or 'standard lobectomy' method. With this strategy one decides within which lobe the focus resides, and then that lobe is removed 'en bloc' with a standardized operation. When dealing with the temporal lobe, the resection routinely involves the anterior 4.5 cm of the left (dominant) and 5.5 cm of the right temporal lobe. This resection is done without electrocorticography or functional cortical mapping. However, in many cases the patients have already undergone extensive electrophysiological monitoring with intracortical depth electrodes, thus precluding the need for electrocorticography. The obvious advantages to this approach are: (1) it is done under general anesthesia, (2) the total operating time is less, and (3) a large block of tissue is obtained that can be studied in the pathology laboratory. The disadvantage is that intraoperative 'tailoring' of the resection site is not done. Therefore one must have faith that the focus will be within the confines of the standard resection margin (a fact which is not always the case). Recently Spencer *et al.* (1984) have found that 20 percent of their patients with unilateral temporal lobe foci who were studied by depth electrodes had foci located in posterior hippocampus (i.e. caudal) to the usual limits of the standard 'en bloc' temporal lobectomy. As a result they modified their operation as follows. A standard 4.5 cm anterior lobectomy is conducted. Then the anterior aspect of the temporal horn is entered, and the lateral temporal cortex is elevated so that the posterior hippocampus can be resected 'en bloc'. They feel this provides more precise removal of the epileptogenic cortex while sparing important lateral temporal cortex which has many important contributions to memory.

When the focus has been demonstrated (by intracranial electrode studies) to reside solely within the hippocampus or mesial portion of the temporal lobe, an alternative approach has been reported by Wieser and Yasargil (1984). The surgical procedure has been termed 'selective amygdalohippocampectomy', because the surgeon removes the amygdala and hippocampus without removing the lateral temporal cortex. The surgery is done through a peritonal approach, much the same as used by Yasargil for approaching anterior circulation aneurysms. The Sylvian fissure is split and the medial side of the temporal tip is entered. The mesial portion of the temporal lobe is then dissected in a subpial fashion, removing only hippocampus and amygdala. These authors report that 116 patients operated on with this technique have enjoyed excellent results. What is more impressive is that they have demonstrated minimal postoperative memory deficits as a result of temporal lobe surgery.

At our epilepsy center we do not tend to use only one of the above approaches. For example, although we used to believe that cortical mapping was always an essential part of surgery, our present results have indicated that, in most routine cases, that is not needed. Thus I have chosen to do all cases under general anesthesia. By limiting the lateral extent of cortex resected from the temporal lobe while maximizing the amount of hippocampus resected, the results can be exceptionally good. Thus I have used a mixture of the techniques described by both Spencer (1984) and Weiser and Yasargil (1984). As yet, we have not needed to place the electrode grids described by Goldring (1984) for the purposes of speech mapping.

The temporal lobe is the most common site of epileptogenic foci. The frontal lobe is the second most common location, followed by the parietal lobe. In my own series I have encountered only 10 foci in occipital lobe. The approach to foci outside the temporal lobe is handled in much the same manner as described above. However, as a general rule the more uncommon the location of the focus, the more need to approach its removal with the 'tailored' approach.

Case report

A 13-year-old right-handed white male was referred for consideration of surgery because of complex partial seizures that were refractory to Dilantin, Tegretol, Mysoline, and Depakene alone or in combination. His seizures had begun 3 years earlier. His growth and development had been normal. The family history was negative for epilepsy. His past medical history was negative for any factors contributory to the development of epilepsy.

His initial evaluation at the time of the onset of his seizure disorder included a normal physical and neurological examination, a normal CT scan, a normal lumbar puncture, normal routine blood analysis, and an EEG which showed some epileptiform discharges arising from the right temporal region.

He was admitted to the Epilepsy Center EEG/video monitoring ward, scalp electrodes were placed and sphenoidal electrodes inserted. His anticonvulsant medications were withdrawn. Three typical complex partial seizures were recorded. In each case the seizures clearly began from the right sphenoidal and anterior temporal electrodes on the right side. His neuropsychological evaluation was indicative of right temporal dysfunction. He and his family were offered the option of resection of his right temporal epileptogenic focus.

At surgery direct EEG recording from the right temporal lobe revealed only delta and theta activity from the lateral aspect with some epileptogenic spiking from the most mesial portions near the hippocampus. Immediately upon resection of the lateral portions of the temporal tip a tumour was found. This tumor was removed grossly, as was the hippocampus. Pathologic examination determined the tumour to be an oligodendroglioma.

Since surgery the patient has been seizure-free at 1 year follow-up. The patient will undergo repeat MRI scans every 6 months to follow the tumor for recurrence. At present there is no evidence for tumour progression.

Results of focal resections

If all major modern surgical series are combined, the results of cortical resections indicate that approximately 81 percent of people undergoing temporal lobectomy are improved from surgery, and many can eventually be withdrawn completely from drugs. Because the results of any one of these series can be influenced by different selection biases, it is impossible to determine if superior results are derived from the 'tailored' versus the 'en bloc' approaches. In Weiser and Yasargil's series of 102 patients they report that 93 percent of patients who were operated for conditions other than malignant tumor benefited from their selective amygdalohippocampectomy. This may represent a significant improvement in surgical approach, or it may represent a highly selected group of patients with restricted foci only within the mesial temporal lobe. In either case these results are excellent. Few surgical series have been confined to a pediatric sample until recently. Meyer, Marsh, Laws, and Sharbough (1986) reported a series of 50 children with temporal lobe epilepsy who were operated on at a mean age of 15.8 years (having had seizures for an average of 7.5 years). They report 54 percent seizure-free, 24 percent had occasional auras without loss of consciousness, 10 percent had fewer seizures, and 12 percent were unchanged. Therefore 78 percent were essentially seizure-free and 88 percent benefited significantly from the operation. Although they had no systematic measures, they reported significantly improved social outcome in most patients whose seizures were controlled by the surgery. They also reported that the shorter the gap from onset of epilepsy to surgery, the greater the gain in postoperative IQ.

Some surgeons have felt that the results of temporal lobe surgery are superior to resections which involve frontal, perirolandic, and parietal lobe (Talairach *et al.*, 1974). For epileptogenic foci outside the frontal or temporal lobe the results of surgery are not as good as temporal lobe surgery, with only about 55 percent of patients benefiting (Rasmussen, 1975).

The results of any surgical series are heavily influenced by the criteria used for selecting patients. For example, any surgeon who selects patients (1) who have foci in nondominant hemisphere, (2) with only focal discharges that never spread to involve the contralateral side, (3) who are of average intellegence, and (4) who are between the ages of 20 and 30 years, will have a series of patients that will demonstrate an excellent outcome from surgery. However, what do we do with the patients who have less than excellent odds for benefiting from surgery? For example, how should one proceed if depth EEG demonstrated a seizure origin near Wernicke's speech area, but propagation and maintenance of the seizure discharge always seemed to depend critically on mesiobasal limbic structures? Obviously the focus in such a case is located in an area of cortex which cannot be surgically removed without major deficits. In this example a mesial resection stands a reasonable chance of decreasing (but not totally controlling) the patient's seizures.

Recently, Wieser and Yasergil (1984) have introduced the term 'palliative' (vs. 'causal') resections. This term refers to cases in which the medically intractable seizures represent a severe handicap, and in which the surgery offers only a limited chance of possible amelioration and not complete cure.

Amost all surgical series have such patients included in them, and these cases 'dilute' the results. Two major points should therefore be made. First, after a comprehensive surgical workup patients can be identified as either good or poor candidates to have their seizures controlled or 'cured' with surgery. Therefore some patients will have a much better than average chance of successful surgery, whereas others will not. This should be considered prospectively in future surgical series so that accurate statistics can be generated as to the results of seizure surgery. Second, because some patients can be shown to be excellent candidates for surgery, this option should be given to them as soon as it is apparent that the major anticonvulsants have failed to achieve reasonable control of their seizures.

The morbidity associated with focal cortical excisions has been mild. Ablation of the nondominant temporal lobe results in subtle deficits in pattern recognition, visual and spatial memory, and some mild discrimination of tonal patterns. After dominant lobe resections there are often some mild word finding problems. In about 28 percent of my own patients I have found a degree of a quadrantanopsia, if the temporal resection is taken posterior to the tip of the ventricle. There is a small incidence of permanent hemiplegia after temporal lobectomy, and the incidence is probably less than 5 percent. (In many cases this is due to vasospasm of the middle cerebral artery.) The mortality rate from cortical resection is less than 1 percent. The morbidity associated with focal resections in other regions of brain is directly related to the function subserved by cortex removed. In general there is little morbidity with frontal resections; in fact a patient's performance may improve somewhat after successful removal of an active focus.

Hemispherectomy

In some patients epileptiform activity will not be confined to one lobe or focal region, but will be spread diffusely throughout an entire hemisphere. In some of these cases a hemispherectomy may be indicated. In my own series the most frequent indication is a patient with medically refractory seizures that were the sequelae of infantile hemiplegia. Removal of the entire hemisphere was introduced by Krynauw in 1950. However, complete hemispherectomy had a serious complication, a syndrome of superficial cerebral hemosiderosis (Oppenheimer and Griffith, 1966), and which occurred in about 25 percent of patients followed for 5 years. Although this complication can be treated by permanent ventriculoatrial shunt, it does increase the morbidity and mortality of the surgery. Preservation of a small portion of the hemisphere (i.e. occipital lobe) appears to prevent this complication (Rasmussen, 1975). In several of my own cases of infantile hemiplegia I have left the entire pre- and postcentral gyri.

Rasmussen (1975) reported a series of patients who underwent a complete hemispherectomy: 59 percent of patients were seizure-free after some early attacks, 26 percent were markedly improved, whereas 15 percent had a less good result. In that series (from 1952 through 1968), two of the patients operated early in this series died of progressive encephalopathy. Since that complication can be minimized by leaving some cortex behind, the mortality rate of this procedure can now be minimized.

Rasmussen also reported a series of 48 patients (from 1937 to 1972) who had removal of at least three lobes of the brain. In this series of subtotal hemispherectomy 45 percent were seizure-free (some after early attacks), 25 percent significant reductions in seizures, and 30 percent had only a 'moderate or less reduction of seizure tendency'. There was one postoperative death in their series of 48 patients. Thus, at least 70 percent of these patients were benefited by surgery.

Case report

A 13-year old white female was referred for consideration of surgery because of seizures which were not controlled with any of the standard anticonvulsant medications. She had three types of seizures. (1) She had frequent spells that were absence-like; i.e. she would simply stop and stare but had no automatisms nor movements. These spells would last for approximately 10 seconds with a short period of mild confusion afterwards. (2) She also had frequent myoclonic-like jerks during the day, and sometimes these were strong enough to cause her to fall. (3) The third type of seizure would begin with a blank stare and then progress to fumbling movements of the hands for several seconds before generalizing to a full tonic–clonic convulsion. She had two or three of these seizures per week under her best control with a combination of Tegretol and Dilantin.

Her family history was negative for epilepsy. Her birth had been uneventful. At age 7 months she had a febrile episode and had suddenly developed a permanent left hemiplegia. Her subsequent growth and development had been normal.

A CT scan demonstrated a cystic infarction of the right cerebral hemisphere in the distribution of the middle cerebral and posterior portions of the anterior cerebral arteries. CCTV/EEG monitoring with sphenoidal electrodes demonstrated frequent epileptiform discharges from both the right frontal pole and anterior temporal regions. At craniotomy direct cortical EEG recordings revealed areas of epileptogenic spiking emanating from the mesial temporal lobe and mesial frontal lobe. The frontal, temporal, and portions of the parietal lobe were resected, leaving the occipital pole intact. The patient has remained seizure-free for the 5 years of postoperative follow-up. In addition, she has been removed from all anticonvulsant drugs during the past 2 years.

Corpus callosum

Van Wagenen and Herren (1940) were the first to introduce the technique of corpus callosal section for treatment of epilspsy. Their rationale for performing this type of surgery was based on their observation that a patient with a tumour which had invaded the corpus callosum had a decreasing seizure frequency as the tumour grew and destroyed the callosum. Since then, many small surgical series have been reported in which the corpus callosum with or without other midline tracts such as the fornix, massa intermedia, anterior commissure and hippocampal commissure have been sectioned. The results in terms of morbidity and mortality have been variable (Bogen and Vogel, 1962; Gates, Leppik, Yap, and Grumnit, 1984; Geoffroy, Laffonde, and Delise, 1983; Huck *et al.*, 1980; Luessenhop, de la Cruz, and Fenichel, 1970; Rayport, Ferguson, and Corrie, 1983; Wilson, Reeves, and Gazzaniga, 1982). Early operations sectioned many of the midline tracts and often required more than one operation. As a result the morbidity was high, with complications such as hydrocephalus occurring in 50 percent of patients. Therefore, more limited operations have recently been proposed in which only the callosum is sectioned. Recent series with the more moderate surgical approach have demonstrated very acceptable morbidity with excellent psychosocial and cognitive outcome (Ferrell, Culver, and Tucker, 1983).

The indications for this surgery are not entirely clear. This is partly due to a lack of sufficiently large series of patients with clear diagnosis. Most published series are small and have a poorly defined group of patients. Gates *et al.* (1984) reported a group of six patients with epilepsy with generalized discharges and falling attacks who underwent total callosal section. Although no significant change in the number of generalized discharges could be found between the pre- and postoperative EEGs there was a significant decrease in the number of falling attacks. Spencer *et al.* (1984) have reported 'excellent' control of generalized seizures in most of 17 patients. However, in five of those patients more intense (although not necessarily more frequent) focal seizures occurred postoperatively. This occurred primarily in patients with EEG evidence of bilateral, bifrontal, independent, and asymmetrical foci.

If one combines all reports on this procedure, the concensus is that callosal section results in a significant reduction in generalized seizures in the majority of patients. Which types of generalized seizure disorders benefit the most is difficult to determine with precision, for those data are not available. However, this surgery does not benefit patients who suffer from true petit-mal epilepsy. In my own practice I have retained this procedure for patients with generalized discharges without any defined focus, and who have tonic, atonic, tonic–clonic, or clonic seizures. Patients with complex partial, or atypical, absence attacks and generalized discharges do not do well from this operation. The results have been quite satisfactory in significantly decreasing the numbers of attacks. However, the percentage of seizure-free patients is much less then from focal cortical resections.

Case report

An 8-year-old white female was referred for consideration of surgery. Her birth, growth, and development had been normal until age 9 months. She had been given a DPT immunization which had resulted in a severe neurological complication. She had total arrest on her neuropsychological development with the onset of tonic, tonic–clonic seizures and frequent drop attacks. Her drop attacks occurred so frequently during each day that she had to be confined to a protected environment. In addition, her drop attacks were regularly causing her head and facial injury. Because of this she had become a major management problem for the family. This, in turn, was having a negative effect upon the other two children in the family.

A CT scan was normal. CCTV/EEG monitoring demonstrated very frequent bilateral and synchronous spike and spike-wave discharges over the entire scalp distribution without any focality. She underwent sectioning of the anterior two-thirds of the corpus callosum. Postoperatively she had an approximately 80 percent reduction in seizure occurrence. Repeat EEGs showed frequent epileptiform discharges, but now they were not bilaterally synchronous in the anterior portions of the scalp. In addition to the improvement in seizure frequency she became more alert and was able to walk unassisted. Because of the persistence of some seizures it was elected to complete the callosum sectioning 9 months after the first sectioning. Since then she has had a further reduction, but still has two or three small seizures a week.

Although the patient is not entirely seizure-free, the frequency of seizures has been lowered by approximately 90 per cent with a decrease in severity of those that remain. A further benefit has been the improvement in alertness, a decrease in physical injury, and normalization of family interactions. Therefore, although the patient is not seizure-free, there has been a tremendous benefit to both patient and family from surgical intervention.

SUMMARY

The previous sections have shown that there are several surgical approaches available for treating a variety of different types of partial and generalized seizure disorders. For complex partial seizures of temporal lobe origin there is: (1) standard en bloc resection, (2) the 'tailored' resection, and (3) the selective amygdalohippocampectomy for those patients who have been shown to harbor an epileptogenic focus only in their mesial temporal lobe. For patients with extratemporal foci, variations on the 'tailored' resection are available. For patients with various types of primarily generalized epilepsies, the corpus callosum section has been refined so that it now provides excellent seizure reduction with acceptable morbidity. With increased use of prolonged EEG/ video monitoring more precision is being obtained in the preoperative localization of epileptogenic foci. For the patients with more difficult foci to localize, the techniques of intracranial depth electrodes or the newer subdural 'strip' electrodes are available, which can provide extremely valuable data upon which rational surgical decisions can be based. The introduction of CT scanning a little over a decade ago resulted in more accurate identification of pathological structural lesions that previously would not have been diagnosed with angiography and pneumoencephalography. The identification of such lesions has helped localize many epileptogenic lesions, and should improve the outcome of epilepsy surgery. It is too soon to determine the impact that MRI scanning will have upon seizure surgery, but one can predict that it will be positive. It is predicted that MRI scanning may well identify subtle structural lesions associated with temporal lobe foci, such as mesial temporal sclerosis and chronic mesial temporal herniation. With increasing diagnostic accuracy for localizing and classifying epileptogenic foci, we should see an increase in postoperative success. But we should also see an improvement in patient selection. For as pointed out by Spencer *et al.*, (1984), the use of intracranical recordings is also useful for determining the presence of multifocal diseases which will not respond to surgical excision.

In addition to improved diagnostic methods there have been many advances in surgical techniques. The increased use of the operating microscope has brought the introduction of new operative procedures such as the selective amygdalohippocampectomy which was unknown a decade ago. The use of the microscope for routine resection of mesial temporal structures, or for dividing the corpus callosum, as examples, has resulted in a decrease in the morbidity associated with surgery. The use of intraoperative neuropsychological testing will allow larger resections in some dominant temporal lobes with minimal postoperative deficits.

The mortality associated with craniotomy for epilepsy is extremely small and much less than 1 percent. This is due to several factors. First, the patients being operated upon are usually healthy and not suffering from an acute disease process (which is commonly the case with other neurosurgical operations). Second, the patients are usually young and do not have many secondary problems such as hypertension or diabetes which may predispose to complications. Third, many of the operations are done under local anesthesia, thereby precluding a major risk factor. The fact is that the mortality of this type of surgery is less than for many common abdominal surgeries.

Even though the results and morbidity of surgery have been improving, there is still a reluctance by many neurologists to refer patients for surgery. The reasons are many, but most hinge around the risk of surgery compared to medication. However, the risk of medications is not insignificant, and can be just as great as surgery if the patient suffers irreversible bone marrow suppression or liver destruction. And just as surgery is not reversible, neither is cerebellar degeneration from phenytoin toxicity. In addition, patients who do not have their seizures controlled are at higher risk for (1) sudden death (Wannamaker, 1985); (2) neuronal deterioration; and (3) adverse neuropsychological effects from multiple drugs. The fact is that surgery is three times more effective in controlling seizures in patients who have been refractory to medication. Moreover, criteria for identifying prospectively those patients who are candidates for 'palliative' or 'causal' resections has increased considerably. As a consequence, it may be that in good surgical candidates the chances of an excellent result may approach the 93 percent level reported by Wieser and Yasergil. If this is the case then one is no longer justified in keeping the option of surgery from good candidates, for the results of surgery become far better than the chances that further combination of drugs will control the seizures. Even for those patients in whom it is most likely that only a 'palliative' resection can be done, the morbidity and mortality of modern epilepsy surgery is acceptable to the point that surgery should not be considered as the last of all options to be tried.

REFERENCES

Bancaud, J., Talairach, J., Bonis, A., Schaub, C., Szikla, G., Morel P., and Bordas-Ferrer, M. (1965). *La stereo-electroencephalographie dans l'epilepsie*. Masson, Paris.

Bogen, J.E., and Vogel, P.J. (1962). Cerebral commissurotomy in man. *Bulletin of the Los Angeles Neurological Society*, **27**, 169–172.

Dodrill, C.B., Wilkus, R.J., Ojemann, G.A., Ward, A.A. Jr, Wyler, A.R., van Belle, G., and Tamas, L. (1986). Multidisciplinary prediction of seizure relief from cortical resection surgery. *Annals of Neurology*, **20**, 2–12.

Dodrill, C.B. (1986). Correlates of generalized tonic-clonic seizures with intellectual, neuropsychological, emotional, and social function in patients with epilepsy. *Epilepsia*, **27**, 399–411.

Ferrell, R.B., Culver, C.M., and Tucker, G.J. (1983). Psychosocial and cognitive function after commissurotomy for intractable seizures. *Journal of Neurosurgery*, **58**, 374–380.

Gates, J.R., Leppik, I.E., Yap, J., and Gumnit, R.J. (1984) Corpus callosotomy: clinical and electroencephalographic effects. *Epilepsia*, **25**, 308–16.

Geoffroy, G.M., Lassonde, F., and Delise, M. (1983). Corpus callosotomy for control of intractable epilepsy in children. *Neurology*, **33**, 891–897.

Goldring, S., and Gregorie, E.M. (1984) Surgical management of epilepsy using epidural electrodes to localize the seizure focus. Review of 100 cases. *Journal of Neurosurgery*, **60**, 457–66.

Hauser, W.A., Annegers, J.F., and Elveback, L.R. (1980) Mortality in patients with epilepsy. *Epilepsia*, **21**, 399–412.

Huck, F.R., Radvany, J., Avila Jo Pires de Camargo, C.H., Marino, R. Jr, Ragazzo, P.C., Riva D., and Arlant, P. (1980). Anterior callosotomy in epileptics with multiform seizures and bilateral synchronous spike and wave EEG pattern. *Acta Neurochirurgica* (Suppl.), **30**, 127–135.

Krynauw, R.A. (1950) Infantile hemiplegia treated by removing one cerebral hemisphere. *Journal of Neurology, Neurosurgery and Psychiatry*, **13**, 243–267.

Luessenhop. A.J., de la Cruz, T.C., and Fenichel, G.M. (1970). Surgical disconnection of the cerebral hemispheres for intractable seizures. Results in infancy and childhood. *Journal of the American Medical Association*, **213**, 1630–1636.

Meyer, F.B., Marsh, W.R., Laws, E.R., and Sharbough, F.W. (1986). Temporal lobectomy in children with epilepsy. *Journal of Neurosurgery*, **64**, 371–376.

Oppenheimer, D.R., and Griffith, H.B. (1966) Persistent intracranial bleeding as a complication of hemispherectomy. *Journal of Neurology, Neurosurgery and Psychiatry*, **29**, 229–240.

Penfield, W., and Jasper, H. (1954). *Epilepsy and the Functional Anatomy of the Human Brain*. Little, Brown & Co. Boston, MA.

Rasmussen, T. (1975). Surgery for epilepsy arising in regions other than the temporal and frontal lobes. In D.P. Purpura, J.K. Penry, and R.D. Walter (eds), *Advances in Neurology*, vol. 8, Raven Press, New York, pp. 207–226.

Rayport, M., Ferguson, S.M., and Corrie, W.S. (1983). Outcomes and indications of corpus callosum section for intractable seizure control. *Applied Neurophysiology*, **46**, 47–51.

Rosenbaum, T.J., Laxer, K.D., Vessely, M., and Smith, B.W. (1986). Subdural electrodes for seizure focus localization. *Neurosurgery*, **19**, 73–81.

Spencer, S.S., Spencer, D.D., Glaser, G.H., Williamson, P.D., and Mattson, R.H. (1984). More intense focal seizure type after callosal section: the role of inhibition. *Annals of Neurology*, **16**, pp. 686–93.

Spencer, D.D., Spencer, S.S., Mattson, R.H., Novelly, R.A., and Williamson, P.D. (1984). Access to the posterior temporal lobe structures in the surgical treatment of temporal lobe epilepsy. *Neurosurgery*, **15**, 667–671.

Spencer, S.S. (1981). Depth electroencephalography in selection of refractory epilepsy for surgery. *Annals of Neurology*, **9**, 207–214.

Sperling, M.R., Mendius, J.R., and Engle, J. Jr (1986). Mesial temporal spikes: a simultaneous comparison of sphenoidal, nasopharyngeal, and ear electrodes. *Epilepsia*, **27**, 81–86.

Sperling, M.R., Wilson, G., Engel, J. Jr, Babb, T.L., and Croudall, P. (1986). Magnetic resonance imaging in intractable partial epilepsy: correlative studies. *Annals of Neurology*, **20**, 57–62.

Talairach, J., Bancuad, J., Szikla, G. *et al.* (1974) Approache nouvelle de lar neurochirugie de l'epilepsie. Methodologie stereotaxique et resultats therapeutiques. *Neurochirurgie*, Suppl. 20, 1–240.

van Wagenen, W.P., and Herren, R.Y. (1940). Surgical division of commissural pathways in the corpus callosum. Relation to spread of an epileptic attack. *Archives of Neurology*, **44**, 740–759.

Wada, J., and Rasmussen, T. (1952). Intracarotid injection of sodium Amytal for the lateralization of speech dominance. Experimental and clinical observations. *Journal of Neurosurgery*, **17**, 266–282.

Wannamaker, B.B. (1985). Autonomic nervous system and epilepsy. *Epilepsia*, **26**, Suppl. 1, S31–39.

Wilson, D.H., Reeves, A.G., and Gazzaniga, M.S. (1982). 'Central' commissurotomy for intractable generalized epilepsy: series two. *Neurology (NY)*, **32**, 687–97.

Wieser, H.G., and Yasargil, G. (1984). Selective amygdalohippocampectomy as a surgical treatment of mediobasal limbic epilepsy. *Surgical Neurology*, **17**, 445–457.

Wyler, A.R., Ojemann, G.A., Lettich, E. and Ward, A.A. Jr (1984). Subdural strip electrodes for localizing epileptogenic foci. *Journal of Neurosurgery*, **60**, 1195–1200.

Chapter 12

Behavioral Medicine Approaches to Enhancing Seizure Control in Children with Epilepsy

David E. Schotte and M. Andrew DuBois

The importance of establishing seizure control in children with epilepsy, particularly at the outset of treatment, is highlighted by the fact that the occurrence of seizures may predispose to further seizures, and that early effective treatment may be essential in averting the development and psychosocial concomitants of chronic, more intractable epilepsy (Shorvon and Reynolds, 1982). Thus, the primary goal for the treatment of children with epilepsy is the early establishment of maximal seizure control. Unfortunately, remission of seizures is difficult to obtain (Trachtenberg, 1983) and research suggests that anticonvulsant medication is ineffective in achieving complete remission of seizures in approximately two-thirds of those with epilepsy (DeVivo, 1983).

The purpose of the present chapter is to present an overview of the potential contributions of behavioral medicine approaches as adjunctive strategies for enhancing seizure control in children with epilepsy. In particular, we will discuss research in behavioral medicine which focuses on enhancing patient compliance to complex treatement regimens and recent advances in adjunctive behavioral approaches (i.e. relaxation and biofeedback) to seizure control.

COMPLIANCE

Poor adherence to medical regimens is a problem common to the pharmacologic management of all medical disorders, both acute and chronic. For example, patients with chronic illnesses miss from 20 to 50 percent of scheduled physician appointments, and approximately 50 percent of patients with chronic illnesses do not take their medication in accord with physician instructions (Sackett, 1976). Even in disorders such as epilepsy, where nonadherence may

Childhood Epilepsies: Neuropsychological, Psychosocial and Intervention Aspects
Edited by B. Hermann and M. Seidenberg

result in clear aversive consequences (i.e. seizure activity), compliance may be poor. In fact, poor compliance appears to be the most frequent cause of non-therapeutic serum anticonvulsant levels (Masland, 1982).

Unfortunately, research suggests that physicians overestimate the degree of compliance among their patients, and that they are unable to accurately predict the likelihood of a patient adhering to treatment recommendations (Caron and Roth, 1968; Mushlin and Appel, 1977). Gilbert, Evans, Haynes, and Tugwell (1980), for example, found that physicians were unable to predict compliance to digoxin therapy in cardiology patients at levels better than chance, even in patients who they had known for more than 5 years. Attempts by physicians to predict the compliance of children to acute medication regimens on the basis of perceived characteristics of the mother result in equally low levels of prediction (Charney *et al.*, 1967). Physicians once tended to ascribe such poor compliance to patient personality characteristics. However, research has failed to obtain a relationship between levels of patient adherence and patient personality variables (Haynes, Taylor and Sackett, 1979).

Although questioning the patient may provide a face valid means for assessing adherence to the prescribed medication regimen, it is important to note that patient interviews tend to overestimate compliance. For example, Haynes *et al.* (1976) were able to identify only 50 percent of poor compliers in a hypertensive treatment program by interview, and Park and Lipman (1964) found that only half of noncompliers were willing to admit this to the prescriber. Research on the relationship between pill counts and patient self-reports further suggests that inaccurate reporting is most frequent for minor deviations from prescribed regimens (Rickels and Briscol, 1970). Those who admit to poor adherence, however, may be particularly responsive to programs aimed at improving compliance (Sackett, 1979).

Despite the limited amount of literature available on compliance to medication regimens among those afflicted with epilepsy, it appears that poor adherence to anticonvulsant regimens is common. For example, in a large sample of adolescents and adults with temporal lobe epilepsy treated at the London Hospital, 3 percent reported having discountinued their medication against medical advice despite ongoing seizure activity, and 75 percent admitted to 'irregular' compliance (Currie, Heathfield, Henson, and Scott, 1971).

Similarly, in a study of teenaged and young adults with epilepsy, Peterson, McLean and Millingen (1982) found that nearly 50 percent reported missing at least one dosage of antiepileptic medication each month, and 5 percent had no detectable anticonvulsant in their blood. In general, patients with generalized tonic–clonic seizures or frequent seizure activity appeared to be more compliant with their medication regimens than were patients with focal or less frequent seizures. When patients were questioned about noncompliance with medication prescriptions, the reasons reported most frequently were the 'inconvenience' of taking medication and 'forgetfulness.'

From a behavioral perspective the likelihood that a behavior (e.g. medication-taking) will be engaged in is determined by its antecedent conditions, characteristics of the behavior itself, and the nature and temporal sequencing of the consequences of the behavior. Thus, characteristics of the patient's medical condition, of the medication prescribed, and of the treatment regimen itself can be expected to influence the level of patient adherence. For example, the chronicity of the disorder or its treatment, the complexity of the treatment regimen, the saliency of cues for taking medication, the presence or absence of aversive side-effects of the medication, and the occurrence, valence, and temporal sequencing of the consequences for taking medication can be important factors in determining patient compliance (Zifferblatt, 1975).

Disorders and treatments which require chronic adherence to medication regimens (e.g. epilepsy) are likely to result in poor compliance among significant numbers of patients, especially if such nonadherence is associated with only sporadic aversive consequences (Haynes *et al.*, 1976). For example, in the Peterson *et al*, (1982) study, the patients with less frequent or less pronounced seizures (e.g. those with either infrequent or focal seizures) had the lowest rates of compliance. From a behavioural perspective this is not surprising, as there are the patients for whom the negative consequences of not taking medication, when they occur, are the least aversive.

In addition, more complex treatment regimens, such as those requiring multiple daily dosages or multiple medications, can also be expected to result in poorer compliance, particularly in the absence of salient cues for taking the medication (Epstein and Cluss, 1982). Thus, if a patient is required to take multiple medications at a number of times throughout the day, such as is typically the case in epilepsy, then the patient is more likely to inadvertently miss required doses. In such cases the absence of salient stimuli which remind the patient to take medication (e.g. aversive interoceptive events, such as pain, or salient environmental cues or prompts) make missed doses more likely.

In addition, because anticonvulsants do not tend to alleviate ongoing aversive stimuli, and are not generally associated with pleasant physiological effects, as are some medications (e.g. minor tranquilizers or analgesics), their reinforcement value, either positive or negative, is low. Compliance with anticonvulsant regimens, therefore, may be improved by increasing the reinforcing value of taking medication. In the child this can be accomplished through the use of programs whereby appropriate medication usage results in the delivery of external reinforcers.* At the outset of such programs the reinforces (e.g. points or tokens which may be exchanged for toys or money) should be delivered immediately, and prompts to take medication at the appropriate time may be required. As time on the program progresses, and when good control over the behavior has been established, prompts may be

* A useful parent guide with a summary and explanation of procedures for implementing operant programs to shape children's behavior is available from Research Press (see Patterson, 1975).

gradually faded out and reinforcers may be more delayed, or can be gradually replaced with social reinforcers, such as praise. Punishment for failure to take medication(s) should *not* be a part of such programs, as research suggests that punitive approaches are associated with lower rates of compliance among children on anticonvulsant regimens (Hauck, 1972). Often, the use of a publicly displayed chart, documenting medication taking and reinforcers earned, can heighten the effects of reinforcement programs and can serve as a salient environmental cue for prompting the parents to maintain the program. In addition to increasing compliance with the medication regimen, such programes can provide a useful and effective mechanism for training the child in medication self-management.

Careful assessment of potential barriers to medication compliance can be accomplished through interviews with the parent(s) and child. Such interviews can be used to identify concerns about the medication or its side-effects, and to explicate other perceptions on the part of the parent(s) or child which might make them reluctant to follow the prescribed regimen. Discussion of these issues can also be used to identify erroneous beliefs about epilepsy or its treatment which might be held by the parent(s) or child. The physician should not assume that the parent(s) or child hold the same values regarding the purpose and goals or treatment, or that they understand the importance and benefit of effective early management. Rather, the physician should utilize such discussions as a forum for education and reassurance of parent(s) and child. Provision of written material detailing educational topics is also recommended as this will aid patient retention of information.

Increasing the salience of environmental cues, such as through the use of specialized medication containers or medication diaries may serve to promote better adherence to such complex medication regimens (c.f. Zifferblatt, 1975). Low-cost medication containers with built-in alarms which signal the time at which doses are to be taken are now available at most pharmacies (e.g. the Electronic Pill Box Timer, Alaron Incorporated, Troy, MI). In addition, medication diaries can be fabricated easily and kept on hand for distribution to patients. When medication diaries are used, however, it is important that both the parent(s) and the prescriber review the diary regularly, to ensure that its salience and usage continue to be maintained. The child should complete the diary at the time at which medication is taken, and should record at the end of the day the occurrence of any missed doses. Having the child also note seizure activity in the diary can provide useful information to the physician, and may serve to provide the child with regular feedback on the importance of taking medication.

Adherence to complex schedules may also be increased by pairing medication-taking with salient routines in the child's daily activities, such as tooth brushing, eating meals, or other regular events (Zifferblatt, 1975). When this approach is used, it is important that the events selected occur on a regular and predictable basis which is in accord with the pharmacologic requirements of the medication(s) prescribed. The events themselves also need to be sufficiently salient to ensure that they serve as effective antecedents to medication taking. Simply recommending such an approach to the parent or child is not sufficient. Instead, the prescriber or an assistant will need to work with the patient to develop an appropriate schedule, to monitor subsequent adherence to the schedule over time, and to modify the program as needed.

Multiple medications also increase the probability of unpleasant side-effects (Reynolds and Travers, 1974), thereby resulting in negative consequences for medication ingestion. In the absence of positively or negatively reinforcing events which precede or outweigh unpleasant side-effects (e.g. response-contingent pleasant effects or the cessation of ongoing, unpleasant interoceptive stimuli), such iatrogenic effects of medication taking tend to decrease the likelihood of good adherence. Thus, minimizing side-effects through careful titration of medication dosages, and using the fewest possible medications, are crucial to promoting effective compliance with drug therapies.

A number of researchers (c.f. Epstein and Cluss, 1982) have demonstrated that such relatively simple techniques can improve the level of patient adherence to chronic medication regimes. Peterson, McLean, and Millingen (1984), for example, were able to halve seizure frequency and increase plasma medication levels among outpatient teenagers and adults with epilepsy through a program which included patient education, self-monitoring of medication intake and seizure frequency, usage of a daily medication container, and mailed reminders to patients who did not refill prescriptions as expected. In their program, patient counseling included education about the importance and goals of anticonvulsant medication and the importance of regular compliance with medication schedules. Patients were also assisted in matching their medication schedule to salient aspects of their daily routine. In addition, patients were provided with a specialized medication container which allowed them to check each evening for compliance during the day. They were asked to examine their medication container for unused medication each night, to record their adherence in a daily medication log, and to report on the occurrence of seizure activity during the preceding 24 hours. To facilitate medication prescription refills, the dates on which patients were scheduled to refill their prescriptions were determined, and patients who had not refilled them through the hospital pharmacy by that date were mailed a reminder. Mailed reminders were also used to improve attendance at scheduled clinic appointments. The interested reader may obtain copies of all materials used in this study by contacting the investigators (see Peterson, McLean and Millingen, 1984).

Increasing patient adherence to anticonvulsant medication regimes is one of the most promising and cost-effective approaches to reducing seizure frequency in the epileptic child. Such programs, if incorporated routinely into patient care, can maximize the efficacy of pharmacologic management of epilepsy. In addition, behavioral techniques such as those we have described may be used to teach the child medication self-management skills.

Unfortunately, research in this area has been limited to adolescent populations and may not, therefore, generalize to the younger child or to those with developmental disabilities. Research on medication self-management in diabetics (e.g. Epstein *et al.*, 1981; Lowe and Lutzker, 1979), whose medication regimens may be similarly complex, however, suggests that the techniques we have described may be suitable for the preteen. In the case of very young children, or those with moderate to profound mental retardation, compliance programs should target the caregiver.

RELAXATION AND BIOFEEDBACK

Virtually all neuroelectrical events that can be recorded have now been used in the operant conditioning paradigm (Elbert and Rockstroh, 1984). In the effort to control epileptic seizures, biofeedback studies have focused most frequently on increasing voluntary control of the 'sensory-motor' rhythm (SMR: Feldman, Ricks, and Orren, 1983). SMR is a 12–15 Hz frequency signal assumed to originate in the lateral thalamic nuclei. SMR is most clearly observed during periods of alert relaxation and is also apparent during slow-wave sleep as the sleep spindle or mu rhythm (Sterman, 1984).

In early research with animals, Sterman and his colleagues (Sterman, 1976, 1977; Sterman, Goodman, & Kovalesky, 1978) demonstrated that operantly conditioned increases in SMR were associated with increased resistance to drug-induced seizures. Other investigators have replicated these findings in animals (c.f. Lubar, 1984) and recent research suggests that SMR training may be an effective adjunctive approach to increasing seizure control in humans (Finley, 1976; Finley, Smith, and Etherton, 1975; Mostofsky and Balaschak, 1977; Feldman *et al.*, 1983; Sterman, 1984).

Finley and his colleagues (Finley, 1976; Finley *et al.*, 1975), for example, provided SMR biofeedback training to a 13-year-old boy with a high frequency of atonic seizures which had proven refractory to pharmacologic management. During feedback training the presence of SMR activity (12 ± 1 Hz) was indicated by a tone and a blue light, and the boy was reinforced with points, exchangeable for monetary reward, for every 5 seconds of continuous SMR activity. As training progressed, additional feedback was provided on the presence of epileptiform activity through the use of a red light. Biofeedback training resulted in marked increases in SMR activity, dramatic reductions in seizure frequency (from approximately 75 to less than 10 per 10 hour wake period), and significant reductions in epileptiform activity. In a subsequent single-blind withdrawal phase, during which sham biofeedback was instituted, SMR activity decreased, seizures became more frequent, and epileptiform discharges increased. Thus, providing false feedback appeared to result in a substantial reduction in treatment effects. A subsequent return to active treatment, however, resulted in the reinstatement of treatment gains. Non-specific effects of treatment (e.g. expectancies), therefore, did not appear to be responsible for the observed improvements in seizure control.

Sterman (1984) has demonstrated that significant reductions in the frequency of psychomotor seizures can also be obtained through SMR biofeedback training. Using an ingenious feedback paradigm, Sterman was able to reduce seizure frequency by 53 percent in 24 drug-refractory patients who presented with stable, long-term seizure histories. In his training procedure, SMR conditioning was accomplished through the use of a video soccer game operated by the patient's own somatosensory EEG. During the game the patient could advance the soccer ball toward the opposing goal, and thereby score points, by maintaining 12–15 cps EEG activity. When 4–7 cps activity was registered (in the absence of muscle artifact or spike-waves), however, the opposition would score. The game was divided into four 7-minute quarters, with 1-minute rest periods between quarters, yielding a 31-minute training session.

The entertaining nature of Sterman's (1984) procedure suggests that it might be ideally suited to the special requirements of biofeedback training with children. In addition, Lantz and Sterman (1988) have recently provided evidence that biofeedback-induced improvements in seizure control are accompanied by enhanced cognitive and motor funcion. Thus the beneficial effects of focused behavioral treatment may generalize to other aspects of central nervous system functioning.

It is not clear, however, that the efficacy of such approaches is dependent on the use of biofeedback technology *per se*. In fact, Wyler (1984) has suggested that the increases in SMR which occur during biofeedback training may result from the decreases in afferent thalamic activation which accompany muscular relaxation. If this is the case, then increases in SMR and enhanced seizure control should be attainable through muscular relaxation training alone.

In accord with Wyler's (1984) hypothesis, several groups of investigators (Dahl, Melin, Brorson, and Schollin, 1985; Rousseau, Hermann, and Whitman, 1985) have demonstrated that relaxation training is effective in reducing seizure frequency and that cue-controlled relaxation may be used to preempt seizure onset in those whose seizures are preceded by predictable physical sensations (Ince, 1976; Wells, Turner, Bellack, and Hersen, 1978).

Ince (1976), for example, used training in cue-controlled relaxation to treat a 12-year-old boy who had a 4-year history of grand- and petit-mal seizures which were poorly controlled by medication. A tape-recorded relaxation procedure (described as pseudo-hypnotic) was used and the child was instructed to repeat the word 'relax' ten times at the end of each practice episode. The child was then instructed to use the word 'relax', a conditioned stimulus for inducing relaxation, whenever he experienced prodromal seizure symptoms (i.e. whenever he felt the onset of a seizure approaching). Training included therapist-guided practice within sessions and twice-daily home practice. Sessions were conducted once each week over a 3-month period. Prior to treatment the child was experiencing nine to ten grand-mal and 25 to 26 petit-mal seizures per week. Seizure frequency decreased rapidly during the course of treatment, and by the end of therapy grand mal seizures were controlled and petit-mal episodes had been reduced to three or four per week. Petit-mal seizures subsided during follow-up and at last evaluation the boy had been free of seizures of either type for 9 months. Parenthetically, additional behavioral treatment (i.e. systematic desnsitization) was highly successful in reducing sceondary symptoms of social anxiety and school phobia arising from the boy's seizure history.

Rousseau *et al.* (1985) have also reported on the enhancement of seizure control through relaxation training. In their series of cases, Rousseau *et al.* treated eight patients (aged 19–32 years) who, despite the use of anticonvulsants, had evidenced at least six seizures during a 3-week baseline period. Both therapist-guided relaxation procedures and a commercially available audio-tape (Goleman, 1976) were used to train patients in Bernstein and Borkovec's (1973) differential relaxation procedure. The training itself consisted of only one session with the therapist, followed by 3 weeks of twice-daily home practice with the audio-tape. This minimal cost intervention resulted in a 53 percent reduction in mean seizure frequency. Unfortunately, no follow-up data are reported.

The use of a broader-based behavioral treatment program to treat children with medication-refractory epilepsy has been reported by Dahl *et al.* (1985). These investigators used self-monitoring of seizures and antecedent conditions (e.g. prodromal signs) to identify seizure precursors and to provide situations for teaching the child, through role playing, to relax in the presence of early-warning signals. In addition, Dahl *et al.* worked with the parents and teachers to reduce inadvertent operant reinforcement of seizures. This was accomplished by teaching the child's parents and teachers to deal with seizures in an emotionally neutral fashion. This 6-week program resulted in substantial reductions in a combined measure of seizure frequency and duration. Untreated children in waiting list and attention-placebo control groups, however, did not display significant improvements in seizure control. Furthermore, follow-up assessment data demonstrated that treatment gains were well-maintained over time.

Wells *et al.* (1978) have obtained similarly positive gains in seizure control through cue-controlled relaxation training with a 13-year-old girl of 'borderline' intelligence whose seizures were poorly controlled by medication. Behavioral treatment conducted in a group format, however, does not appear to be effective in reducing seizure frequency (Tan and Bruni, 1986). Thus, such approaches appear to be most effective when training is conducted on an individual basis. Individual therapy also allows for a more detailed assessment of triggering events, which can then be used to tailor the treatment to the patient's needs.

At the present time, long-term follow-up data (i.e. greater than 1 year) on the maintenance of treatment effects is lacking. In addition, although relaxation programs for younger children, and children with special needs, are available (e.g. Cautela and Groden, 1978), studies of biofeedback and relaxation training for control of epilepsy have not tended to include younger children. Research directed toward remediation of these limitations would probably serve to increase the acceptance and use of these techniques as adjuncts to traditional pharmacologic approaches.

SUMMARY

The primary goal for treatment of children with epilepsy is the early establishment of maximal seizure control. Unfortunately, significant numbers of patients are unable to achieve satisfactory remission of seizures through pharmacotherapy alone. Recent research suggests that, in such cases, behavioral techniques may serve as useful adjuncts to anticonvulsant medication.

Noncompliance with anticonvulsant medication regimens appears to be one of the most common causes of poor seizure control, and the research we have discussed here suggests that behavioral programs for improving patient adherence can be highly effective in reducing seizure frequency. Such programs, if incorporated routinely into patient care, can maximize the efficacy of pharmacologic management of epilepsy. In addition, these techniques provide a useful means for teaching the child medication self-management skills.

Even the compliant patient, however, may prove refractory to medication management. In this case clinical research suggests that adjunctive behavioral therapies, such as relaxation or biofeedback training, are effective in reducing seizure frequency. Although no comparative studies are available, it appears that positive results may be obtained using either relaxation or biofeedback treatments. Thus, relaxation training may be the more cost-effective, adjunctive strategy.

Focused behavioral programs for enhancing seizure control may contribute to functional improvements in other areas, including cognitive and motor function. In addition, behavioral techniques can be used to alleviate secondary conditions (e.g. social anxiety or school phobia) which limit the child's social or educational functioning. Taken together, the findings discussed in this chapter support the utility of broad-based behavioral assessment and treatment of children with epilepsy.

REFERENCES

Bernstein, D.A., and Borkovec, T.D. (1973). *Progressive Relaxation Training: A Manual for the Helping Professions*, Research Press, Champaign, IL.

Caron, H.W., and Roth, H.P. (1968). Patients' cooperation with a medical regimen. *Journal of the American Medical Association*, **203**, 922–926.

Cautela, J.R., and Groden, J. (1978). *Relaxation: Comprehensive Manual for Adults, Children, and Children with Special Needs*, Research Press, Champaign, IL.

Cerkoney, A.B., and Hart, K. (1980). The relationship between the health belief model and compliance of persons with diabetes mellitus. *Diabetes Care*, **3**, 594–598.

Charney, E., Bynum, R., Eldredge, D., Frank, O., MacWhinney, J.B., McNabb, N., Scheiner, A., Sumpter, E.A., and Iker, H. (1967). How well do patients take oral penicillin? A collaborative study in private practice. *Pediatrics*, **40**, 188–192.

Currie, S., Heathfield, K.W.G., Henson, R.A., and Scott, D.F. (1971). Clinical course and prognosis of temporal lobe epilepsy: a survey of 666 patients. *Brain*, **94**, 173–190.

Dahl, J., Melin, L., Brorson, L., and Schollin, J. (1985). Effects of a broad-spectrum behavior modification treatment program on children with refractory epileptic seizures. *Epilepsia*, **26**, 303–309.

DeVivo, D.C. (1983). How to use other drugs (steroids) and the ketogenic diet. In P.L. Morselli, C.E. Pippenger, and J.K. Penry (eds), *Antiepileptic Drug Therapy in Pediatrics*, Raven Press, New York, pp. 283–292.

Ebert, T., and Rockstroh, B. (1984). Classification and overview of CNS electrical activity tested on operant conditioning. In T. Ebert, B. Rockstroh, W. Lutzenberger, and N. Birbaumer (eds), *Self-regulation of the Brain and Behavior*, Springer, Heidelberg.

Epstein, L.H., and Cluss, P.A. (1982). A behavioral medicine perspective on adherence to long-term medical regimens. *Journal of Consulting and Clinical Psychology*, **50**, 950–971.

Epstein, L.H., Beck, S., Figueroa, J., Farkas, G., Kazdin, A.E., Daneman, D., and Becker, D. (1981). The effects of targeting improvements in urine glucose on metabolic control in children with insulin dependent diabetes. *Journal of Applied Behavior Analysis*, **14**, 365–375.

Feldman, R.G., Ricks, N.L., and Orren, M.M. (1983). Behavioral methods of seizure control. In T.R. Browne and R.G. Feldman (eds), *Epilepsy: Diagnosis and Management*, Little, Brown, Boston, MA, pp. 269–279.

Finley, W.W. (1976). Effects of sham feedback following successful SMR training in an epileptic: follow-up study. *Biofeedback and Self-Regulation*, **1**, 227–235.

Finley, W.W., Smith, H.A., and Etherton, M.D. (1975). Reduction of seizures and normalization of the EEG in a severe epileptic following sensorimotor biofeedback training: Preliminary study. *Biological Psychology*, **2**, 189–203.

Gilbert, J.R., Evans, C.E., Haynes, R.B., and Tugwell, P. (1980). Predicting compliance with a regimen of digoxin therapy in family practice. *Canadian Medical Association Journal*, **123**, 119–122.

Goleman, D. (1976). *Deep Relaxation*, Psychology Today (cassette), New York.

Hauck, G. (1972). Sociological aspects of epilepsy research. *Epilepsia*, **13**, 79–85.

Haynes, R.B., Sackett, D.L., Gibson, E.S., Taylor, D.W., Hackett, B.C., Roberts, R.S., and Johnson, A.L. (1976). Improvement of medication compliance in uncontrolled hypertension. *Lancet*, **1**, 1265–1268.

Haynes, R.B., Taylor, O.W., and Sackett, D. (1979) (eds), *Compliance in Health Care*, Baltimore, Johns Hopkins University Press.

Ince, L.P. (1976). The use of relaxation training and a conditioned stimulus in the elimination of epileptic seizures in a child: a case study. *Journal of Behavior Therapy and Experimental Psychiatry*, **7**, 39–42.

Lantz, D., and Sterman, M.B. (1988). Neuropsychological assessment of subjects with uncontrolled epilepsy: effects of EEG feedback training. *Epilepsia*, **29**, 163–171.

Lowe, K., and Lutzker, J.R. (1979). Increasing compliance to a medical regimen with a juvenile diabetic. *Behavior Therapy*, **10**, 57–64.

Lubar, J.F. (1984). Applications of operant conditioning of the EEG for the management of epileptic seizures. In T. Ebert, B. Rockstroh, W. Lutzenberger, and N. Birbaumer (eds), *Self-regulation of the Brain and Behavior*, Springer, Heidelberg, pp. 107–205.

Masland, R. (1982). The nature of epilepsy. In H. Sands (ed.), *Epilepsy: A Handbook for the Mental Health Professional*, Brunner/Mazel, New York, pp. 5–57.

Mostofsky, D.I., and Balaschak, B.A. (1977). Psychobiological control of seizures. *Psychological Bulletin*, **84**, 723–750.

Mushlin, A.I., and Appel, F.A. (1977). Diagnosing patient noncompliance. *Archives of Internal Medicine*, **137**, 318–321.

Park, L.C., and Lipman, R.S. (1964). A comparison of patient dosage deviation reports with pill counts. *Psychopharmacologie*, **6**, 299–302.

Patterson, G.R. (1975). *Families: Applications of Social Learning to Family Life*, Research Press, Champaign, IL.

Peterson, G.M., McLean, S., and Millingen, K.S. (1982). Determinants of patient compliance with anticonvulsant therapy. *Epilepsia*, **23**, 607–613.

Peterson, G.M., McLean, S., and Millingen, K.S. (1984). A randomized trial of strategies to improve patient compliance with anticonvulsant therapy. *Epilepsia*, **25**, 412–417.

Reynolds, E.H., and Travers, R.D. (1974). Serum anticonvulsant concentrations in epileptic patients with mental symptoms. *British Journal of Psychiatry*, **124**, 440–445.

Rickels, K., and Briscol, E. (1970). Assessment of dosage deviation in outpatient drug research. *Journal of Clinical Pharmacology*, **10**, 153–160.

Rousseau, A., Hermann, B., and Whitman, S. (1985). Effects of progressive relaxation on epilepsy: Analysis of a series of cases. *Psychological Reports*, **57**, 1203–1212.

Sackett, D.L. (1976). The magnitude of compliance and non-compliance. In D.L. Sackett and R.B. Haynes (eds), *Compliance with Therapeutic Regimes*, Jossey-Bass, San Francisco, pp. 189–215.

Sackett, D. (1979). The hypertensive patient: 5. Compliance with therapy. *Canadian Medical Association Journal*, **121**, 259–261.

Shorvon, S.D., and Reynolds, E.H. (1982). Early prognosis of epilepsy. *British Medical Journal*, **285**, 1699–1701.

Sterman, M.B. (1976). Effects of brain surgery and EEG operant conditioning on seizure latency following monoethyhydrazine intoxication in the cat. *Experimental Neurology*, **50**, 757–765.

Sterman, M.B. (1977). Sensorimotor operant conditioning: experimental and clinical effects. *Pavlovian Journal of Biological Science*, **12**, 63–90.

Sterman, M.B. (1984). The role of sensorimotor rhythmic EEG activity in the treatment of generalized motor seizures. In T. Ebert, B. Rockstroh, W. Lutzenberger, and N. Birbaumer (eds), *Self-regulation of the Brain and Behavior*, Springer, Heidelberg, pp. 11–19.

Sterman, M.B., Goodman, S.J., and Kovalesky, R.A. (1978). Effects of sensorimotor EEG feedback training on seizure susceptibility in the Rhesus monkey. *Experimental Neurology*, **62**, 735–747.

Tan, S., and Bruni, J. (1986). Cognitive-behavior therapy with adult patients with epilepsy: a controlled outcome study. *Epilepsia*, **27**, 225–233.

Trachtenberg, M.C. (1983). Basic mechanisms of epilepsy. In T.R. Browne and R.G. Feldman (eds), *Epilepsy: Diagnosis and Management*, Little, Brown, Boston, MA, pp. 11–20.

Wells, K.C., Turner, S.M., Bellack, A.S., and Hersen, M. (1978). Effects of cue-controlled relaxation on psychomotor seizures: an experimental analysis. *Behavior Research and Therapy*, **16**, 51–53.

Wyler, A.R. (1984). Operant conditioning of single neurons in monkeys and its theoretical application to EEG operant conditioning in human epilepsy. In T. Ebert, B. Rockstroh, W. Lutzenberger, and N. Birbaumer (eds), *Self-regulation of the Brain and Behavior*, Springer, Heidelberg, pp. 85–94.

Zifferblatt, S.M. (1975). Increasing patient compliance through the applied analysis of behavior. *Preventive Medicine*, **4**, 173–182.

Chapter 13

Vocational and Psychosocial Interventions for Youths, with Seizure Disorders

Robert T. Fraser and David C. Clemmons

INTRODUCTION

The focus of this chapter is on psychosocial and vocational interventions that can abet the successful life adjustment of the child or adolescent with epilepsy. In contrast to rehabilitation efforts for adults with epilepsy, early intervention or, in fact, preventative efforts to counter psychosocial maladjustment in youth with epilepsy, have been grossly underemphasized. Earlier interventions are being emphasized today for other developmentally disabled populations, but the needs of young people with epilepsy continue to be largely overlooked. It is hoped that this chapter may highlight the vocational and psychosocial adjustment concerns for the child or adolescent with epilepsy and spur greater efforts toward intervention.

The initial emphasis of this chapter will be on the identification of those young people who might best profit from psychosocial or vocational intervention efforts. This will be followed by a review of known research and clinical efforts in this area, and finally a discussion of the implications of these efforts with clinical and program recommendations.

YOUTHS WITH EPILEPSY AT GREATEST RISK FOR PSYCHOSOCIAL DIFFICULTY

Resources in epilepsy rehabilitation have been relatively limited as compared to other developmentally disabled groups (Commission for the Control of Epilepsy and its Consequences, 1978). It is critical that lobbying efforts be maintained until state developmental disability boards provide the necessary funds for the prevention of psychosocial difficulties. Until these monies become more readily available, service administrators and providers need to carefully consider the manner in which present funds are allocated.

Childhood Epilepsies: Neuropsychological, Psychosocial and Intervention Aspects
Edited by B. Hermann and M. Seidenberg

A review of the literature suggests consistent themes common to those young people with epilepsy who are more likely to have problems. These critical variables may be categorized in a number of different ways, but for the sake of simplicity we will divide them into two groups: those specific to the young person with epilepsy and those specific to his/her environment. There are also, of course, interactions between these variables which have not been clarified, but can intensify the difficulties experienced by these young people.

Several research efforts have underscored variables that are specific to the young person or to the medical treatment of the youngster's seizure condition (Goldin *et al.*, 1977; Stores, 1978; Ferrari, Barabas, and Matthews, 1983; O'Leary *et al.*, 1983; Sillanpää, 1983; Corbett, Trimble, and Nichol, 1985; Fraser, Clemmons, Trejo, and Temkin, 1985) which may predispose the child to adjustment difficulties. A list of these variables includes the following:

1. early age of onset (prior to age 6) (O'Leary *et al.*, 1983);
2. additional disability(ies) such as other neurological problems or physical handicaps (Goldin *et al.*, 1977);
3. associated neuropsychological impairment (Corbett *et al.*, 1985);
4. more severe and/or frequent seizure activity (Fraser *et al.*, 1985);
5. long-term, complex anticonvulsant medication regiment (Ferrari *et al.*, 1983)
6. male gender (Stores, 1978; Fraser *et al.*, 1985)

Other researchers (Appolone, 1978; Goldin *et al.*, 1977; Romeis, 1980; Curley *et al.*, 1987) have addressed the environmental variables that increase the risk of psychosocial maladjustment. As Ziegler (1981) emphasized, regardless of the degree of control provided by the medication, loss of control as a psychological concern may remain. An individual's experiences in his/her daily environment are what make the difference relative to that person's sense of control over his/her life. The following variables have been implicated in the psychosocial maladjustment of children with epilepsy:

1. parental fears (Appolone, 1978);
2. divisive or dysfunctional parenting styles (Curley *et al.*, 1987);
3. special education (Goldin *et al.*, 1977);
4. limited socialization and recreation (Goldin *et al.*, 1977);
5. poor relationships with parents and siblings (Goldin *et al.*, 1977);
6. intrusive and disruptive grandparenting styles (Romeis, 1980).

The entire area concerning the relationship of risk factors to the psychosocial maladjustment of children with epilepsy deserves considerably more research attention. Many of those with more obvious seizure-related impairments are referred for psychosocial services. There are others, however, who are simply not identified as 'at risk' for psychosocial dysfunction. The presence or absence of these types of factors should be systematically reviewed by high-school counselors, epilepsy association case workers, or medical clinic social workers to ensure that those most in need of services have their needs met. For this purpose, epilepsy associations could sponsor educational campaigns to educate neurologists, school nurses, teachers and families of young people with epilepsy about the 'high-risk' factors for maladjustment. It should be emphasized, however, that all youths having epilepsy should be screened for further psychosocial evaluation and intervention needs. Lobbying efforts should continue for funding support of this type of early screening and intervention, because remediation can do much to prevent the later development of more involved psychosocial difficulties.

In a recent study, Curley *et al.* (1987) restricted their study of risk factors to psychosocial maladjustment (behavioral disturbances) to a sample of boys ($N=60$) because they observed that boys seemed to be having more adjustment difficulties than girls (Stores, 1978). In this study, neuropsychological impairment, divisive parenting styles, and number of lifetime seizures accounted for approximately half the variance relative to the boys' behavioral disturbances—28 percent due to neuropsychological impairment and 13 percent due to each of the other variables. Young boys with difficulties in these areas may be the subgroup that will have the greatest adjustment difficulties.

A REVIEW OF PSYCHOSOCIAL INTERVENTION EFFORTS FOR CHILDREN AND ADOLESCENTS WITH EPILEPSY

Although a considerable amount has been written about the general psychosocial intervention needs of youth with epilepsy and their families, as reviewed by Appolone (1978), few intervention efforts have actually been described in the literature. In this section of the chapter an effort will be made to summarize the available literature in this area.

Working with parents

In her work at the Pediatric Neurology Clinic at Bowman Gray, Appolone (1978) describes four areas of intervention emphasis with parents: (a) exploring fantasies and fears about epilepsy, (b) interpreting facts about this disorder, (c) aiding parents to establish reasonable behavioral expectations for the child, and (d) enabling parents to disclose information about the child's condition in a manner beneficial to the child.

In her article, Appolone stresses the need to address the parents' fantasies and fears (specifically about the youngster's death) that are commonly experienced by parents. This author's discussion of the interpretation of facts about the disorder is also important because many young patients and their families do not fully understand the physician's discussion of medical information, or are hesitant to take the physician's time to seek clarification. Continued explanation of medical facts by the social worker, the encouragement of parents in their questioning of the physician, and distribution of relevant pamphlets to the parents, can increase their understanding of the disability. With better understanding of epilepsy, medication mechanisms, and the use of blood-level data, proper compliance with an anticonvulsant regimen is more likely to occur.

The final two areas of concern, as addressed by Appolone, include behavioral management of the child and appropriate disclosure of seizure information. It can be very difficult for parents not to overprotect their child and to set realistic daily expectations—particularly if they are overly fearful of seizures or if the 'sick child' status is reinforced by other family members. The social worker can be very helpful in clarifying reasonable activity goals and diffusing parental fears.

Finally, the disclosure of information about epilepsy can be a particular area of difficulty. Parents may feel uncomfortable in their lack of knowledge or fear the disclosure's effect upon teachers, friends, and family members. Appolone emphasizes that parents' abilities to discuss their children's seizure conditions clearly and succinctly should improve their self-confidence and provide positive feelings about educating others. A well-informed medical social worker can provide basic medical information and offer feedback to the parents during disclosure rehearsal sessions. Appolone indicates that in some instances it may be more beneficial for the social worker to discuss the seizure condition with family members (e.g. grandparents) when emotional complications make it difficult for the parents themselves to present the information.

Young adult groups: clinical reports

There is little empirical work in the literature on the effectiveness of different psychosocial intervention formats for young people with epilepsy. The clinical experiences of Appolone and Gibson (1980), working with young adults, however, suggest guidelines that in our experience are very relevant for youth:

1. Group interventions seem to be more effective in aiding the young patient to surrender a 'sick' or dependent role. This is much more difficult in one-to-one counselling. When offered several counseling options, most young people choose a group setting.
2. Young members who make an initial commitment to counseling often fail to appear. Scheduling a large group, therefore, allows for 'dropouts.' Appolone and Gibson schedule twice as many clients as needed. Dropout rates are not an important consideration for inpatients.
3. Group meetings are structured over 12 sessions with membership being closed once the group begins.

4. The group moves through several definable stages: (a) *group identity*, members share their background and seizure information while being reinforced by the group leader; (b) *goal exploration*, members begin to discuss 5-year goals while the group leader begins to confront them and model confrontation for other group members; (c) *modifying behavioral patterns*, group members confront each other using a 'hot-seat' approach that focuses on their current behaviors as relevant to goals; and (d) *progress assessment*, the final two meetings review progress toward goal attainment.

Young adult groups: empirical study

As previously discussed, the existence of empirical psychosocial intervention studies is sparse. Wallace (1979) attempted concurrent group psychotherapy for adolescents aged 12–18 and their parents, as a means of improving psychosocial adjustment. Of 40 families contacted, 13 were interested in involvement; eight youngsters between 12 and 18 years old, and their parents, were subsequently assigned a group psychotherapy, and five families assigned to a control group. Treatment involved a model which was psychoanalytically oriented. The adolescents and their parents were assigned to separate groups.

During the 25-session treatment phase the adolescents tended to focus on issues such as their disability, control of anger and aggression, fear of death, family concerns, and sexual issues. The parents' (mostly mothers) topical concerns were quite different. Their sessions emphasized concerns such as resentment, and parental inadequacy, family overprotectiveness, and offspring dependency.

On seven outcome measures, the adolescents indicated significant change only on self-concept (as measured by the Piers Harris Inventory). None of the other measures (locus of control, depression, a family adjustment measure, medication compliance, seizure frequency, and EEG findings) indicated any significant difference.

Wallace was troubled about the lack of responsiveness to this type of group psychotherapy approach. Although this may have been a selective sample, the results were minimal for this type of effort. It should be emphasized that 66 percent of those contacted refused involvement. A more didactic, fixed-duration treatment might be offered to families who reject a group psychotherapy approach.

Working with family members

Other researchers have assessed the value of treating the significant individuals in the lives of children with epilepsy as an approach to facilitating their medical and psychosocial adjustment (Shope, 1980; Rassel, Tonelson, and Appolone,

1981). Shope found that 70 (35 percent) of 201 pediatric seizure patients at the Epilepsy Center of Michigan were judged to be non-compliant with their medication regimen. The mothers of these patients were randomly assigned to an experimental group (N=28) or a control group (N=39). Three mothers were dropped from the study due to their children's medication changes. All mothers in the experimental group received a letter and phone call encouraging them to attend two discussion groups. Regardless of actual group attendance, the experimental group who had been contacted seemed to respond positively to the contact. On follow-up, medication compliance in the intervention group was significantly greater than in the control group.

It is of interest that in the experimental group no differences could be established between discussion group attenders and non-attenders. Shope emphasized that a group intervention may not be appropriate for everyone, and that timely phone contacts or individual counseling interventions at the time of clinic visits may be more appropriate for a substantial group of patients. Shope hypothesizes that short letters and clinic phone contact may indicate clinic staff interest and support, while also serving as a reminder. A number of mothers indicated work conflicts and other time constraints that made attendance difficult.

Interventions with teachers

Rassel *et al.* (1981) developed an educational program for teachers to help teachers better understand epilepsy and have less fears when a pupil has a seizure. As compared to a control group, the teachers involved in the intervention understood significantly more factual information about the disability, and had more positive attitudes toward dealing with a student having epilepsy then did the controls. This study did not assess whether the teachers' actual classroom behavior was affected by the workshop participation.

Vocational/prevocational interventions

Vocational or prevocational interventions for persons with epilepsy in the schools are, with few exceptions, non-existent. Demonstration projects involving information dissemination and needs assessment studies appear to be the most frequent school-initiated research undertakings related to the concerns of youth with epilepsy (Hartlage and Green, 1972; Martin, 1974; Richardson and Stanford, 1974; Usinger, 1978; Ryan, 1981). While these endeavors have probably had the positive effect of disseminating information about epilepsy, they do not constitute intervention. They may, explicitly or implicitly, project the image that all persons with epilepsy are 'just like everybody else' except when they are having seizures, minimizing or ignoring the possible presence of underlying cerebral dysfunction, and the need for specialized services.

One of the few documented efforts is the work by Freeman *et al.* (1984). This project was supported by city and state governments to comply with Public Laws 94–142 and 94–484. The project provided a number of service components to 333 students (mostly urban black) which included: assessment, counseling, work experience, training, epilepsy education, and placement. Seventy percent of the students had psychosocial difficulties in addition to their seizure condition.

This intensive program had an individual orientation and some very positive results. The program decreased the non-promotion rate to less than half of local school system rates, and reduced by 50 percent the number of youths unemployed or not in vocational training 1 and 2 years after graduation. The cost per pupil averaged only 10 percent greater than the expenditures the school system was already making on its pupils. It appears that a key factor in the success of the project was that it enabled school personnel to develop individualized programs for its disabled students under Public Laws 94–142 and 94–484. In our experience at the University of Washington, the cooperation of school personnel is vital in effecting a successful intervention with young people.

This section of the chapter reviews our studies of psychosocial interventions for youths with epilepsy. Although some gains have been made in relation to program development, there is limited empirical data. It became obvious that this area is fertile ground for further research and program demonstration efforts.

RELEVANT WORK AT THE UNIVERSITY OF WASHINGTON EPILEPSY CENTER

At the University of Washington Regional Epilepsy Center much of our work has focused on reasons for intervention with adolescents and the possible emphases of that intervention. It is of interest that in a study of parents of young adults ($N=24$) at our center (Sutton, Smith, and Fraser, 1979), parents endorsed the following concerns in relation to their child (ratings were 1=least bothersome through 6=most bothersome):

(a) not knowing how to encourage independence in their child, mean rating=4.7;
(b) having difficulty finding a job, mean rating=3.9;
(c) son/daughter has no overall life goals, mean rating=3.6.

Concerns about medical care were not highly endorsed by these parents. Medical issues may have been resolved, or parents had become accustomed to them by the time these young adults reached their early 20s. Concerns about independent living, and finding and maintaining jobs, were prominent.

Clemmons (1985) reviewed the case histories of 343 adults referred to the Vocational Unit at our Center, and found that the mean age for seizure onset was approximately 14 for both males and females. By age 19, about 75 percent of the sample were experiencing seizures.

Other work by our group (Fraser *et al.*, 1985) suggests that male outpatients with major motor seizures and/or early onset were 'at risk' for having a restricted range of vocational and academic interests. Although there were generally lower General Occupational theme and Special Interest scores on the Strong Campbell Interest Inventory (SCII) for this group, significantly lower scores were found on the Investigative and Academic Orientation scales. These males tended to show less scientific interest (need to understand the physical world) than the SCII norm group (Campbell and Hansen, 1981). Additionally, they scored significantly lower on the SCII special scale, Academic Orientation, which assesses interest in pursuring a range of subjects in a school setting.

Clemmons and Dodrill (1983, 1984) conducted follow-up studies which examined the neuropsychological and intellectual test scores of adolescents 4½ years after high school graduation. Both studies reviewed the vocational status of an initial group of 51 adolescents referred for neuropsychological evaluation an average of 6½ years previously. It was found that measures such as the Wechsler Adult Intelligence Scale Full Scale IQ and the total number of neuropsychological tests outside normal limits successfully discriminated between individuals able to obtain full-time employment and those unable to do so. These studies underscored the possible utility of neuropsychological tests as predictors of later life performance. Such measures could be useful for the early identification of adolescents with epilepsy who may benefit from specialized or intensive vocational intervention.

The 1983 study also reviewed aspects of subjects' vocational and economic status at follow-up. They found that 31 percent of 42 subjects (N=13) were receiving Supplemental Security income within 4 years of high school graduation, while only 29 percent (N=12) of the subjects were working on a full-time basis. Thirteen individuals (31 percent) reported entering employment through the intervention of family or friends at some time during the 5 years after high school graduation. Thirty-six percent of the sample (N=15) reported receiving state vocational rehabilitation services, although only two of these (14 percent of those receiving services) entered employment. This latter finding is congruent with other literature reviewed by Fraser *et al.* (1985) that suggests state agency vocational rehabilitation services are not fully or effectively used by persons with epilepsy.

Dodrill and Clemmons (1984) conducted a follow-up study on adolescents examined at our Center, which more thoroughly examined subjects' neuropsychological status with respect to later life functioning. Subjects' work and social histories were available for analysis, as well as neuropsychological, intellectual, and psychological testing. The study was conducted at an average of 5.9 years (SD=1.86 years) after subjects' initial neuropsychological evaluation which included an expanded Halstead–Reitan Battery, a Wechsler Adult Intelligence Scale (WAIS), and a Minnesota Multiphasic Personality Inventory (MMPI). Subjects were 16–19 years old at the time of testing (chi-square=17.26, SD=0.94 years) and the average age of seizure onset was 7.47 years (SD=5.12). Subjects were divided into two groups, labeled 'Fully Functioning' (N=12) and 'Deficient Functioning' (N=27) using a rating scale which included measures of employment and independent living status. MMPI results were not useful in discriminating between the two groups. Following control for multiple comparisons, a number of test measures discriminated between the two groups at a statistically significant level. These included global measures, such as the Halstead impairment index and the WAIS Verbal and Performance IQs, as well as several individual neuropsychological tests, such as the Seashore Rhythm and total errors on the Aphasia Screening test. This latter measure proved to be the most sensitive in discriminating between the two groups ($t=-6.19$, $p< 0.05$). The authors hypothesized that this finding underscored the importance of language use in successful social functioning. Scores obtained in this study were entered into a discriminant function analysis which was able to discriminate between the two groups with a high degree of accuracy. The authors concluded that this study suggested that young persons with epilepsy who will have later problems in life functioning may be identified at an early age.

None of the studies reviewed found a significant relationship between type of frequency of seizures and employment status. This is consistent with program evaluations conducted on adults at our Center, as well. It should be noted that all the studies discussed above were conducted with an epilepsy rehabilitation population. Typically, this is a population of persons with increased seizure frequency, increased psychosocial dysfunction, and more problems with respect to intellectual and neuropsychological status than would be expected in the general population of persons with epilepsy.

Work by Clemmons (1985) and Clemmons, Fraser, and Trejo (1987) suggests that the assessment of vocational aptitudes using instruments standardized in general populations may present a number of special problems. School and rehabilitation institutions frequently make use of assessment tools developed for the general population, such as the General Aptitude Test Battery (GATB) (United States Department of Labor, 1970). Clemmon's research indicated that the relationship between tested aptitudes as measured by the GATB and employability was tenuous at best for adults with epilepsy. The validity of the GATB with special populations, such as adolescents with epilepsy, may be questionable. These are important considerations, since the GATB is frequently used in vocational assessment 'packages' provided in connection with high school career counseling programs.

The poorest predictors of outcome were found among the motor coordination and dexterity scores on the GATB: Motor Coordination (K), Finger Dexterity (F), Manual Dexterity (M). It was a frequent occurrence to find subjects with dexterity and coordination scores one or two standard deviations below published cut-off scores for the occupation in which they were successfully employed. The precise reasons for this phenomenon are unclear. It may be a function of the effects of brain impairment, anticonvulsant side-effects, the interaction of these variables, or the timed nature of the test for young people lacking experience with 'hands-on' activities. Nevertheless, the fact remains that they were able to perform adequately on the job, and this standardized aptitude assessment did not adequately predict their performance.

In summary, research at our Center suggests the following:

1. Parents perceive independent living skills and vocational direction and attainment as salient potential problems for adolescents with epilepsy.
2. Early, specialized vocational rehabilitation efforts should occur for many adolescents with epilepsy to improve their eventual employment status and reduce dependence on public subsidy.
3. Boys with early-onset and major motor seizures may be particularly 'at risk' vocationally and academically. They may benefit from specific interventions (supportive counseling, pro-social experiences and involvement with 'hands-on' and exploratory types of tasks around the home). Supportive counseling in the school setting and educational programs concerning epilepsy for their peers might also be helpful to the boys' school adjustment.
4. Neuropsychological assessment should be standard practice for adolescents who have had a substantial number of generalized tonic–clonic seizures, have a history of status epilepticus, or have known neurological trauma, to establish their patterns of neuropsychological strength and deficit. Such information would be of value for educational and vocational planning.
5. The best gauge of employability for adolescents with epilepsy will often be a situational job assessment instead of the use of standardized vocational tests in an agency context. Volunteer jobs within hospitals or federal agencies can be used for this purpose, as well as temporary work provided by community employers.

Clinical experience and suggestions for working with youths with epilepsy

High school students seeking vocational services through our Epilepsy Center have generally responded well to three types of services: (1) the presentation of general information about epilepsy-related medical and vocational issues, (2) vocational evaluation activities examining their aptitudes and interests, and (3) small group counseling experiences directed at vocational, as well as general life adjustment, goals.

Receiving adolescent referrals who can profit from these services from parents or the schools can be a basic problem. It is not completely understood, but there appears to be a complex issue related to parent and school protectionism, i.e. the perception that the referral of high school students is premature, or that only those who are more obviously disabled need to be referred. Certainly the work by Clemmons and Dodrill (1983) emphasizes the need for early intervention. Examination of the risk factors for significant maladjustment as discussed earlier is also helpful in referral considerations. There is clearly a need for educational programs for parents and school personnel. While there are definitely a number of youngsters with epilepsy who do not require psychosocial intervention, most (particularly those requiring the specialized medical or neuropsychological services at an epilepsy center) could profit from a time-limited, structured vocational group intervention.

Neuropsychological assessment has been particularly helpful in vocational evaluation and planning. This testing can be costly, and it is therefore helpful to families if the neuropsychological testing is requested by a physician because then it is more likely that these costs will be borne by medical insurance plans. Another viable method for securing payment is through a school system's special services. Neuropsychological testing can aid in framing a student's individual educational plan (IEP), and, at times, avoid an inappropriate special education placement. Neuropsychological testing performed in adolescence also provides benchmark data for each client, and can be reviewed after future testing to establish areas of progress or decrement. The IEPs, however, need to be developed without a total dependence on standardized testing, because neuropsychological testing or the GATB will tend to underestimate life performance capabilities.

A work trial or volunteer job station experience within a hospital, federal agency, or university can be helpful in establishing actual capabilities and areas of remediation to be addressed in the IEP. Establishment of these work experience programs is discussed in Chapter 306:11–2 of our government's Federal Personnel Manual (United States Office of Personnel Management, Appendix, F, 1982).

Many adolescents with epilepsy are extremely naive about the work world, due to parental sheltering, lack of normal interactions with peers, reduced expectations for household maintenance and repair activities, and so forth. It is not always in the young client's best interests to directly confront his/her goals about, for instance, computer programming, when these goals are unrealistic. As a response to the naive young client's specific job goal, it can be helpful to reframe their interests into two or three general job categories or potential work environments. A volunteer job experience in a related work area as a data entry person, a computer tape librarian aide, or even a custodian, may be acceptable to young people if they feel they will learn more about their ideal goal and have a start in the desired direction. These experiences place the youngster in a realistic position to learn about the job demands of such a position, while being oriented to the work demands and benefits of less complex jobs that exist in large numbers in the labor market.

A grant awarded to us from the National Institute of Neurological and Communicative Disorders and Stroke (NINCDS, No. NS21706–01) has allowed us to synthesize a number of years of clinical experience in the development of a group-oriented curriculum which addresses several concerns central to the needs of young people with epilepsy. The curriculum consists of an information dissemination/problem-solving format with applications of the material through behavioral rehearsal or 'role play.' Specific topics of a six-session group program include: indentifying job goals, activities affecting job-getting (alcohol and recreational drugs, driving considerations, etc.), discussing specific seizure conditions with employers, general employment interview skills, job-getting resources and employer contact telephone scripts, and a final general review and practice. This program involved six 2-hour sessions with homework assignments specific to the topics.

One of the most useful features of the groups has been providing young persons with epilepsy the opportunity to meet each other in a non-threatening environment to discuss epilepsy-related issues. Nearly every group member, for example, has reported embarrassment over seizures, or over the possibility of having a seizure at school, yet few had seen an epileptic seizure or talked with a person having epilepsy. In a similar vein, group members frequently indicated concerns relating to issues such as dating or being perceived as different by classmates, while tending to express surprise in learning that others had similar concerns. The groups appear to serve a remedial socialization or 'normalization' function. The co-ed nature of the groups seems to enhance the social sharing and discussion among members, although it sometimes made it difficult to adhere strictly to a specific format. Group members appeared to lag behind their peers without epilepsy in social skills and experience relating to the opposite sex. They were interested in the group meetings as a vehicle for approaching these issues. The post-high school vocational outcome of those who attended these groups is currently being evaluated. A copy of the vocational group curriculum is available from the authors.

SUMMARY AND RECOMMENDATIONS

It is acknowledged that not every adolescent with epilepsy will require a psychosocial or vocational intervention. Most, however, could generally profit from vocational or some of the interventions reviewed in this chapter. A review of risk factors for psychosocial maladjustment suggests that youngsters with earlier age of onset, males, those with more active and complex seizures conditions, or those having additional disabilities including neuropsychological impairment, will be more prone to adjustment difficulties. Family or extended family difficulties, special education placement, and limited socialization and recreational opportunities also complicate the adjustment process. A greater effort should be made to reach out to these youngsters, and their parents, who demonstrate one or more of the risk factors complicating their adjustment process.

Our recommendations, and those of Goldin *et al.* (1977), suggest that the following policy and service considerations be incorporated into comprehensive early service delivery models:

(a) Outreach

Physicians need to be contacted to ensure that young people who could profit from an intervention are referred. Social work interviews at epilepsy or neurology clinics, or by intake workers at epilepsy associations, can facilitate the identification of those needing early intervention. Early outreach to parents can enable a social worker or medical professional to open dialogue in sensitive areas before parental defenses are well established. Parents can also be assisted to establish reasonable expectations for their child for completion of home tasks, participation in school activities, and community/social group involvement to promote patterns of independence. O'Donohoe (1983) provided some general guidelines for parents relative to sports and school participation.

(b) Integration of resources

In order to maximize a youngster's potential for adjustment, it is important that all available resources are utilized in an integrated manner. Community rehabilitation or social service representatives can work closely with parents, teachers, and even recreational specialists at significant development points. Negative experiences in one area may be countered by coordinated efforts in other areas, or may at least be prevented from causing damaging interactions with other life activities, e.g. school performance difficulties affecting the client's willingness to interact socially with peers. Goldin *et al.* reinforced the need for coordinated efforts by epilepsy associations, developmental disability councils, and other youth agencies to improve the socialization of the more severely or multiply disabled persons with epilepsy.

(c) Form of psychosocial intervention

Goldin *et al.* recommended that different group vs. individual intervention approaches need to be examined for their usefulness with youngsters having epilepsy, to a large degree because of the pro-social nature and efficiency of the group format. These approaches, in our opinion, are very helpful, particularly when oriented to the specific needs, established by pre-group survey, of the youngsters or their parents. Although there has been no definitive experimental work in this area, time-limited, structured groups involving six to 12 sessions appear to be the most reasonable.

Suggested guidelines have been presented by the authors for vocational groups, and by Appolone and Gibson (1980) for more general psychosocial groups. These groups seem to offer a mix of didactic approaches, personal sharing, and confrontation among group members, and *in vivo* social skill and network building. Time-limited, structured group activities facilitate the involvement of more youngsters and their parents, and can be more comfortable for youngsters with social skill deficits and single parents.

It should be noted that to improve certain problem areas for youngsters having seizures (e.g. anticonvulsant compliance), letters and phone calls to mothers were as effective as involving the mothers in group interventions (Shope, 1980). Targeted efforts of this type might be contrasted with more labor-intensive group interventions as related to definable objectives that should aid in a young person's social adjustment (e.g. increasing a youngster's social activities or making contact with vocational rehabiliation).

(d) School educational efforts

It seems likely that epilepsy education efforts within the schools are beneficial to youngsters with epilepsy, and may positively affect the attitudes and beliefs of other students and teachers. Specific changes in school performance of the student with epilepsy, or in interactions between the student and teachers or peers that result from these efforts, have yet to be established.

(e) Independent living skills training

Since dependency can be a prominent concern for youngsters with epilepsy (particularly the more severely or multiply handicapped), it can be beneficial for epilepsy associations, centers, or other community agencies to provide independent living skills training. Fraser and Smith (1982) emphasized that competence in independent living not only contributes to self-esteem and life satisfaction, but is supportive of job procurement and maintenance. These skills have been taught within a variety of settings: day centers, epilepsy associations, group homes, or in private homes. These courses can be taught in groups from two or three to twelve, depending on the complexity of the material. Individuals should be assigned to these groups based on personalized assessment of needs, enrolled with clearly articulated goals, and supported throughout the training with specific exercises.

Courses in independent living have included training in grooming and physical appearance, clothing selection, living alternatives, home equipment and furniture selection, housekeeping and home maintenance, financial management, food shopping and nutrition, food preparation, use of transportation, and health care/medical management. In the national day centers of Denmark, these classes involve 5–6 hours of instruction and are taught 2 days per week (Lund and Randrup, 1972). Obviously, some courses such as cooking, which can be more complex, or shopping, which involves field trips, may required more time.

There are a number of programs available for the implementation of an independent skills training program. Neistadt and Marques (1984) developed 12 modules of behaviorally oriented coursework for multiply disabled clients. Modules were also developed for advocacy and recreation management. The number of classes in each module ranged between three and 15, based on complexity and breadth of the material. The program is tightly structured. Clients sign a contract outlining attendance, homework, and other responsibilities before participation. Pre- and post-module examinations and regularly scheduled class tests are given to ensure that the students meet competency criteria. Participants are involved in between 112 and 132 hours of instruction over approximately 7 months.

Vogelsberg, Williams, and Bellamy (1982) offer an expanded description of independent living skills curricula that are tailored to the needs of those with epilepsy and more involved cognitive and neuropsychological deficits. Under community survival, for instance, there is a complete domain of skills which include negotiating intersections. These authors contributed substantially to the delineation of the variables important in establishing individual objectives for each student. These include specific environmental considerations, community mobility, the need to maintain present living setting, age, student preferences, unique learner characteristics, and parent or guardian preferences.

(f) Vocational interventions

The time-limited, structured vocational group intervention, which had been evaluated at our center, appears to show promise in vocationally and psychosocially assisting adolescents with epilepsy toward competitive employment, but ultimately the adolescent with a seizure condition (particularly those with more active or complicated conditions) will best profit from a school-to-work transition program. Clemmons and Dodrill (1983) observed that a third of their high-school students were receiving long-term federal subsidy within 5 years of graduation. United States Department of Labor (1984) data suggest that sheltered work settings competitively place only 12 percent of these clients and only 34 percent of these facilities have a full-time placement specialist. To avoid long-term subsidy or a sheltered work placement, which is inappropriate for many of these young people, the transition to work is best accomplished at the secondary school level.

School-to-work programs usually contain the following basic components: a linkage with an outside agency, private sector consultation and support (e.g. through a local employers' council), job readiness curricula about employment interviewing and other job-seeking skills, and job placement assistance. In our experience the involvement of an agency external to the school system and private sector advisement are critical components of these school-to-work transition programs. Otherwise the work-oriented goals of the student can be co-opted by the schools' needs for on-site census, teachers' needs to focus on academic coursework that may not be in the student's best vocational interests, and so forth.

Okolo and Sitlington (1986) present a model for a school-to- work transition program for learning-disabled adolescents that has applicability for adolescents with more severe seizure conditions or other associated disabilities. The program modules are taught by special educators with the consultation of vocational educators. Vocational education teachers help provide direction to the program and are particularly in the final transition to competitive employment. Based upon their review of relevant research, these authors conclude that the ideal program modules would include the following:

1. occupational awareness, exploration, and diverse in-school and community work experience;
2. in-depth career/vocational assessment;
3. instruction in job-related academic skills relevant to a learner's vocational training program or targeted jobs areas;
4. instruction in job-related interpersonal skills that have been empirically validated (Greenan, 1984; Matthews, Whang, and Fawcett, 1980);
5. support services for other professionals, such as vocational educators or community agency representatives by the special educators;
6. post-school placement and follow-up vocational educators and liason vocational rehabilitation staff.

It is hoped that these types of programs will become more prevalent in our secondary school systems. For many young people with involved seizure conditions, associated disabilities, or a high degree of work-world naiveté, it will take this type of effort to enable them to make a successful transition to competitive employment. In some instances the use of vocational rehabilitation on-the-job training funds, other forms of employer subsidy, or the use of an on-site job coach will be necessary to ensure the success of the final placement. The use of the job coach for on-site skill training or job site advocacy is a form of 'supported employment' which will be appropriate for a subgroup of these youngsters.

CONCLUSION

This chapter reviewed risk factors for psychosocial and vocational maladjustment for youngsters with seizure conditions. It summarized the diverse psychosocial and vocational interventions that have been attempted in the epilepsy field, with specific discussion of research and clinical efforts at the University of Washington Regional Epilepsy Center. The final section of the chapter synthesizes information from the initial sections and related areas of research and/or project demonstration efforts in the form of recommendations. It is hoped that this information is helpful to epilepsy service providers in considering and devising interventions that will prevent psychosocial problems and facilitate life adjustment for young people with epilepsy. This areas of service deserves considerably more attention than it is currently receiving.

REFERENCES

Appolone, C. (1978). Preventive social work intervention with families of children with epilepsy. *Social Work in Health Care*, **4**,(2), 139–148.

Appolone, C., and Gibson, P. (1980) Group work with young adult epilepsy patients. *Social Work in Health Care*, **6**(2), 23–32.

Campbell, D.P., and Hansen, J.C. (1981). *Manual for the SVIB-SCII: Form T325 of the Strong Campbell Vocational Interest Blank*, 3rd edn, Stanford University Press, Stanford, CA.

Clemmons, D.C. (1985). Assessment of vocational aptitudes of epileptics in a rehabilitation setting. Doctoral dissertation, University of Washington, Seattle, Washington.

Clemmons, D.C., and Dodrill, C.B. (1983). Vocational outcomes of high school students with epilepsy, *Journal of Applied Rehabilitation Counseling*, **14**(4), 49–53.

Clemmons, D., and Dodrill, C.B. (1984). Vocational outcomes of high school students with epilepsy and neuropsychological correlates with later vocational success. In R.J. Porter *et al. Advances in Epileptology*, vol, 15. Raven Press, New York, pp. 611–614.

Clemmons, D.C., Fraser, R.T., and Trejo, W.R. (1987). The general aptitude test battery: implications for vocational counseling and employment in epilepsy rehabilitation, *Journal of Applied Rehabilitation Counseling*, **18**(3), 33–38.

Commission for the control of Epilepsy and Its Consequences (1977). *Plan for Nationwide Action on Epilepsy*. United States Department of Health, Education and Welfare, Washington, DC.

Corbett, J.A., Trimble, M.R., and Nichol, T.C. (1985). Behavioral and cognitive impairments in children with epilepsy: the long-term effects of anticonvulsant therapy, *Journal of the American Academy of Child Psychiatry*, **24**,(1), 17–23.

Curley, A.D., Delaney, R.C., Mattson, R.H., Holmes, G.L., and O'Leary, D.K. (1987) Determinants of behavioral disturbance in boys with seizures. Presented at the Annual Convention of the American Psychological Association, New York.

Dodrill, C.B., and Clemmons, D. (1984). 'Use of neuropsychological tests to identify high school students with epilepsy who later demonstrate inadequate performances in life, *Journal of Consulting and Clinical Psychology*, **54**,(4), 520–527.

Ferrari, M., Barabas, G., and Matthews, W.S. (1983). Psychologic and behavioral disturbance among epileptic children treated with barbiturate anticonvulsants, *American Journal of Psychiatry*, **140**,(1), 112–113.

Fraser, R., Clemmons, D., Trejo, W., and Temkin, N.R. (1983). Program evaluation in epilepsy rehabilitation, *Epilepsia*, **24**, 734–746.

Fraser, R.T., and Smith, W.R. (1982) Adjustment to daily living. In H. Sands (ed.), *Epilepsy: A Handbook for the Mental Health Professional*, Brunner/Mazel, New York, pp. 189–224.

Fraser, R., Trejo, W., and Blanchard, W. (1984). Epilepsy rehabilitation: evaluating specialized versus general agency outcome. *Epilepsia*, **25**, 332–337.

Fraser, R., Trejo, W., Temkin, N., Clemmons, D., and Dodrill, C. (1985). Assessing the vocational interests of those with epilepsy, *Rehabilitation Psychology*, **30**, 29–33.

Freeman, J.M., Jacobs, J., Vining, E., and Rabin, S. (1984). Epilepsy and the inner-city schools: A school-based program that makes a difference, *Epilepsia*, **25**, 438–442.

Goldin, G.J., Perry, S.L., Margolin, R.J., Stotsky, B.A., and Foster, J.C. (1977). *Rehabilitation of the Young Epileptic*, D.C. Heath, Lexington, MA.

Greenan, J.P. (1984) The construct of generalizable skills for assessing the functional learning abilities of students in vocational technical programs, *Journal of Students and Technical Careers*, **2**, 91–104.

Hartlage, L.C., and Green, J.B. (1972). The relation of parental attitudes to academic and social achievement in epileptic children, *Epilepsia*, **13**(1), 21–26.

Lund, M., and Randrup, J. (1972). A day centre for severely handicapped people with epilepsy, *Epilepsia*, **13**(1), 245–247.

Margalit, M. and Heiman, T. (1983). Anxiety and self-dissatisfaction in epileptic children, *International Journal of Social Psychiatry*, **29**(3), 220–224.

Matthews, R., Whang, P., and Fawcett, S. (1980). *Behavioral Assessment of Job Related Skills: Implications for Learning Disabled Yound Adults*, University of Kansas Institute for Research in Learning Disabilities, Lawrence, KA.

Neistadt, M.E., and Marques, K. (1984). Independent living skills training program, *American Journal of Occupational Therapy*, **38**(10), 671–676.

O'Donohoe, N.V. (1983). What should the child with epilepsy be allowed to do?, *Archives of Disease in Childhood*, **58**, 934–937.

Okolo, C.M., and Sitlington, P. (1986). The role of special education and ld adolescents' transition from school to work, *Learning Disability Quarterly*, **9**, 141–155.

O'Leary, D.S., Lovell, M.R., Sackellares, J.C., Berent, S., Giordani, B., Seidenberg, M., and Boll, T.J. (1983). Effects of age of onset of partial and generalized seizures on neuropsychological performance in children, *Journal of Nervous and Mental Disease*, **171**,(10), 624–629.

Rassel, G., Tonelson, S., and Appolone C. (1981). Epilepsy workshop for public school personnel, *Journal of School Health*, January, 48–50.

Richardson, D.W., and Standford, B.F. (1974). Psychosocial problems of the adolescent and patient with epilepsy, *Clinical Pediatrics*, **13**, 121–126.

Romeis, J.C. (1980). The role of grandparents in adjustment to epilepsy, *Social Work in Health Care*, **6**(1), 37–43.

Ryan, R. (1981). *Attitudes and Knowledge Regarding Epilepsy: A Survey of Employees of the Beaverton School District, Beaverton, Oregon*, Good Samaritan Hospital, Portland, OR.

Shope, J.T. (1980). Intervention to improve compliance with pediatric anticonvulsant therapy, *Patient Counseling and Health Education*, **3**, 135–141.

Sillanpää, M. (1983) Medico-social prognosis of children with epilepsy, *Acta Paediatrica Scandinavica*, **62**, Suppl. 237.

Stores, G. (1978). School children with epilepsy at risk for learning and behavior disorders, *Developmental Medicine and Child Neurology*, **20**, 502–508.

Sutton, D., Smith, W.R., and Fraser, R.T. (1979). A comparative study of parent counseling approaches. Paper presented at Thirtieth Annual Western Institute Symposium on Epilepsy, Portland, Oregon.

United States Department of Labor, Manpower Administration (1970). *Manual for the USES General Aptitude Test Battery, Section III: Development*, Government Printing Office, Washington, DC.

United States Department of Labor (1984). *Sheltered Work Study: A Nationwide Report of Sheltered Work and Employment of Handicapped Individuals*, Government Printing Office, Washington, DC.

United States Office of Personnel Management (1982). *Federal Personnel Manual*, U.S. Government Printing Office, Washington, DC.

Usinger, J. (1978) One in fifty—a guide for the in-service training of teachers, nurses, and other school personnel Washington State Office of Public Instruction, Education Services District No. 121.

Vogelsberg, R.T., Williams, W., and Bellamy, G.T. (1982). Preparation for independent living. In B. Wilcox and G.T. Bellamy (eds), *Design of High School Programs for Severely Handicapped Students*, Brooks Publishing, Baltimore, pp. 153–173.

Wallace, S.M. (1979). *Efficiacy of the Use of Group Psychotherapy with Adolescents Who Have a Seizure Disorder*, University of Pittsburgh, Pittsburgh, PA.

Ziegler, R.G. (1981) Impairments of control and competence in epileptic children and their families, *Epilepsia*, **22**, 339–346.

Chapter 14

Childhood Epilepsy and Mental Retardation

Janusz J. Zielinski

Mental retardation (MR) and epilepsy are among the most common developmental disabilities. Epilepsy, like MR, in many cases tends to become a chronic condition, significantly influencing the psychosocial development of an afflicted child. Such children frequently become a challenge for parents, siblings, and all family members. The coexistence of MR and epilepsy makes the raising, teaching, and training of the child significantly more difficult in comparison to children suffering only from MR or epilepsy. A child with such a double disability can achieve his or her maximum level of social functioning only if provided with a comprehensive, interdisciplinary approach. It requires careful planning and full cooperation among parents, teachers, doctors, psychologists, and all other professionals involved in the long-term treatment program.

Numerous textbooks have been written on mental retardation, but epilepsy is only briefly discussed, if touched on at all. Similarly, in textbooks on epilepsy the problem of mental retardation is usually mentioned only marginally. Therefore, the main goal of this chapter is to review our current state of knowledge concerning the medical needs of children with both mental retardation and epilepsy. The frequency of the problems will be illustrated by means of epidemiological estimates. Furthermore, the basic and most important clinical syndromes will be discussed in order to help the reader improve his/her knowledge of the complexity of needs of these multiply handicapped children and to better the medical treatment of this demanding population. Difficulties in the differential diagnosis between seizures and other episodic behaviors in mentally retarded children, as well as the potentially devastating side-effects of anticonvulsants, will also be discussed.

DEFINITIONS

MR, especially when severe, may become evident in early childhood, but milder cases may not be diagnosed until later, for instance, in pre-teen or

Childhood Epilepsies: Neuropsychological, Psychosocial and Intervention Aspects
Edited by B. Hermann and M. Seidenberg

adolescent years. DSM-III (1986) defines MR as significantly subaverage general intellectual functioning, resulting in, or associated with, deficits or impairments in adaptive behavior, with onset before the age of 18. Four types of MR are recognized:

1. Mild MR (MIMR) with an IQ range from 70 to 50, representing about 80 percent of all people with a diagnosis of MR.
2. Moderate MR (MOMR), IQ range 49–35: about 12 percent of diagnosed cases.
3. Severe MR (SEMR): IQ range 34–20: about 7 percent of diagnosed cases.
4. Profound MR (PMR): IQ below 20: about 1 percent of diagnosed cases.

MIMR is frequently referred to as 'educable,' while MOMR is referred to as 'trainable.' MOMR, SEMR, and PMR are frequently discussed together as 'severe' MR (IQ <50).

Epilepsy is defined as a chronic brain disorder of various etiologies characterized by recurrent epileptic seizures (Gastaut, 1973). As discussed in Chapter 1, epileptic seizures are classified into three fundamental categories: partial, primary generalized, and unclassified. Partial seizures without impairment of consciousness are named simple partial. They can manifest themselves via a wide variety of motor, somatosensory, autonomic, and psychic signs and symptoms. The hallmark of a complex partial seizure is disturbance of consciousness. Complex partial seizures can present with impairment of consciousness only (and then occasionally can be difficult to differentiate from absence seizures) or can be associated with purposeless movements or activities. Both simple and complex partial seizures can evolve into a secondarily generalized tonic–clonic seizure (previously called 'grand mal'), or its incomplete form (tonic or clonic). As reviewed in Chapter 1, one seizure type can evolve into another; for example, simple partial or complex partial into tonic–clonic, simple partial into complex partial into tonic–clonic, and so on.

Partial seizures tend to predominate, particularly in the adult population with epilepsy, while in children younger than 15, over 50 percent present with primarily generalized seizures (Gastaut *et al.*, 1975). The latter category covers a variety of seizures associated with a loss of consciousness from the very onset, no partial manifestations, and various motoric manifestations, i.e. tonic, clonic, tonic–clonic, and/or myoclonic. Atonic seizures are characterized by a loss of muscle tone, while with absence seizures no gross motoric disturbances are seen (patients are usually motionless, occasionally 'staring' or 'eye-blinking').

There is no generally accepted classification of epilepsy. The recent proposal of the Commission of the International League Against Epilepsy (ILAE) (Dreifuss *et al.*, 1985) introduced the term 'epileptic syndrome,' defined as 'an epileptic disorder characterized by a cluster of signs and symptoms customarily occurring together.' There are numerous syndromes which may occur especially or exclusively in childhood and adolescence, and some of these will be discussed later in this chapter.

EPIDEMIOLOGY OF MENTAL RETARDATION (MR) AND EPILEPSY

MR

Although the prevalence of MR is generally accepted to be around 1 percent of the general population, a more exact estimation of its frequency is difficult. These difficulties are due to various methods of case-ascertainment and definitions ('administrative' vs. 'psychometric,' known cases versus those non-registered) which have been utilized in the literature. Cases with severe MR (IQ <50) are easier to diagnose and prevalence rates are estimated to be about 3–4 per 1000 inhabitants. In longitudinal studies there is a little variation in annual age-specific prevalence rates for nonspecific MR. For instance, in Salford (England) the prevalence of severe MR cases among children aged 5–9 and 10–14 years was, respectively, 3.06 and 2.74 in 1970, and 3.14 and 4.91 per 1000 in 1980. However, prevalence rates of MR associated with Down's syndrome among children aged 5–9 years fell from 1.52 in 1967 to 0.71 in 1980 (Fryers, 1984).

Epilepsy

Several epidemiologic studies have revealed that the highest prevalence rates of epilepsy occur in children. In a British national survey of 5000 births, over 2 percent of the children experienced a seizure before the age of 2 (Cooper, 1965). Another birth cohort study in Great Britain revealed that of the 15,500 children followed at the age of 7 and 11 years, 103 were suspected of having recurrent seizures. In 64 of these children the diagnosis of epilepsy was confirmed (prevalence rate 4.1/1000), whereas in another 39 epilepsy 'was reported by doctors but not substantiated' (Ross, Peckham, West, and Butler, 1980). This tendency to overdiagnose epilepsy was also found in the Warsaw study by Zielinski (1974a, 1986). In 20 percent of the cases this diagnosis could not be confirmed. In a cohort of children born in San Francisco, 1 percent had an afebrile seizure before the end of 5 years (Van den Bergh and Yerushalmy, 1969). The Collaborative Perinatal Project conducted by National Institutes of Health included a birth cohort of over 39,000 childen, and 218 of them (5.6/1000) suffered from recurrent nonfebrile seizures before the age of 7 years (Ellenberg, Hirtz, and Nelson, 1984).

Epilepsy and MR combined

The coexistence of epilepsy and MR is usually measured by estimating the prevalence rate of MR among children with epilepsy, or the prevalence rate of epilepsy among children with MR. Unfortunately, only a few epidemiological surveys have covered both these disorders. Among all children (9–11 years) living on the Isle of Wight (England), two or more seizures occurred in 16.4 percent of those with MR, compared to only 1.4 percent of the control group (Rutter, Tizard, and Whitmore, 1970). Among 150 children (up to 14 years of age) living in East London with an IQ below 50, 32 percent had a history of seizures (Corbett, 1983). In Warsaw, 7.2 percent of known cases of epilepsy up to 15 years of age were diagnosed as severely MR (Zielinski, 1974a).

A cohort of MR individuals born in a British city was followed until the age of 22, and a total of 27 percent had a history of at least one seizure. However, seizures were reported in 47 percent of those with an IQ below 50, 29 percent of those with an IQ of 50–59 experienced seizures, and only 20 percent with IQ of more than 60 had seizures. Among controls without MR a history of seizures occurred in only 4 percent. Of children with severe MR, 69 percent had seizures during the first year of life, but only 20 percent of those with IQ greater than 60 (Richardson, Keller, and Katz, 1980). In contrast, children with neurological or developmental abnormalities who were evaluated by the Collaborative Perinatal Project during the first year of life did not have their first seizure earlier than children without such abnormalities. However, an abnormality in the first year of life, before the onset of seizures, was associated with an increased rate of MR and cerebral palsy (Ellenberg *et al.*, 1984).

Further studies on a representative sample of 192 MR inhabitants (aged 16–22) of a British city found epilepsy in 10 percent and behavioural disturbances in 38 percent. Epilepsy was noted most often among those with profound MR (45 percent). Among those with an IQ of 20–29 this percentage was 16, IQ 50–59=11 percent, IQ 60–69=7 percent, and among those with an IQ above 70 only 2 percent had epilepsy (Richardson, Keller, Katz, and McLaren, 1984).

Jacobson and Janicki (1983) listed individuals with mental retardation, autism, cerebral palsy, and epilepsy in all counties of New York State, who: (1) were enrolled in preschool, school, and adult habilitative programs, who lived in a variety of out-of-home residential care situations (including group homes and institutions); or (2) were living at home and participating in or requesting services of programs providing health care, social services, recreation, and other forms of generic services. They found 43,692 inhabitants, 95 percent of whom suffered from MR (22 percent MIMR, 24 percent MOMR, 22 percent SEMR, and 32 percent PMR). This distribution was significantly different from that cited in DSM-III, mostly because of a different case-ascertainment procedure. Specifically, many MIMR cases would not be considered as DD individuals. Of those studied, 33 percent were 21 years old and younger. All together, 23 percent of the children had epilepsy, 23 percent had cerebral palsy, and the average number of conditions per person was 1.44. The authors calculated the chance of coexistence of another disability if one was already present. Among those with MR (up to age 21 years) 23 percent also had epilepsy, and 16 percent had CP. Among those diagnosed with epilepsy, 88 percent also had MR, and 32 percent had CP. Epilepsy as the only handicap was found in 9 percent of the developmentally disabled population up to 21 years of age. Moreover, the frequency of both epilepsy and CP increased along with the severity of MR: in MIMR, 9 percent each; in MOMR, 11 and 8 percent; in SEMR, 20 and 13 percent; and in PMR, 43 and 29 percent respectively.

In summary, both MR and epilepsy belong to the most prevalent mental/neurological disorders among children. If the prevalence of children with an IQ of less then 50 varies between three and four per 1000, then the prevalence of mild MR (extrapolated from DSM-III estimates) will be around 15–20 per 1000. Thus, as many as 1.8–2.4 percent of children in the general population are mentally retarded. Over six children among every 1000 will present with epilepsy, and the more severe the mental retardation, the higher the proportion of those also suffering from epilepsy. If one remembers that the frequency of cerebral palsy also correlates with the severity of MR, an increase in multiple and complex needs of these children becomes obvious.

ETIOLOGICAL FACTORS

Any brain injury suffered during the pre-, peri- or postnatal period can be considered as 'causative' for epilepsy, MR, and/or CP. There is also a lengthy list of diseases and conditions associated with MR and epilepsy, including metabolic errors, storage disorders, and chromosomal defects. Some of these factors will be briefly discussed in a review of the more important epileptic syndromes which are often associated with MR. It should be mentioned, however, that many factors which are generally considered causative for epilepsy and MR (shorter gestation, prolonged labor) have not been verified in properly designed studies, while eclampsia, severe brain injury, and a family history of epilepsy have been more consistently observed (Leviton and Cowan, 1982). Finally, in well over half of cases, 'causative' factors for both MR and epilepsy remain unknown.

EPILEPSIES AND EPILEPTIC SYNDROMES FREQUENTLY ASSOCIATED WITH MENTAL RETARDATION

Although the ILAE classification proposal (Dreifuss *et al.*, 1985) has not yet been accepted in final form, it seem useful for clinical–social considerations. Generally, the presence of MR with or without neurological abnormalities before the onset of epilepsy indicates that the epilepsy is 'symptomatic' in terms of this classification in contrast to the 'idiopathic' epilepsies and syndromes in which MR usually does not occur.

Generally the ILAE classification covers four major groups of epilepsies and epileptic syndromes which are subdivided in terms of coexisting signs of brain disorder other than epilepsy, specific disorders associated with seizures, and etiological or triggering factors. This classification is as follows:

1. Localization-related epilepsies and syndromes (focal):
   idiopathic with age-related onset (e.g. Rolandic epilepsy);
   symptomatic, comprising types based on their anatomical localization, seizure type, and etiological factors.
2. Generalized epilepsies and syndromes:
   idiopathic;
   idiopathic and/or symptomatic;
   symptomatic: nonspecific etiology and specific syndromes.
3. Epilepsies and syndromes undetermined as to whether they are focal or generalized.
4. Special syndromes: febrile convulsions, seizures related to other identifiable situations such as sleep deprivation, alcohol withdrawal, toxins; isolated seizures and chronic progressive epilepsia partialis continua of childhood.

Localization-related (focal or partial) epilepsies and epileptic syndromes

Cases in which an epileptogenic focus or foci can be identifed are included here. One of the hallmarks of this class is the occurrence of partial seizures. In Gastaut *et al*'s (1975) series of children with epilepsy, partial seizures were diagnosed in 45 percent (including complex partial seizures in 21 percent and secondarily generalized seizures in 16 percent). The frequency of partial seizures in children with MR is unknown. Because of inadequate or no verbal communication on the part of the patient, a variety of non-epileptic motoric manifestations (varying from tics and mannerisms to spasticity and tremors), and the frequent coexistence of abnormal neurological findings (especially among those with severe MR), the diagnostic accuracy in seizure classification is significantly compromised. Therefore, the occurrence of partial seizures can be underestimated, and many cases are probably included among the generalized epilepsies. This may, in part, explain the beneficial results of therapy with antiepileptic drugs (AEDs) especially effective for partial seizures.

Generalized epilepsies and syndromes

The hallmark here is the presence of primarily generalized seizures, while partial seizures do not occur. Similarly, epileptiform discharges in the EEG are of a generalized type. There are, however, several types of epilepsies which are included in special subgroups, i.e., 'idiopathic and/or symptomatic.' MR frequently coexists in many of these syndromes.

Infantile spasms (IS or West syndrome)

Fortunately, this very severe epileptic syndrome occurs in only a small percentage of children with epilepsy. Incidence rates in the USA are estimated at about 25/100,000 live births followed until the age of 5 years (Van den Berg and Yerushalmy, 1969). Among children with epilepsy, Janz (1969) found 1.8 percent with infantile spasms. In Poland this proportion is estimated at about 3 percent, although in neuropediatric centers it can be much higher (Zielinski, 1976, unpublished data).

IS typically occurs in the first year of life, and up to 70–80 percent of these infants present with some neurological abnormality and/or delayed psychomotor development prior to the onset of seizures. These seizures, also known as 'salaam,' 'jack-knife,' or 'spasm in flexion' attacks, occur frequently in a series. Initially they can be very mild and difficult to recognize, and they are occasionally misdiagnosed as colic attacks. Gradually, the frequency and severity of the seizures increase while at the same time an arrest of development and apparent psychomotor regression may be noted. In the majority of children a typical EEG pattern occurs, consisting of chaotic, high-voltage discharges of a particular spike and slow wave complex (hypsarrhythmia).

Infants who did not show any neurological or psychomotor signs prior to the onset of the seizures are considered to suffer an 'idiopathic' IS and to have a somewhat better prognosis. Others with 'symptomatic' IS and an early age of onset have a poorer prognosis regarding their further psychomotor development. Pre- or perinatal brain injury, mostly of an ischemic–anoxic type, seem to be the most common etiological factor. More rarely, other neurological disorders and syndromes may be diagnosed such as infections (especially cytomegalovirus), tuberous sclerosis, brain malformations, including Aicardi syndrome, phenylketonuria and others (Bellman, 1983; Aicardi, 1986). The psychomotor deterioration can become persistent even when IS subside, and may be more frequent and severe in 'symptomatic' cases. Although treatment with ACTH or steroids can be very effective in arresting the seizures, it does not seem to have a major influence upon the psychomotor sequelae.

Hormonal treatment, however, is associated with a high risk of severe side-effects, including infections, arterial hypertension, electrolyte imbalance, and other problems. Therefore, some authors (Aicardi, 1986) suggest that hormonal treatment should be used only in the 'idiopathic' cases, which have a better prognosis for further psychomotor development. 'Symptomatic' cases can only suffer from the side-effects of this therapy, with little hope for any benefit. Anticonvulsants should be used in all cases: most effective are benzodiazepines, and especially nitrazepam (Mogadon) in monotherapy or in combination with valproic acid. Other AEDs seem of little, if any, value in the treatment of IS.

As mentioned before, the overall prognosis in IS is poor, with a fatality rate of around 20 percent. In survivors, up to half become neurologically handicapped and about 80 percent will suffer from MR. Cases from the 'idiopathic' group have a better prognosis, but over half of the survivors will develop epilepsy, frequently of the Lennox–Gastaut type or with temporal lobe seizures. Underlying cerebral abnormality is the most important factor influencing prognosis. There are no convincing data that early treatment can substantially influence the prognosis (Aicardi, 1986; Holmes, 1987).

Lennox–Gastaut syndrome (LG)

Epidemiological data regarding the incidence of this type of epilepsy are scarce. Janz (1969) estimates its frequency at around 1 percent of the childhood epilepsies, while Gastaut *et al.* (1975) found over 10 percent of such cases among 'classifiable' private patients up to the age of 15 years. These discrepancies are probably related to varying definitions of the syndrome and biases in case-series selection. This epileptic syndrome probably consists of several overlapping disorders (Holmes, 1987). Diagnostic criteria include the occurrence of more than one type of primarily generalizied seizure (e.g. atonic, tonic, myoclonic), mental retardation, and a characteristic EEG pattern. Onset of the seizures generally occurs between 2 and 5 years of age, occasionally later. Similar to IS, there is no single etiological factor and some cases of IS evolve to LG. 'Idiopathic' and 'symptomatic' forms of LG have been proposed (Aicardi, 1986), and the etiological factors are similar to those in IS, aslthough brain malformations occur less often. Tuberous sclerosis is frequently associated with LG.

A variety of clinical seizure types are typically seen in association with LG. Atonic seizures, associated with a sudden loss of muscle tone, vary in their clinical appearance from 'head drops' to sudden heavy falls, frequently resulting in head injuries which can occasionally be severe in nature. The patients frequently appear with numerous scars over their eyebrows, nose, under the chin, and in the occipital area. Atonic seizures are usually very brief, with fast recovery, but can occur in series and, in some cases, appear daily. Brief myoclonic seizures can occur occasionally and may also be associated with a rapid fall. Tonic seizures, which are usually symmetric, can be prolonged. Fully developed tonic–clonic seizures are less frequent. Rarely, typical absences may also occur. As a rule, seizures in LG are frequent and difficult to control.

The EEG usually reveals slow background activity with superimposed atypical spike and wave discharges (usually 1.5–2.5 Hz), and they are usually generalized with a preponderance over the anterior head regions ('petit-mal variant').

As mentioned before, seizures in LG are usually intractable or poorly controlled. Valproate monotherapy, or in combination with benzodiazepines (nitrazepam, clobazam, clonazepam) seems most effective in LG. Other AEDs are rarely helpful. In addition, sedation and drowsiness in patients with LG can precipitate the occurrence of seizures (Papini, Pasquinelli, Armellini, and Orlandi, 1984). Sedative antiepileptic drugs, such as phenobarbital, can thus contribute to an increased frequency of seizures. Finally, carbamazepine has been found to occasionally increase the occurrence of myoclonic, atonic, and absence seizures in children (Snead and Hosey, 1985; Shields and Saslow, 1983). Other side-effects of sedative AEDs and phenytoin will be discussed later.

The prognosis in LG seems to be associated mostly with the underlying etiology. The proportion of severe MR among those with a symptomatic etiology reaches over 72 percent versus some 20 percent of 'primary,' idiopathic cases (Aicardi, 1986). Early onset, similar to IS, is associated with poorer prognosis both in terms of the seizures and psychomotor development.

Symptomatic generalized epilepsies of specific etiologies.

These are frequently associated with MR (mostly genetically transmitted). Only diseases and syndromes in which the epileptic seizures are among the prominent symptoms, and in which MR frequently occurs, are listed below. More complete information will be found in more recent and comprehensive reviews (Aicardi, 1986; Holmes, 1987).

Cerebral malformations:
Aicardi syndrome: females only, agenesis of corpus callosum, early onset, frequently IS, severe MR, survival rarely beyond 20 years
Phacomatoses
- tuberous sclerosis
- meningofacial angiomatosis (Sturge–Weber syndrome)

Neonate infant metabolic errors
- myoclonic encephalopathy
- phenylketonuria
- ceroid lipofuscinosis

Child and adolescence:
Lafora disease: tonic, clonic, myoclonic seizures, ataxia, rapidly progressive MR: average survival 5.5 years
Progressive familial myoclonic epilepsy without Lafora bodies (Unverricht–Lundborg): tonic–clonic and myoclonic seizures, cerebellar ataxia, photosensitivity: MR usually mild, slowly progressing course. A variant of this

form of epilepsy, also of familial type but associated with deafness, is known as May–White syndrome (May and White, 1968)

Rett's syndrome: females only, after a period of normal development, arrest and regression of psychomotor function occurs. Loss of motoric skills of the hands, autism, ataxia, and seizures frequently appear in this syndrome (Rett, 1977; Verma, Chheda, Nigro, and Hart, 1986; Rett Syndrome Diagnostic-Criteria Work Group, 1988).

Other genetically transmitted disorders and chromosomal defects associated with MR will not be discussed here, either because of their very low incidence rate (e.g. juvenile Huntington's disease), or the relatively low frequency of cases with coexisting seizures (e.g. Down's syndrome).

Epilepsies and syndromes undetermined as to whether they are focal or generalized.

It seems that many cases of epilepsy associated with moderate and severe MR can be put in this category. Severe myoclonic epilepsy in infancy, with normal development before the onset of seizures and subsequent arrest of psychomotor development and occurrence of seizures of other types, is considered as a distinct epileptic syndrome.

DIAGNOSING EPILEPSY IN CHILDREN WITH MENTAL RETARDATION

Differential diagnosis

Because of the risk of additional psychosocial complications and chronic anticonvulsant toxicity, the diagnosis of epilepsy in MR children should be made very carefully. All other possible nonepileptic intermittent events should be ruled out. Moreover, such events can occasionally coexist with genuine epileptic seizures. Not infrequently, the differentiation between genuine seizures and other events in childen with MR can be much more difficult than in nonretarded children. Only the most frequent events which run a high risk of being misdiagnosed as epileptic seizures will be discussed below.

Breath-holding spells

This episodic disturbance in breathing pattern is quite frequent in young children, and can be misdiagnosed as tonic seizures. However, these attacks are associated with emotional events and crying, and the child will stop breathing *before* losing consciousness. These spells never occur in sleep and the EEG does not reveal paroxysmal discharges. It is unknown whether children with MR suffer from breath-holding spells more often than children with normal IQs.

Tics

These involuntary, intermittent, spasmodic but habitual movements occur frequently in children and are usually enhanced by an emotional stress. Only rarely can they be misdiagnosed as simple partial motor seizures, but more complex tics can arouse suspicion of psychomotor seizures. Tics are not associated with impairment of consciousness or paroxysmal EEG activity.

Startle responses

These are complex, physiological responses to sudden unexpected stimuli like a loud noise. A good example of such a reaction is Moro response in small children. Usually spasmodic, involuntary movements can be misdiagnosed as a tonic or myoclonic event. In some children (considered to be 'oversensitive') a startle disease may be diagnosed. An episodic hypotonia with a fall or startle reaction without any apparent stimulus can occur.

Startle responses should be differentiated from a startle seizure, i.e. a partial or generalized epileptic seizure (frequently of tonic type) triggered by unexpected stimuli. This type of startle epilepsy occurs more often in children with MR and other neurological handicaps (Anderman and Anderman, 1986).

Night terrors

These usually occur in a child in a deep sleep. The victim suddenly wakes up with a terrified cry and looks extremely frightened. Periods of a restlesness may be as long as 10 minutes, but then the child falls asleep again. The frequency of night terrors in MR children in unknown, and episodes can be mistaken for psychomotor seizures.

Episodic rage attacks (dyscontrol syndrome)

These are not infrequently seen among MR children with or without epilepsy. They are usually triggered by minor events that may even be unnoticed by a witness and will become recognized only after a careful history of the event is obtained. Such patients present with poorly organized violent behavior (spitting, kicking, thrashing, etc.) which is sometimes associated with crying or shouting. Occasionally, violent behavior may be transformed into direct physical aggressiveness against other persons (not necessarily those who 'triggered' the reaction) or into self-abuse, which at times can be dangerous (i.e. head-banging). Rage attacks are sometimes suspected to be of epileptic origin (psychomotor seizures), but are actually rarely of such origin. However, the presence of a triggering factor, violent behavior (unusual in psychomotor seizures), a changing pattern of motoric behavior from one event to another, and frequently disturbed interictal behavior allow for an accurate differentiation between these two possibilities. If an EEG record can be obtained during the event (i.e. by means of a portable cassette recorder), no paroxysmal activity is seen. There is no loss of consciousness during the episode, although some confusion and/or post-event drowsiness and sleep can occur.

Seizures versus pseudoseizures in MR—particular difficulties in differential diagnosis

Pseudoseizures are not infrequent in children, especially among teenagers, and can occur in those with or without epilepsy. Pseudoseizures or psychogenic seizures can be defined as episodes of a particular behavior which are usually triggered by emotional factors. It is probable that not all of these episodes are produced purposefully. Pseudoseizures vary in their clinical appearances from patient to patient and occasionally from event to event. They may consist of simple motor body movements ('thrashing'), but also of more or less organized purposeless or semi-purposeless movements and activities. In an MR population pseudoseizures are usually less organized and can manifest themselves via sudden falls, shakiness, unresponsiveness or 'staring'. Differentiation of these behaviors from genuine seizures may be very difficult even with the use of modern equipment (EEG-videomonitoring), because a substantial amount of cooperation from the patient is needed for such evaluations. Moreover, the patients should not be sedated and should be capable of remaining under close supervision with scalp electrodes for a considerable time. Although with an uncooperative MR patient this method can be of limited value, videomonitoring can be very helpful in identifying the epileptic vs. nonepileptic origin of particular behaviors in children with epilepsy and MR (Holmes, McKeever, and Russman, 1983; Neil and Alvarez, 1986).

There are two other factors which make the differentiation between genuine and psychogenic seizures in those with MR even more difficult. In profoundly MR patients, especially with coexistent CP, seizures and pseudoseizures can be very subtle, and genuine seizures quite atypical. Finally, emotional and behavioural disturbances can be associated with prolonged episodes of hyperventilation, which in turn may precipitate seizures.

Thus, in an MR population with epilepsy, genuine seizures can occasionally be erroneously diagnosed as psychogenic (false negative), while psychogenic spells are sometimes considered to be genuine (false positive). Even the most careful monitoring of these episodes, and most detailed descriptions provided by family members or workers, may sometimes be insufficient for proper differentiation, even in children with known epilepsy and interictal paroxysmal discharges in the EEG (Neil and Alvarez, 1986). Significant elevations of serum prolactin level after a seizure, especially of the tonic–clonic type, can be helpful in differentiating seizures from pseudoseizures, although elevations of prolactin may occasionally occur after heavy physical exercise or pseudo-seizures with massive muscle movements (Oxley, Roberts, Dana-Haeri, and Trimble, 1981; Pritchard, Wannamaker, Sagel, and Daniel, 1985). An additional problem comes from the fact that some of the children with profound MR can continue their tasks despite continuous paroxysmal discharges in their EEG.

Self-induced seizures

The frequency of this phenomenon is unknown, but it seems to occur more often among mentally retarded children with epilepsy than among their peers with normal mental development. Most often these seizures are of a minor variety (although the occurrence of tonic–clonic seizures is occasionally seen). Self-induction is often associated with photosensitive epilepsy documented by a photoconvulsive response in the EEG to photic stimulation. Children usually look into a bright light and begin waving a hand rhythmically (occasionally with fingers spread) against their eyes. In my experience I had the opportunity of seeing only two such cases. Both were males, 7 and 11 years old, mildly MR with behavioral problems and otherwise infrequent seizures of a primary generalized variety. Self-induction seems to occur less often among those with severe MR. Rare cases of triggering seizures by the blinking of eyelids or watching a TV screen up close have also been reported. A more detailed review of this phenomenon can be found in Aicardi's book (1986). According to Aicardi, self-induced seizures occur more often than is currently thought.

There are several important clinical features regarding self-induced seizures. First, they frequently are not properly diagnosed. Second, children may need treatment only if non-induced seizures also occur (which happens in the majority of cases). Third, the frequent occurrence of self-induced seizures may result in either overmedication or classifying those cases as 'intractable epilepsy.' If properly diagnosed, children with self-induced seizures can be successfully helped by means of non-medical measures (avoiding bright lights, wearing dark glasses, watching TV from a distance, etc.). The drug choice in these cases is valproate.

Behavioral problems

There is no doubt that behavioral problems can produce significant difficulties in the diagnosis and treatment of epilepsy in children with MR. Some of the most important problems will be briefly discussed below.

The frequency of behavioral problems seems to be inversely correlated with the level of mental functioning. Even among nonretarded children with epilepsy, those with poor neuropsychological function manifest significantly more aggression and less social competence compared to children with good neuropsychological performance (Hermann, 1982). In a strictly selected group of 100 children with temporal lobe epilepsy (Lindsay, Ounsted, and Richards, 1979a), almost 25 percent presented with a Verbal IQ below 70, and 85 percent with psychological problems (26 percent hyperkinetic, 29 percent with catastrophic rage). At the end of follow-up (among 87 survivors), 10 percent had 'overt schizophreniform psychosis,' 12 percent had antisocial behavior, and 5 percent had neurotic syndrome or depression (Lindsay, Ounsted, and Richards, 1979b). Among 155 severely MR children Corbett (1975) identified 13 percent with self-injurious behavior; half of them were head-banging. An epidemiological study in a British city (Richardson *et al.*, 1984) revealed 192 persons aged 16–22 years with various levels of MR. Behavioral disturbance including emotional problems, aggressiveness, and self-injurious behavior were identified in 38 percent of the sample. The frequency of such disturbances among the mildly, moderately, and severely retarded varied between 32 and 36 percent; only among the profoundly retarded was this frequency slightly higher, i.e. 40 percent. Interestingly enough, among individuals with epilepsy 40 percent presented with behavioral problems. This percentage is similar to the average for the total group (38 percent).

There is no doubt that behavioral problems can produce significant difficulties in the diagnosis and treatment of epilepsy in children with MR, and some of the most important problems will be briefly discussed below.

Urinary incontinence

Most children with MR present with primary enuresis, i.e. they have never achieved sufficient bladder control. Incontinence can occur only during sleep (bed-wetting) and less often during the daytime. After ruling out the potential organic causes of urinary incontinence (including UTI), a question should be raised whether incontinence might be associated with the occurrence of a seizure. This suspicion can be very essential in cases with relatively infrequent episodes of incontinence, especially during the night. Children should then be carefully watched and other findings suggestive of a nocturnal seizure should be explored (bitten tongue; saliva, especially bloody, on the pillow; falling out of bed). It is quite obvious that the treatment of incontinence in such cases is targeted against the primary cause—seizures, and not against bed-wetting as such. Moreover, bed-wetting secondary to seizure occurrence may be tentatively used in recording the frequency of nocturnal seizures which otherwise might be overlooked. Similarly, urinary incontinence during the day may be associated with seizures, especially of a generalized variety, including typical and atypical absences. It cannot be emphasized enough that children who experience seizures during their sleep should not have pillows in their beds, since there is a risk of suffocation during or immediately after the seizure if the child turns and 'sinks' her or his face in the pillow.

Stool incontinence associated with seizures occurs less often, and happens usually among the severe MR. Children with incontinence of urine and/or stool which is not associated exclusively with seizures are usually placed on special programs. Unfortunately, in some cases the urinary incontinence occurs both with and without seizures. These children should be started on appropriate programs along with attempts to improve the effectiveness of their antiepileptic treatment. It is worth remembering, however, that sedative antiepileptic drugs can contribute significantly to nocturnal enuresis by deepening sleep.

Disturbed sleeping pattern

There are no reliable data regarding the frequency of this problem among children with MR and epilepsy, but it is generally accepted that sleep disturbances occur often, especially in children with MR and CP (Hall, 1984). Frequent awakening during the night, or a tendency toward reversal of a circadian rhythm—especially if prolonged, can reduce the level of alertness during the daytime. This in turn will impair the child's attention span and increase his/her hyperactivity. Moreover, sleep deprivation and drowsiness can precipitate the occurrence of seizures (Aird, 1983), especially in some epileptic syndromes such as Lennox–Gastaut syndrome (Papini *et al.*, 1984). Sleep deprivation can also be iatrogenic. For example, when a child is started on a program to control incontinence, this may include waking him or her several times during the night. A temporary sleep disturbance may also be associated in rare cases with phenobarbital withdrawal syndrome (Zielinski and Rader, 1987).

Hyperventilation

Episodic and especially prolonged periods of overbreathing may occur not infrequently in severe MR cases, but may also be occasionally seen among the mildly retarded. Usually these episodes are triggered by emotional stimuli. If prolonged, hyperventilation will produce respiratory alkalosis and thus trigger a seizure (Aird, 1983). In some cases, periods of overbreathing appear intermittently with breath-holding spells.

Vomiting, regurgitating, and rumination

These abnormal behaviors occur more often in severe MR, especially complicated by CP (Hall, 1984), and can significantly reduce the effectiveness of medical treatment. In addition, some AEDs have irritative properties to the stomach (valproate, carbamazepine, phenytoin) which, although mild, may be sufficient to trigger episodes of vomiting or regurgitation. If vomiting occurs shortly after an AED is administered, one can never be certain what proportion of the dose remained in the stomach. Adjustment of doses in such cases can be very difficult, and in extreme conditions the patients might have to be treated with phenobarbital i.m. once a day. Most often, however, the problem can be solved by giving medications with a small amount of the child's favorite food, and employing behavior modification measures. However, in every child with epilepsy and MR, vomiting should be suspected if serum levels of the AED vary despite an unchanged dose, or if a therapeutic serum concentration cannot be achieved. Numerous other factors can also play a role, including medical noncompliance and drug interactions. Habitual vomiting and rumination in extreme cases can be life-threatening.

Pica

Swallowing of inedible objects and substances occurs most often in severe MR, and occasionally results in serious problems. One is the risk of lead encephalopathy secondary to eating paints containing lead. Nowadays this risk can also be associated with swallowing various chemicals. One of my own patients managed to swallow a large plastic trash bag, and required a surgical procedure to remove it from the gut. In the meantime, the patient presented with serious nutritional problems along with a significant increase in seizure frequency secondary to impaired absorption of AEDs. Ingestion of hair or clothes can also result in intestinal obstruction.

Self-injurious behavior (SIB)

It is important to differentiate this type of behavior from other stereotyped or manneristic motoric activities like rocking or hand-clapping, which may occur in about 30 percent of children with MR (Corbett, 1975). SIB is usually defined as intentional activity, and hard enough to cause tissue damage. In a special program for MR patients with SIB in England, 89 percent were severely retarded, and higher rates occurred in children and adolescents. SIB has been identified in 12 percent of institutionalized MR cases compared to only 3 percent of noninstitutionalized cases (Oliver, Murphy, and Corbett, 1987). A higher rate of SIB in institutions is related to case-selection, i.e. those with SIB were more often referred to hospitals and institutions. Special syndromes such as the Lesch–Nyhan syndrome occur very seldom. About half of those with SIB present with head-banging, either against hard structures (wall, floor, furniture, etc.), or hand-hitting. This type of behavior is frequently related to emotional outbursts or to attention-seeking. If hard enough it may result in severe brain injury, including intracranial bleeding and cerebral tissue damage. It is quite obvious that in cases with a coexisting seizure disorder this may aggravate the course of the epilepsy. Drug treatment is usually ineffective and behavior modification programs are the treatment of choice (Hall, 1984). In extreme cases aversion methods can be employed, but they should be used very carefully and only by experienced and reliable staff (Corbett, 1975; Council on Scientific Affairs, 1987). A mist of cold water to the face seems a relatively safe and effective method.

Irritability, aggressiveness

An increase in irritability prior to a seizure, and relaxation afterwards, is a well-known phenomenon. On the other hand, aggressiveness only rarely occurs as an ictal event, and even then is usually provoked by external stimuli (i.e. attempts to restrain a child during a complex partial seizure). This problem has been extensively reviewed recently by a special committee (Special Report, 1981) in nonretarded, mostly adult patients with epilepsy. In those with MR, aggressiveness not related to seizures seems to occur more frequently, but no exact statistics are available.

A negative influence of sedative AEDs on cognitive functions and behavior is discussed in other chapters of this book. It should be mentioned here, however, that patients with epilepsy and MR have been known for a long time to be 'oversensitive' to anticonvulsant drugs. In 1940 Williamson reported the frequent occurrence of severe side-effects of phenytoin in a group of MR patients, including disturbances of consciousness and an increase in seizure frequency. The case fatality rate in this series was as high as 20 percent.

Phenobarbital is well known for causing irritability in children, and phenytoin for producing behavioral problems (Rivinus, 1982; Sheard, 1984). In my own series of 151 mentally retarded patients with epilepsy, in whom sedative AEDs were discontinued, almost 80 percent presented with excessive irritability and 65 percent with physical aggressiveness. Of those, up to 80–90 percent were significantly improved after sedative AEDs were finally discontinued (Zielinski and Rader, 1987). The frequency of SIB in this series was not analyzed, but family and/or group home staff members reported a decline in SIB along with an increase in alertness and activity level in many patients after the discontinuation of sedative AEDs.

Medical diagnosis

The initial medical diagnosis in children with MR and epilepsy does not differ from the routine steps taken with nonretarded children. Important for both groups are the family and individual history, detailed description of seizures, general and neurological examination, EEG, CT head scan, and psychological evaluation if needed. A complete neuropsychological evaluation in addition to special laboratory tests aimed towards the detection of metabolic and chromosomal anomalies, and occasionally angiography or MRI in special syndromes (such as phacomatoses), are needed in the medical evaluation of MR children with a seizure disorder.

Furthermore, additional coexisting problems (e.g. CP, autism, skeletal abnormalities) must be evaluated in detail and a comprehensive, multidisciplinary treatment program should be developed covering immediate and long-range goals. The development of close and regular cooperation between the physician, parents, and other persons involved in a comprehensive care and treatment program is of vital importance.

ANTICONVULSANT TREATMENT AND FOLLOW-UP

Indications for the initiation of treatment and AED choice do not differ from the routine practice in the treatment of childhood epilepsy (American Association of Pediatrics, 1985). It should be kept in mind, however, that patients with MR may be more sensitive to the various side-effects of AEDs. In addition, clinical signs of AED side-effects/toxicity can be distorted or masked by preexisting neurological abnormalities and delays in mental development. Therefore, one should avoid (if possible) AEDs known to have adverse effects on the nervous system, even in so-called 'therapeutic' serum concentration (Reynolds, 1982).

In a comprehensive review of the long-term effects of anticonvulsant therapy in mentally retarded children with epilepsy (Corbett *et al.*, 1985), intellectual deterioration of those treated with phenobarbital and phenytoin was widely discussed. The problem of phenytoin-induced cerebellar atrophy in mentally retarded children has also been surveyed by Iivanainen, Vinkari, and Helle (1977). More research is needed on this topic. Similarly, phenytoin-induced peripheral neuropathy in children has been reported (Mochizuki *et al.*, 1981). Behavioral side-effects of AEDs in MR patients have been studied using an operant behavior method (Gay, 1984) and operant tasks appeared to be sensitive to AEDs. Patients on phenobarbital most frequently exhibited frustration during testing, whereas those on valproate responded at rates comparable to controls. A review of the current bulk of literature, including extensive monographs (Hall, 1984; Holmes, 1987; Aicardi, 1986), indicates that drugs of first choice in epilepsy are valproate, carbamazepine, and ethosuximide. Sedative AEDs, including clonazepam, are indicated only if other AEDs are ineffective. The use of phenytoin might be limited because of its side-effects to which multiply handicapped, mentally retarded children seem to be especially sensitive.

As a rule, treatment should be started using a single AED. If ineffective in sufficient serum concentration, an alternate drug should be tried. Use of multiple drugs significantly increases the risk of chronic toxicity secondary to drug–drug interactions. However, the use of more than two AEDs might sometimes be necessary in treating refractory cases (Theodore, Schulman, and Porter, 1983).

Comedication with psychotropic drugs is usually not effective in alleviating behavioral problems. Even more problematic is the fact that many psychotropic drugs tend to lower the seizure threshold, and in turn might result in an otherwise unnecessary increase in AED dose/serum level to achieve sufficient seizure control (James, 1986). Finally, a pharmacodynamic type of interaction between lithium (occasionally used for the treatment of behavioral problems) and phenytoin and carbamazepine can produce lithium toxicity within a 'therapeutic' serum concentration. Thus, with few exceptions, the use of sedatives and tranquilizers should be regarded as an evil and very temporary 'holding device' in the treatment of associated behavioral disturbances (Kirman, 1975).

Keeping a routine record of seizure frequency may be helpful in the treatment of a seizure disorder, but it is especially essential in children with MR who have frequent seizures and who are not capable of reporting their own seizure frequency. Such a record (if systematic and reliable) can be of major importance in making choices about and adjusting doses of AEDs, especially over a prolonged period of time. Comparing records from consecutive months and years can provide useful information including the most effective medication regimen. Moreover, further diagnostic procedures (repeated neuropsychological evaluation, EEG, or head CT scan) might be necessary when there is a change in the clinical appearance of the seizures, or when there is a change in the pattern and frequency of the seizures (assuming serum levels of AEDs remain the same). Change in a seizure pattern in a child with chronic epilepsy may be indicative of the appearance of a new problem (drug toxicity, brain tumor, chronic subdural hematoma).

The clustering of seizures can sometimes indicate the possibility of medical noncompliance. However, if this is not the case, the use of temporary measures to extinguish a cluster (i.e. Valium p.r.n.) can be considered instead of increasing the daily doses of an AED.

Because children with MR seem more sensitive to the side-effects of AEDs, monitoring of serum levels should be done more often, especially if new manifestations of uncertain origin appear. Otherwise, in asymptomatic children with epilepsy, frequent repetition of AED serum levels—and especially blood tests and screening for AED-induced liver, blood, or renal damage—seem to be of little value (Camfield, Camfield, Smith, and Tibbles, 1986). Similarly, in poorly controlled epilepsy, repeated EEG records are of limited, if any, clinical value (Theodore, Sato, and Porter, 1984). Thus major attention should be focused on observing the child and reducing drug treatment to a necessary minimum. Once again, the physician's role in preparing the parents or other caregivers to adequately supervise and observe the MR child with epilepsy is of crucial importance for achieving maximum therapeutic effects and avoiding potentially dangerous situations.

PROGNOSIS AND THERAPEUTIC CONSIDERATIONS

The chances of achieving seizure-free status in specific seizure syndromes such as infantile spasms and Lennox–Gastaut syndrome is usually poor, although they might vary depending upon diagnostic criteria and case ascertainment methods. Generally, less than 10 percent of children with 'symptomatic' infantile spasms can achieve seizure freedom, while among those with Lennox–Gastaut 60–100 percent are 'refractory' to treatment (Leviton and Cowan, 1982). Aicardi (1986) considers prognosis in 'symptomatic' infantile spasms to be very poor independent of treatment, and he therefore carefully weighs the serious side-effects of hormonal therapy versus doubtful improvement, which rarely is achieved. In a group of selected children with severe temporal lobe epilepsy, about 33 percent achieved a seizure-free status (Lindsay *et al.*, 1979b). Annegers, Hauser, and Elveback (1979), in a longitudinal Rochester population study, found that among patients with seizure onset in childhood and adolescence, some 60 percent are seizure-free for 5 years within 10 years after the diagnosis of epilepsy, and 70 percent at 20 years. Unfortunately, mental status is not considered by these authors.

A review of the pertinent literature by Aicardi (1986) suggests that mental retardation may be associated with a poorer prognosis regarding seizure freedom. This was also found in the Warsaw study (Zielinski, 1974a), although no separate data for children are available. Schmidt (1985), pooling selected case-series, found that on the average only 14 percent of patients were seizure-free and MR was associated with a high risk of recurrence. However, status epilepticus was rarely, if ever, seen as result of AED discontinuation. On the other hand, several authors have stated that impaired mental status is not necessarily associated with poorer seizure control, and over 60 percent of MR patients can achieve seizure freedom. No differences in outcome as a function of the level of MR were found (Theodore *et al.*, 1983; O'Neil *et al.*, 1977; Shinnar *et al.*, 1985). Thus, a significant percentage of MR individuals with epilepsy have a chance of becoming seizure-free for long periods of time.

Although the frequency of relapse is considered to be about 25–30 percent in those who achieved remission, the percentage does not seem much higher among patients with MR. In my own series, 30 percent of patients who were seizure-free for 6 months prior to discontinuation of sedative AEDs did not suffer any seizures over a 2-year follow-up.

The above data have significant implications for the initiation and maintenance of treatment with AEDs among children with seizures and MR. Keeping in mind the chronic toxicity of anticonvulsants, decisions regarding the initiation of treatment must be taken very carefully. Some authors consider treatment only in cases with frequent or severe seizures, or if improvement can be achieved without major side-effects (Reynolds, 1982; Taylor and McKinlay, 1984). In my own experience I have found patients who have been seizure-free for years who are still being maintained on high doses of anticonvulsants because of the widespread opinion concerning the poor prognosis of seizure control in patients with MR. However, if a pessimist accepts that in most of these cases the risk of relapse is about 30 percent, an optimist points out that there is a 70 percent chance of remaining seizure-free without medication, and that the patient deserves to be given such a chance. Finally, 'persistence of epilepsy *despite* treatment is the surest indication for persisting with treatment,' and 'many patients are kept in treatment despite continuous seizures on the basis of anxieties about what might happen without it' (Taylor and McKinlay, 1984). If discontinuation of treatment cannot be considered, placement of such 'refractory' cases on moderate doses of the least toxic anticonvulsant seems the wisest course of action. Thus, an old saying 'primum non nocere' (first—do not harm) is fully applied to cases in whom seizures can be fully controlled only at the price of severe lethargy or suppression of remaining cognitive functions (Reynolds, 1983; Vining, 1987) or even the loss of locomotion (Iivanainen *et al*. 1977).

Mortality rates

Increased standardized mortality ratios (SMR—proportion of observed to expected number of deaths) and reduced survivorship in patients with epilepsy are well known from the literature (Hauser, Annegers, and Elveback, 1980; Zielinski, 1974b). In Rochester the SMR was calculated at 2.3, but for patients with a 'neurodeficit since birth' the ratio was 11.0 (including 20.0 in first year and 33.3 between 2 and 4 years after diagnosis of epilepsy was made). Patients whose diagnosis was made prior to 1 year of age had a very poor prognosis. In Warsaw the SMR was calculated at 3.5 in the younger age group (0–29 years). In a selected group of 100 children with temporal lobe epilepsy, five died before reaching age of 15 (including three deaths directly related to epilepsy). An additional nine died prior to age of 20 (three of them died of status epilepticus) (Lindsay *et al*., 1979b).

Similarly, higher death rates are noted among mentally retarded persons, especially among those with severe MR. In the Salford area, over a period of 13 years, 118 deaths occurred among the severe MR and 43 among mildly MR citizens. The SMR for MR population was 1.62. However, over 50 percent of the deaths in the general population occurred above 70 years of age, whereas among deaths in the severe MR almost 30 percent occurred by the age of 5 and another 7 percent by the age of 15 years. The above figures were computed by me on the basis of figures presented in the Salford area study by the author (Fryers, 1984). The majority of deaths in those with mild MR occurred after the age of 40. Respiratory diseases were responsible for 40 percent of the deaths among severe MR persons (Fryers, 1984). In Canadian institutions for MR a 17 percent reduction in the number of inpatients was noted over the period between 1966 and 1978. At the same time the median age of inpatients increased and the average age at death increased by 5 years. SMR declined from 2.5 to 2.0, but MR inpatients between 5 and 9 years of age have reduced the expected survival by 22.4 (females), to 26 years (males). However, in 1978 survival was almost twice as long compared to the years 1966–8 (Wolf and Wright, 1987). Thus, the coexistence of epilepsy and MR significantly reduces the expected survivorship of children. In recent years this reduction is clearly declining, and this will result in an increased number of children with epilepsy and MR and their accompanying comprehensive needs.

CONCLUSION

It should be pointed out that recognition of comprehensive needs of children with MR and epileptic seizures no longer is limited to a number of professionals and staff members of various institutions for MR children. The recent policy of transferring developmentally disabled persons (most of whom suffer from severe MR) from institutions to small community settings will result in the appearance of MR children and adolescents in various local health service facilities (pediatric, neuropediatric, and neuropsychological offices). At the same time the network of special schools and rehabilitation centers is expanding. Thus, many more professionals in the areas of health and education will be exposed to the multifacited needs of MR children with epilepsy. These professionals need to improve their knowledge base enabling them to cope with the needs of this occasionally extremely difficult and challenging group of children. Various local organizations dealing with problems of epilepsy, MR, and DD, as well as university hospitals and centers, should be of great help.

REFERENCES

Aicardi, J. (1986). *Epilepsy in Children*, Raven Press, New York.

Aird, R.B. (1983). The importance of seizure-inducing factors in the control of refractory forms of epilepsy, *Epilepsia*, **24**, 567–583.

American Association of Pediatrics, Committee on Drugs (1985). Behavioral and cognitive effects of anticonvulsant therapy, *Pediatrics*, **76**, 644–647.

Anderman, F., and Anderman, E. (1986). Excessive startle syndromes: startle disease, jumping, and startle epilepsy. In S. Fahn, C.D. Marsden, and M.H. Van Woerts (eds), *Advances in Neurology*, vol. 43: *Myoclonus*, Raven Press, New York, pp. 321–338.

Annegers, J.F., Hauser, W.A., and Elveback, L.R. (1979). Remission of seizures and relapse in patients with epilepsy, *Epilepsia*, **20**, 729–737.

Bellman, M. (1983). Infantile spasms. In T.A. Pedley and B.S. Meldrum (eds), *Recent Advances in Epilepsy*, Churchill Livingstone, New York, pp. 113–138.

Camfield, C.C., Camfield, P., Smith, E., and Tibbles, J.A.R. (1986). Asymptomatic children with epilepsy: little benefit from screening for anticonvulsant-induced liver, blood or renal damage, *Neurology*, **36**, 838–841.

Cooper, J.E. (1965). Epilepsy in a longitudinal survey of 5000 children, *British Medical Journal*, **1**, 1020–1022.

Corbett, J.A. (1975). Aversion for the treatment of self-injurious behavior, *Journal of Mental Deficiency Research*, **19**, 79–95.

Corbett, J.A. (1983). Epilepsy and mental retardation—a follow-up study. In M. Parsonage, R.H.E. Grant, A.G. Craig, and A.A. Ward Jr (eds), *Advances in Epileptology, XIVth Epilepsy International Symposium*, Raven Press, New York, pp. 207–214.

Corbett, J.A., Trimble, M.R., and Nichol, T. (1985). Behavioral and cognitive impairment in children with epilepsy: the long-term effects of anticonvulsant therapy, *Journal of the American Academy of Child Psychiatry*, **24**, 17–23.

Council on Scientific Affairs (1987). Aversion therapy, *Journal of the American Medical Association*, **258**, 2562–2566.

Dreifuss, F.E., Martinez-Lage, M., Roger, J., Wolf, P., and Dam, M. (1985) Proposal for classification of epilepsies and epileptic syndromes, *Epilepsia*, **26**, 268–278.

DSM-III (1986). *Diagnostic and Statistical Manual of Mental Disorders*, 3rd edn, American Psychiatric Association, Washington, DC.

Ellenberg, J.H., Hirtz, D.G., and Nelson, K.B. (1984). The age of onset of seizures in young children, *Annals of Neurology*, **15**, 127–134.

Fryers, T. (1984). *The Epidemiology of Severe Intellectual Impairment: The Dynamics of Prevalence*, Academic Press, London.

Gastaut, H. (1973). *Dictionary of Epilepsy. Part I: Definitions*, WHO, Geneva.

Gastaut, H., Gastaut, J.L., Goncalves e Silva, G.E., and Fernandez Sanchez, G.R. (1975). Relative frequency of different types of epilepsy: a study of employing the classification of the International League Against Epilepsy, *Epilepsia*, **16**, 457–461.

Gay, P.E. (1984). Effects of antiepileptic drugs and seizure type on operant responding in mentally retarded persons, *Epilepsia*, **25**, 377–386.

Hall, D.M.B. (1984). *The Child with a Handicap*, Blackwell Scientific Publications, Oxford/Boston.

Hauser, W.A., Annegers, J.F., and Elveback, L.R. (1980). Mortality in patients with epilepsy, *Epilepsia*, **21**, 399–412.

Hermann, B.P. (1982). Neuropsychological functioning and psychopathology in children with epilepsy, *Epilepsia*, **23**, 545–554.

Holmes, G.L. (1987). *Diagnosis and Management of Seizures in Children*, W.B. Saunders, Philadelphia.

Holmes, G., McKeever, M., and Russman, B.S. (1983). Abnormal behavior or epilepsy? Use of long-term EEG and videomonitoring with severely to profoundly mentally retarded patients with seizures, *American Journal of Mental Deficiency*, **87**, 456–458.

Iivanainen, M., Viukari, M., and Helle, E.P. (1977). Cerebellar atrophy in phenytoin-treated mentally retarded epileptics, *Epilepsia*, **18**, 375–385.

Jacobson, J.W., and Janicki, M.P. (1983). Observed prevalence in multiple developmental disabilities, *Mental Retardation*, **21**, 87–94.

James, D.H. (1986). Neuroleptics and epilepsy in mentally handicapped patients, *Journal of Mental Deficiency Research*, **30**, 185–189.

Janz, D. (1969). *Die Epilepsien*, Georg Thieme, Stuttgart.

Kirman, B. (1975). Drug therapy in mental handicap, *British Journal of Psychiatry*, **127**, 545–549.

Leviton, A., and Cowan, L.D. (1982). Epidemiology of seizure disorders in children, *Neuroepidemiology*, **1**, 40–83.

Lindsay, J., Ounsted, C., and Richards, P. (1979a). Long-term outcome in children with temporal lobe seizures. I. Social outcome and childhood factors, *Developmental Medicine and Child Neurology*, **21**, 285–298.

Lindsay, J., Ounsted, C., and Richards, P. (1979b). Long-term outcome in children with temporal lobe seizures. III. Psychiatric aspects in childhood and adult life, *Developmental Medicine and Child Neurology*, **21**, 630–636.

May, D.L., and White, H.H. (1968). 'Familial myoclonus, cerebellar ataxia and deafness, *Archives of Neurology*, **19**, 331–338.

Mochizuki, Y., Suyehiro, Y., Tanizawa, A., Ohkubo, H., and Motomura, T. (1981). Peripheral neuropathy in children on long-term phenytoin therapy, *Brain and Development*, **3**, 375–383.

Neill, J.C., and Alvarez, N. (1986). Differential diagnosis of epileptic versus pseudoepileptic seizures in developmentally disabled persons, *Applied Research in Mental Retardation*, **7**, 285–298.

Oliver, C., Murphy, G.H., and Corbett, J.A. (1987). Self-injurious behavior in people with mental handicap: a total population study, *Journal of Mental Deficiency Research*, **31**, 147–162.

O'Neill, B.P., Ladon, B., Harris, L.M., Riley, III H.L., and Dreifuss, F.E. (1977). A comprehensive interdisciplinary approach to the care of the institutionalized persons with epilepsy, *Epilepsia*, **18**, 243–250.

Oxley, J., Roberts, M., Dana-Haeri, J., and Trimble, M. (1981). Evaluation of prolonged 4-channel EEG taped recordings and serum prolactin levels in the diagnosis of epileptic and non-epileptic seizures. In M. Dam, L. Gram, and J.K. Penry (eds), *Advances in Epileptology. XIIth Epilepsy International Symposium*, Raven Press, New York, pp. 343–355.

Papini, M., Pasquinelli, A., Armellini, M., and Orlandi, D. (1984). Alertness and incidence of seizures in patients with Gastaut–Lennox syndrome, *Epilepsia*, **25**, 161–167.

Pritchard, III, P.B., Wannamaker, B.B., Sagel, J., and Daniel, C.M. (1985). Serum prolactin and cortizol in evaluation of pseudoepileptic seizures, *Annals of Neurology*, **18**, 87–89.

Rett, A. (1977). Cerebral atrophy associated with hyperammonemia, *Handbook of Clinical Neurology*, **29**, 305–329.

Rett Syndrome Diagnostic-Criteria Work Group (1988). Diagnostic criteria for Rett syndrome, *Archives of Neurology*, **23**, 425–428.

Reynolds, E.H. (1982). The pharmacological management of epilepsy associated with psychological disorders', *British Journal of Psychiatry*, **141**, 549–557.

Reynolds, E.H. (1983). Biological factors in psychiatric disorders associated with epilepsy. In M. Parsonage, R.H.E. Grant, A.G. Craig, and A.A. Ward (eds), *Advances in Epileptology. XIVth Epilepsy International Symposium*, Raven Press, New York, pp. 155–164.

Richardson, S.A., Koller, H., and Katz, M. (1980). Seizures and epilepsy in a mentally retarded population over the first 22 years of life, *Applied Research in Mental Retardation*, **1**, 123–138.

Richardson, S.A., Koller, H., Katz, M., and McLaren, J. (1984). Patterns of disability in a mentally retarded population between ages 16 and 22 years. In J.M. Berg (ed.), *Perspectives and Progress in Mental Retardation*, Vol.II: *Biomedical Aspects*, IASSMD, pp. 25–37.

Rivinus, T.M. (1982). Psychiatric effects of the anticonvulsant regimens, *Journal of Clinical Psychopharmacology*, **2**, 165–192.

Ross, E.M., Peckham, C.J., West, P.B., and Butler, N.R. (1980). Epilepsy in childhood: findings from the National Child Development Study, *British Medical Journal*, **1**, 207–210.

Rutter, M., Tizard, J., and Whitmore, K. (1970). *Education, Health and Behavior*, Longman, London.

Schmidt, D. (1985). Discontinuation of antiepileptic drugs. In R.J. Porter and P.L. Morselli (eds), *The Epilepsies*, Butterworths, London, pp. 227–241.

Sheard, M.H. (1984). Clinical pharmacology of aggressive behavior, *Clinical Neuropharmacology*, **7**, 173–183.

Shields, W.D., and Saslow, E. (1983). Myoclonic, atonic and absence seizures following institution of carbamazepine therapy in children, *Neurology*, **33**, 1487–1489.

Shinnar, S., Vining, E.P.G., Mellits, E., D'Souza, B.J., Holden, K., Baumgardner, R.A., and Freeman, J.M. (1985). Discontinuing antiepileptic medication in children with epilepsy after two years without seizures, *New England Journal of Medicine*, **313**, 976–980.

Snead, III, O.C., and Hosey, L.C. (1985). Exacerbation of seizures in children by carbamazepine, *New England Journal of Medicine*, **313**, 916–921.

Special Report (1981). The nature of aggression during epileptic seizures, *New England Journal of Medicine*, **305**, 711–716.

Taylor, D.C., McKinlay, I. (1984). When not to treat epilepsy with drugs. *Developmental Medicine and Child Neurology*, **26**, 822–827.

Theodore, W.H., Schulman, E.A., and Porter, R.J. (1983). Intractable seizures: long term follow-up after prolonged inpatient treatment in an epilepsy unit, *Epilepsia*, **24**, 336–343.

Theodore, W.H., Sato, S., and Porter, R.J. (1984). Serial EEG in intractable epilepsy, *Neurology*, **34**, 863–867.

Van den Berg, B.J., and Yerushalmy, J. (1969). Studies on convulsive disorders in young children. Part I. Incidence of febrile and nonfebrile convulsions by age and other factors, *Pediatric Research*, **3**, 298–304.

Verma, N.P., Chheda, R.L., Nigro, M.A., and Hart, Z.W. (1986). Electroencephalographic findings in Rett's syndrome, *Electroencephalography and Clinical Neurophysiology*, **64**, 394–401.

Vining, E.P.G. (1987). Cognitive dysfunction associated with anti-epileptic drug therapy, *Epilepsia*, **28** (Suppl. 2), 18–22.

Williamson, B.A.M. (1940). Severe toxic effects of sodium diphenylhydantoin in mentally defective epileptics, *Journal of Mental Sciences*, **86**, 981–987.

Wolf, L.C., and Wright, R.E. (1987). Changes in life expectancy of mentally retarded persons in Canadian institutions: a 12-year comparison, *Journal of Mental Deficiency Research*, **31**, 41–59.

Zielinski, J.J. (1974a). *Epidemiology and Medical–Social Problems of Epilepsy in Warsaw*. Report on Research Program 1-P-58325, Social and Rehabilitation Service, DHEW, Washington, DC and Psychoneurological Institute, Warsaw.

Zielinski, J.J. (1974b). Epilepsy and mortality rates and cause of death, *Epilepsia*, **15**, 191–201.

Zielinski, J.J. (1986). Selected psychiatric and psychosocial aspects of epilepsy as seen by an epidemiologist. In S. Whitman and B.P. Hermann (eds), *Psychopathology in Epilepsy: Social Dimensions*, Oxford University Press, New York and Oxford, pp. 38–65.

Zielinski, J.J., and Rader, B. (1987). Risks and beneficial effects of withdrawal of sedative antiepileptic drugs (SAEDs): long-term follow-up. Paper presented at XVIIth Epilepsy International Congress, Jerusalem, 6–11 September (To be published).

Chapter 15

Treatment of Children with Epilepsy on a Comprehensive Inpatient Unit

Nancy Santilli and Stephen Tonelson

Comprehensive epilepsy programs in the United States developed as an extension of the concept of centers of excellence, and were conceived with the aim of coordinating, advancing, and unifying the efforts directed at understanding, treating, and eliminating seizure disorders by employing both research and service tools (Dreifuss, 1979). The overall objectives of the comprehensive epilepsy programs, known as CEPs, were to develop a program that would maximise the full potential of each individual with epilepsy, and to design a model program that could be translated to other geographic areas or organizational settings. This was possible through the development of research programs that led to a better understanding of the basic mechanisms of the epilepsies and epileptic syndromes, and included ideas to improve methods of treatment. The original five CEPs funded by the National Institute for Neurological and Communicative Disorders and Stroke, developed according to their own inherent strengths and regional characteristics. While most CEPs have many common features, this chapter will focus on the program developed at the University of Virginia.

The CEP at the University of Virginia has three major program areas: service, research, and education. Each major program area interacts with the others to enhance their thinking, and to allow the exchange of experience, ideas, and information. With this close working relationship the lag time between discovery, testing, application, and evaluation of new information and methods is significantly reduced. For the individual who suffers with epilepsy and his family, this up-to-date exchange, as well as the ability to view the person with epilepsy as a whole being, is crucial.

The Commission for the Control of Epilepsy and its Consequences (1977) supported the need for a more service-based multidisciplinary system which they referred to as 'The Epilepsy Family and Individual Resource Team' (EFIRT). They felt these teams should be located at major medical centers

Childhood Epilepsies: Neuropsychological, Psychosocial and Intervention Aspects
Edited by B. Hermann and M. Seidenberg

where technical resources could be shared. The Commission recognized the need for these teams to provide intensive medical diagnosis and treatment, evaluation of neuropsychological aspects of behavior, assistance in coping with socioeconomic problems, educational and vocational evaluations and recommendations, provision for legal and advocacy services, and, at the same time, allow clinical research to improve all aspects of treatment.

Most cases of childhood epilepsy can be treated effectively on an outpatient basis. However, in 10–30 percent of the cases this is not possible. It is these children that need the specialized services available at a comprehensive epilepsy program or exposure to an EFIRT. In the difficult-to-control cases, attention is given to establishing the diagnosis, instituting the appropriate therapy, and developing treatment plans that will produce positive social and educational/vocational outcomes for the child. In these difficult-to-control cases, these principles are achieved most effectively on a comprehensive inpatient unit. Through a multidisciplinary approach, the uncontrolled seizures will have the greatest chance of being controlled without compromising the quality of the child's life.

Comprehensive inpatient units were developed with the understanding that if you could bring a multidisciplinary professional team together in an organized manner to evaluate, monitor, and establish an individualized treatment for a child, his/her chances for a normal life are increased immensely. On these speciality units, the team members work closely with their counterparts in the child's local community from the time of referral to months or years after discharge, depending on the individual needs of the child and family. Thus the process of evaluating, treating, and developing long-term plans for the child on an inpatient unit is a dynamic one from the time the first contact is made until, in some instances, years after discharge.

The specialized inpatient unit at the University of Virginia is located at the Blue Ridge Hospital. The unit consists of 15 beds, with facilities for education, recreation, and activities for daily living. At the same time, the unit provides space for intensive monitoring, comprehensive evaluations, and treatment. Intensive EEG monitoring equipment, which allows for video-recordings of events, is available. Patients are transported to the main Univeristy Hospital approximately 3.5 miles away for tests such as CT and MRI scans. Otherwise, the major portion of the evaluation occurs on site with other specialists being consulted as needed.

Once contact is made regarding a possible referral, the system is set in motion that mobilizes the team. Since individualized care is a cornerstone of the program, the process by which each case is handled varies. The major aspect of care, however, is as follows: evaluation of the referral; initial evaluation and treatment; hospital education; individual and family support; development of self-help skills; epilepsy education programs; and program evaluation.

EVALUATION OF REFERRAL

In most cases, when a child is referred for inpatient evaluation on an epilepsy specialty unit, the child and family have already encountered a large array of health care providers and centers. Most families have not experienced a hospital unit arranged in the fashion of a comprehensive epilepsy inpatient unit. Even though the unit offers the most advanced and sophisticated forms of evaluation and treatment, families are often surprised that this can be accomplished in an environment that permits and promotes the experience of typical life activities (e.g. regular education instruction, recreational activities). Family members are encouraged to participate from the time the initial contact is made. For some children this may mean a family member(s) will be staying with them throughout the hospitalization. For others the family may be able to visit only on weekends. Family participation is encouraged since it is well known that epilepsy impacts upon the whole family. It is important for the family to be involved in all phases of the program, and the establishment of the family's involvement is important to ensure positive outcomes from the hospitalization and to reduce the stress of the hospitalization.

Families receive basic information on epilepsy either on an individual basis or by attending epilepsy education classes. The staff feels it is important for the family to participate in all discussions when treatment plans are being developed. Since most stays are longer than 10 days, and can be extended for several months depending on the difficulty of the case, sharing information about the daily routines and the responsibility of the staff is an integral part of the treatment plan. Each family receives information prior to the hospitalization on what to bring and what to expect during the stay to help make them more comfortable. This means the child shows up with his school books, favorite stuffed toy, and his friends know where to send cards.

The majority of patients admitted to the unit have failed to have their seizures controlled through outpatient treatment and, in many instances, have had multiple hospital admissions. From the beginning the staff makes it clear there are no magical cures. Every case referred for admission to Virginia's inpatient epilepsy unit is evaluated by members of the team to determine the appropriateness and expected outcome for the admission both from the team's and the family's perspective. Not only is it important to gather results from previous diagnostic procedures, as well as psychological, social and educational evaluations, but to begin a dialogue with the family to explore and evaluate their previous experiences with their child's treatment and the family's expectations in coming to a specialized epilepsy program. This dialogue is one of the most important steps in the treatment process, since it provides the team an opportunity to assess the children and their families, prepare them for the experience, and begin to develop a treatment/intervention plan that will be beneficial to all.

INITIAL EVALUATIONS

The principal goals for each child's admission are: (1) to eliminate the seizures, (2) to prevent the seizures from recurring, (3) to prevent/minimize the psychosocial aspects that compromise a normal life, and (4) to accomplish these goals at the least cost (Dreifuss, 1979).

The multidisciplinary team consists of the child and his/her family, epileptologists, electroencephalographer, research fellows in neuroscience, nurses, EEG technician, social worker, pharmacist, psychologist, psychiatrist, rehabilitation counselor, and occupational therapist. Others are consulted as needed (e.g. genetics, neuro-ophthalmology, speech and hearing). The most important members of the team are the child and his/her family. It is their responsibility to share information about themselves, to actively participate in the program, and to assist in the discharge planning. There are several epileptologists involved as team members, and all of them play a major role in making a definitive diagnosis, outlining and initiating the appropriate treatment choices, and evaluating the response. The EEG technician supports the physicians by providing the technical expertise in EEG monitoring. A pharmacist is available to provide detailed information on drug action, interaction, and dosaging.

Each patient and family is assigned a primary nurse prior to admission. The nursing team is responsible for providing nursing care based on their assessment and the assessments of the other team members. In addition they coordinate all the services needed throughout the hospitalization. They are also responsible for all the health education programs.

The psychologist develops, administers, evaluates, and interprets all the neuropsychological testing information. In addition, he or she counsels families about the tests results, and shares this information with the other team members to assist them in treatment planning (e.g. educational programs and intervention). A social worker screens each family to assess their financial status and to evaluate the family's strengths and weaknesses. Beside counselling families, the social worker also works with community resources that can support the family after discharge.

Since most children with difficult seizure management problems have academic difficulties, a special education teacher evaluates each child, then develops and tests a variety of teaching strategies to ensure the best opportunity for learning. After gathering the information, the teacher works with the local school system to establish a similar program that will enhance the child's achievement.

Epilepsy affects all activities of daily living, so the patients are assessed by an occupational therapist and an individual treatment plan is developed accordingly. The therapist initiates and supports group activities to facilitate adaptive recreational activities, provide exercise, and teach skills necessary for activities of daily living.

Each team member has an opportunity to meet with the child and his/her family within the first 2 days of the hospitalization. The purpose of this contact is to gather additional information, supplement the available records, confirm assessments already made, and reassess the child/family. The tests necessary to further evaluate the child are outline at this time. The initial treatment plan is discussed and implemented.

Through their assessments and observation, the team works together to assist the physician in making the appropriate diagnosis and classification of the seizure type. Throughout the hospitalization each staff member, along with the family and child, meticulously describe and record the child's behaviour. This is an extremely important aspect in the diagnosis and management, since it provides careful documentation of possible seizure events. Children can experience a number of episodes that may represent seizures, such as breath-holding spells, night terrors, nocturnal myoclonus, migraine, and temper tantrums. These episodes, when epileptic in nature, may not be recognized as seizure behavior. The staff's observations and child/family's seizure reports are supported by the use of intensive EEG monitoring. This monitoring occurs at various times during the hospitalization, initially to establish and confirm the diagnosis, and later to evaluate the treatment response. The EEG monitoring required is individualized. A wide variety of monitoring techniques are employed, such as routine EEGs, nasopharyngel leads, sleep-deprived recordings, ambulatory cassette, telemetry and closed-circuit television (CCTV/EEG) monitoring.

For children being evaluated for surgical intervention, additional monitoring procedures may be utilized, such as: sphenoidal, depth and subdural–epidural electrodes (these would occur in centers equipped to perform surgery). A Wada test would assist in determining hemispheric dominance for language. In addition to the EEG testing, other neurodiagnostic testing is done to determine the etiology of the seizures and the effects the seizures and treatment have on the child's functioning. Various scanning techniques are employed. CT and MRI scanning are two of the main procedures utilized. MRIs are widely used, since the risk of radiation is limited while providing a clear picture of the brain structures. For children being evaluated for surgical intervention, PET scanning may be utilized to help delineate the area of focus and spread, thereby eliminating the need for more invasive procedures such as depth electrodes.

For all children where medical or surgical management is being pursued, neuropsychological evaluation is essential. This evaluation provides critical information regarding higher cortical function and is of significance in localizing dysfunction. The information provided helps, both from a medical/surgical diagnosis and management perspective, as well as providing valuable information for educational, vocational, and social treatment plans.

HOSPITAL EDUCATION PROGRAM

Although some children with epilepsy do not evidence educational problems, data suggest that children with epilepsy are more at risk of having problems in school than are their normal counterparts (Seidenberg *et al.*, 1986). The majority of the children needing intervention on a comprehensive inpatient unit do experience some difficulties academically. However, it may just be a problem of frequent absenteeism, or of the school restricting the child from participating in gym. The Hospital Education Program provides the specially designed assessment and instruction these children need.

The traumatic experience of hospitalization can be compounded if a child is unable to maintain his/her studies due to an extended absence from school. The inpatient school program provides instructional services to preschool- and school-aged children admitted to the epilepsy unit. Any child hospitalized for 3 or more consecutive days is eligible for enrollment upon receipt of written consent from the parents or legal guardian. The hospital teacher contacts the child's school principal, guidance counselor, and/or classroom teacher to exchange pertinent information. The Hospital Education Program's primary goal is to maintain the academic status of each child. Since many of the children's level of achievement or performance has been altered as a result of the seizure frequency, underlying disease, and/or treatment, an in-depth assessment is conducted to ascertain the child's current performance level so an appropriate instruction plan can be developed. For children who are hospitalized longer than 30 days an Individual Education Program (IEP) is required under P.L. 94–142. The annual goals and short-term objectives encompassing the IEP will be determined from the local school's assignments and the specialized curriculum designed to meet the child's need. The Hospital Education Program has several components; preschool- and school-age programs, a summer enrichment program, and career education.

INDIVIDUAL AND FAMILY SUPPORT

Even though the needs of children with epilepsy are diverse, there are certain components of this disorder that are likely to be manifest in the child, and therefore must be addressed by those working with this population. For example, the psychological and social aspects of epilepsy must be considered. Psychologically the child, family, friends, teachers, and significant others with whom the child comes into contact on a regular basis must adjust to the epilepsy. Socially they must overcome the stigma which surrounds epilepsy, and understand how this disorder can and must be viewed within a social context. A child's epilepsy is rarely cured. Thus the child must learn to live with the disorder. For the majority of cases, seizure can be controlled with medication. While some children may be able to be weaned from all anticonvulsant drugs, others will never be controlled totally. It follows that children with epilepsy must make adjustments for seizures, medications, and for the allied problems associated with the seizures. The child's family, friends, and community can facilitate these adjustments by recognizing and understanding how these variables affect an individual; realizing children do not benefit from pity; and understanding a child with epilepsy should be expected to function according to his ability, regardless of the seizures. The team approaches the child and family in this manner while communicating these ideas to the professionals from the child's local community.

The child and his/her family never know when another seizure will occur. There is often concern associated with long-term use of medication(s) and their possible negative side-effects. In order to ameliorate such fear, all staff coming into contact with the child are equipped to provide appropriate information, care, and acceptance. They also encourage the child and his/her family to ask questions about epilepsy while on the unit and whenever they visit their local care providers. The treatment team must work together to provide support to the child and his/her family. These efforts are coordinated during multidisciplinary rounds, and to other times, through one-to-one communication with appropriate team members.

Other problems often associated with a child's epilepsy pertain to overprotection and physical limitations. Many parents, school personnel, and significant others will be overprotective of the child with epilepsy. While understandable, overprotectiveness is harmful to the developing child. It is well known that children need to make mistakes and to learn from their mistakes. Since experiences in early childhood is the equivalent of learning, the overprotected child is often denied opportunities to experience his environment, and is not allowed to learn. The child with epilepsy must be given age-appropriate opportunities and responsibilities. Every child must learn to be responsible for himself and his environment. This responsibility is best learned when given in age-appropriate, incremental amounts.

The social worker supports the program by assisting the family in gaining better insight into their child's and their own perception of epilepsy. This is accomplished through individual and group counseling sessions. All the disciplines assist the family in developing advocacy skills to help the child obtain that to which he/she is entitled. The staff works with the child in the same manner to teach these necessary skills. This is done by teaching children to ask the doctors, nurses, and schoolteacher questions regarding their treatment, and to speak up during a group meeting, verbalizing their feelings about unit policies. The child and family are kept abreast of all scheduled procedures and medication changes. This is accomplished by meeting daily with the nursing staff, by reviewing a weekly schedule board for scheduled tests, and by using a prepared medication card to keep abreast of all medication changes. For some families, just having the opportunity to meet and to share with others who have similar problems is positive. Many of the relationships developed while hospitalized continue long after discharge. In many instances this is the first time the child has had friends that are totally accepting of his/her epilepsy. For the teenager it may be the first chance to develop a close relationship with someone of the opposite sex.

DEVELOPMENT OF SELF-HELP SKILLS

The nursing staff and occupational therapists work together to teach the hospitalized child independent, age-appropriate skills. These include being responsible for one's living area, clothes, medications, and developing self-sufficient skills such as making a meal. These two disciplines assist the child in learning new recreational skills. Due to overprotectiveness and isolation, many children with epilepsy have had limited or no exposure to swimming, playing ball, or going to public facilities for shopping or entertainment. The staff works with the child and family, not only to provide these new opportunities, but to evaluate future opportunities in a risk/benefit manner to enhance the child's growth and development. In addition, the family is exposed to a variety of activities they can initiate at home that will provide the child valuable learning opportunities with a minimal risk of injury.

EPILEPSY EDUCATION

Many people with epilepsy are ill-formed regarding the nature of their disorder. The Commission for the Control of Epilepsy and its Consequences (1977) recognized the need for greater awareness and understanding of this condition. In their report they stated 'the understanding that an individual has about any disability is directly related to the success the individual has in coping with the disability.' At the Commission's consumer hearings the group heard from people with epilepsy and their families, who knew from bitter experience the problems created by a lack of understanding and knowledge about epilepsy. This lack of knowledge hinders the individual's ability to be a contributing member of the health care team.

Recognizing this need for the individual with epilepsy, the nursing staff created a formal epilepsy education program so that patient and family education is a major focus on the inpatient unit. It has been given special emphasis because we recognize that knowledge about one's health problem will enhance the individual's ability to live a more problem-free existence. The three main goals of the education program are to increase knowledge, to develop positive attitudes and, ultimately, to faciliate behavior changes. Each patient and family is required to attend epilepsy education classes.

There are seven basic areas covered in the program; basic facts and etiology, seizure classification and epileptic syndromes, treatment methods, diagnostic tests, psychosocial aspects, safe living and first aid, and advocacy and legal rights. When appropriate, for the teenager, information on parenting is provided. Children are taught the name of their seizure(s), and their prescribed medication, as well as what first-aid measures should be instituted if a seizure occurs. This ultimately equips them to discuss their epilepsy with peers, teachers, and future employers. The family, also, is provided with a similar, but sometimes more extensive, program, so they too can gain some control over the situation by having basic knowledge about epilepsy and related problems. The program allows the individual one-to-one instruction, if needed, but for the majority of the patients and their families the education is done in a group. The exchange allows the staff more opportunities to assess the child and family, and provides, in many cases, the first chance to share with others in similar situations.

The education program has been standardized to ensure consistency in the information being present. The classes are held at least once daily and on some days two or three times. This allows children and their families ample opportunity to attend. The sessions are brief, 15–30 minutes for the patients, while longer sessions occur for the parents and significant others. All topics can be covered in a 2-week period. The staff encourages patients and their families to attend each class at least twice. Pamphlets, videos, slide–tapes, games, and role playing are just some of the support materials and activites used to enhance learning.

All information presented is reinforced throughout the hospitalization. This is accomplished through unit group sessions, cooking classes, recreational activities on and off the unit, medication administration, and in all activities of daily living. The teaching program has been coordinated with the nursing care plan to assist in assesssing outcome behaviors, e.g. the child will be able to name his/her seizure type, medications, dosage, and to exhibit appropriate judgement in performing activities that could possibly cause an injury.

The children are given recognition for successfully completing the program by giving them a certificate. When each section test covering a topic area is passed (score at least 80 per cent), then the child is excused from attending that particular teaching session. When the child passes all the section tests, he or she is awarded a certificate.

By increasing the childs and family's knowledge about epilepsy, it is hoped ultimately to change attitudes and behaviors in a positive manner. We have been able to document that the education program is successful in improving the child's and family's knowledge about epilepsy, as well as fostering positive attitude changes (Santilli et al., 1984, 1985).

LIAISON WITH LOCAL COMMUNITY SERVICES

In order to maintain and continue the progress made while hospitalized, families are referred to local centers that can complete the necessary drug changes, continue monitoring the child's response, evaluate behavior treatment plans at home and school, and support the family in all aspects of their child's care. This may mean going to a community mental health center, having a public nurse make regular home visits, joining a local epilepsy support group, or follow-up with a local rehabilitation counselor for vocational planning. Team members will send all pertinent information to these referral agencies. When necessary, verbal contact will be made prior to and after discharge. All families leave knowing the center will support them in establishing their treatment plan at home. It is the rare instance when a child would need to return for a second hospitalization.

SUMMARY

The impact of having a child with uncontrolled epilepsy can be significant medically, financially, psychologically, and socially. Uncontrolled seizures and/or crippling side-effects from treatment will drastically alter the quality of the child's and family's life. Evaluation and treatment on an inpatient comprehensive epilepsy program can offer these individuals an opportunity to improve their quality of life if not by totally eliminating the seizures, then by improving their daily existence with a simpler drug regime; and, in both cases, by developing a deeper understanding and ability to live as normal a life as possible. The multidisciplinary integration of evaluation and treatment components has been critical in establishing an effective and successful inpatient program for treating children with epilepsy.

REFERENCES AND FURTHER READING

Commission for the Control of Epilepsy and its Consequences (1977). *Plan for Nationwide Action on Epilepsy*, US Department of Health, Education, and Welfare, DHEW Publication No. 78–276, vol. I.

Dreifuss, F.E. (1979). Development of a comprehensive epilepsy program, In *Epilepsy Updated: Causes and Treatment*, Year Book Medical Publishers; Chicago, Il.

Drury, I., Tonelson, S., Santilli, N., Dreifuss, F.E., Crosby, C., and Ragland, M. (1985). Medical benefits of hospitalization in a comprehensive epilepsy unit. *The Patient's Perspective*, Paper presented to the American Epilepsy Society, New York. NY.

Epilepsy and the School Age Child (1977). Minnesota Comprehensive Epilepsy Program, Minnesota.

Jones, V.R., Ragland, M., Santilli, N., Dreifuss, F.E., and Miller, J.Q. (1978). Longterm hospitalization on a multidisciplinary epilepsy unit, *Proceedings, Epilepsy International Symposium, Vancouver*.

Poche, P. (1978). Educating the child with seizures. In G. Ferriss (ed.), *Treatment of Epilepsy Today*, Oradel, NJ: Medical Economics Company.

Santilli, N., Tonelson, S., Ragland, M., Turner, G., and Crosby, C. (1984). *Health Education Improving Patient Participation in Care*. American Epilepsy Society, San Francisco, CA.

Santilli, N., Tonelson, S., Drury, I., Ragland, M., Crosby, C., and Dreifuss, F.E. (1985). *Patient's Perception of Attitude and Behavior Changes Related to Epilepsy Education*. American Epilepsy Socieity, New York, NY.

Seidenberg, M., Beck, N., Geisser, M., Giordani, B., Sackellares, J.C., Berent, S., Dreifuss, F.E., and Boll, T.J. (1986). Academic achievement of children with epilepsy, *Epilepsia*, **27**, 753–759.

Index